The PTA Handbook

Keys to Success in School and Career
for the
Physical Therapist Assistant

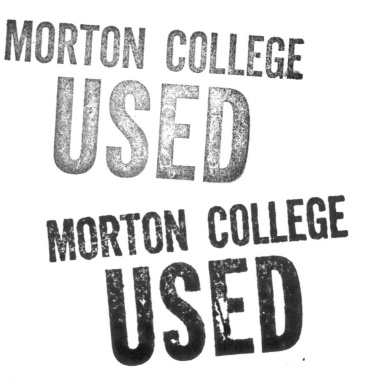

The PTA Handbook

Keys to Success in School and Career
for the
Physical Therapist Assistant

Kathleen A. Curtis, PT, PhD
California State University, Fresno
Fresno, California

Peggy DeCelle Newman, PT, MHR
Oklahoma City Community College
Oklahoma City, Oklahoma

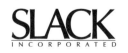

An innovative information, education, and management company
6900 Grove Road • Thorofare, NJ 08086

ISBN-10: 1-55642-621-6
ISBN-13: 978-1-55642-621-6

Published by: SLACK Incorporated
                   6900 Grove Road
                   Thorofare, NJ 08086 USA
                   Telephone: 856-848-1000
                   Fax: 856-853-5991
                   www.slackbooks.com

Printed in the United States of America.

Curtis, Kathleen A.
    The PTA handbook : keys to success in school and career for the physical therapist assistant / Kathleen Curtis, Peggy DeCelle Newman.
       p. ; cm.
    Includes bibliographical references and index.
    ISBN-13: 978-1-55642-621-6 (pbk.)
    ISBN-10: 1-55642-621-6 (pbk.)

    1.   Physical therapy assistants--Vocational guidance. 2.   Physical therapy--Vocational guidance. 3. Physical therapy--Practice.
    [DNLM: 1. Allied Health Personnel. 2. Physical Therapy (Specialty) 3. Career Choice. W 21.5 C979p 2005] I. Newman, Peggy DeCelle. II. Title.

RM705.C873 2005
615.8'2'071173--dc22

                                        2004024265

Last digit is print number: 10 9 8 7 6 5 4 3 2

Dedication

We dedicate this book to:

Harold O. Curtis, PhD...
Who lived with courage, concern for humanity, and an enduring passion for life, science, and the truth.

and

William B. Inverso, PT, PhD...
Whose commitment to excellence in physical therapy education and tenacious advocacy for physical therapist assistant educators is deeply missed. Be well, Bill.

Contents

Acknowledgments

Following the publication of *Physical Therapy Professional Foundations* almost 3 years ago, I have traveled an interesting path while first thinking about and finally writing this book. My search for a coauthor eventually brought me to Peggy Newman, Director of the Physical Therapy Assistant Program at Oklahoma City Community College, a writing partner par excellence, whose enthusiasm for our profession and insight into current issues in physical therapy has added greatly to the depth and breadth of the coverage provided in this text.

The basis for this book is the belief that choosing effective strategies is one choice that we have within our control. Sandra Graham and Bernard Weiner at University of California, Los Angeles initially helped me see the power of strategy through my own doctoral work, applying these choices in the real world of problems and challenges I had experienced early in my career. I continue to appreciate their contributions in helping me find ways to apply attribution theory in my work with practicing health professionals. My ongoing research continues to support the power of conscious choice, reflection, intention, and strategy in fundamentally changing the nature of our lives and career experiences.

My colleagues at California State University, Fresno have provided support, leadership, and encouragement throughout the demanding process of writing this book. Dean Benjamin Cuellar and Associate Dean Andrew Hoff of the College of Health and Human Services, former Provost J. Michael Ortiz, President John Welty, Provost Jeronima Echeverria, Dr. Berta Gonzalez, and Dean Vivian Vidoli, all provide strong leadership to create an academic environment in which creative and scholarly work and long-term projects such as this can thrive and blossom. My interprofessional family and faculty colleagues are never far from me and offer a rich exchange of ideas, thoughts, and experiences.

Carrie Kotlar, Amy McShane, and John Bond at SLACK Incorporated first helped this book come alive through their encouragement and support for these ideas. Christina Buettell continues to be exceptionally helpful in her feedback, suggestions, and contributions to this text. Her own journey illuminates the path for others in so many ways.

On a personal note, I must acknowledge Barclay (the golden retriever puppy I raised to be a service dog) for the hours he lay close by while I sat at the computer, and Behzad Setoodeh for his encouragement. My mother, Therna Curtis, remains a source of never-ending energy and inspiration. Finally, thank you to my colleague, Marilyn Miller, PT, PhD, GCS, for her review of the final manuscript during a very busy academic year.

My gratitude to all,
Kathleen Curtis

What an incredible journey the realization of this work has been! Deliberating the potential need for a textbook of this nature, diligently researching the existing literature and carefully pondering various topics as the manuscript evolved has intensified my conviction that the physical therapist: physical therapist assistant partnership is the most efficient way to deliver quality physical therapy services. This text provides current and future educators and clinicians the tools to foster this relationship.

A special thanks to Lynn Lippert for suggesting me as a potential collaborator on this project. I am ever indebted to Kathy Curtis, from whose incredible scholarship and thoughtful, wise counsel I have learned volumes. This experience has afforded me not only a talented mentor but a dear friend.

I am grateful to Carrie Kotlar, Amy McShane, and John Bond at SLACK Incorporated for being so exceptionally supportive through the personal trials that have occurred since signing on board. I am proud to be associated with such fine individuals!

I want to thank Oklahoma City Community College Provost, Dr. Paul Sechrist; Health Professions Dean, Dr. Jo Ann Cobble; my program faculty, Vicky Davidson, Jennifer Ball, Dee Tipton, and Olivia Feagins; and our students for their support and encouragement without which this project would not have been possible.

Personally, I want to acknowledge my parents, husband and children. To my folks, Donna and Jerry for providing unconditional love, instilling in me the confidence to pursue my dreams and setting the example as to how I should live my life. To my loving husband, Cyrus, for understanding my intense need to actively contribute to many passions and being my refuge along this journey of life. And finally, to my children, David, Becca, and Lizzy, for sharing Mommy with this work and enriching my life so completely.

My deepest appreciation,
Peggy DeCelle Newman

About the Authors

Kathleen A. Curtis, PT, PhD, is a Professor and Director of Research and External Programs in the College of Health and Human Services and former Chairperson of the Department of Physical Therapy at California State University, Fresno. Dr. Curtis received her Bachelor of Science degree in Physical Therapy at Northeastern University, Boston, Massachusetts. She received her Master's degree in Health Science from San Jose State University, and received her PhD in Education at University of California, Los Angeles.

Her background includes a wide variety of experiences in clinical practice, staff development and supervision, clinical research, and clinical and academic teaching in physical therapy. Her academic teaching experience includes graduate courses in physical therapy professional issues, research methods, communication, instructional design, health education, career development, health systems, and psychosocial considerations in health care. She also developed and coordinated an annual Graduate Student Success Seminar for incoming graduate students, a program designed to ensure that they have the skills to succeed in physical therapy professional education.

Her research on interprofessional role conflict, helping behavior, early career development, and role satisfaction has received wide exposure across the health care fields. She coauthored and serves on the Advisory Board of California State University, Fresno's Certificate of Advanced Study in Interprofessional Collaboration. She also developed an interdisciplinary Bachelor of Science program in Interdisciplinary Health and Rehabilitation Sciences, which serves as preprofessional preparation for physical therapy, occupational therapy, and rehabilitation counseling graduate students. She cofounded the interdisciplinary Disability Studies Institute and the Central Valley Health Policy Institute at California State University, Fresno.

She is a well-known speaker and author. She has published extensively in the rehabilitation literature and serves as a manuscript reviewer for several journals. She is a recipient of the California Physical Therapist Faculty Research Award and her books, *The Physical Therapist's Guide to Health Care* and *Physical Therapy Professional Foundations* have been used as texts in a majority of college and university physical therapy professional education programs.

Peggy DeCelle Newman, PT, MHR, is the Physical Therapist Assistant Program Director at Oklahoma City Community College. Peggy received her Bachelor of Science degree from the University of Oklahoma Health Sciences Center and a Master's degree in Human Relations from the University of Oklahoma Norman campus. For 6 years she served as Assistant Professor and Academic Coordinator of Clinical Education at the University of Oklahoma Physical Therapy Program.

She participated in the development of the Normative Model of Physical Therapist Assistant Education (APTA 1999) as a member consultant on curriculum and content. She developed one component and served as invited project reviewer of the PT:PTA Collaboration Module developed by the National Assembly of Physical Therapist Assistants. She serves the Commission on Accreditation for Physical Therapy Education (CAPTE) as an on-site team leader for physical therapist assistant programs.

She has served the Oklahoma Physical Therapy Association as Chapter President, Delegate, and Chief Delegate for multiple terms. She received the Oklahoma Chapter Founder's Award in 2001. She currently serves as an appointed member of the Advisory Panel on Public Relations to the Board of Directors of the American Physical Therapy Association.

She has presented locally and nationally on topics including "Using Support Personnel Effectively," "The Guide to PT Practice: An Introduction," "Fostering Professional Interaction through Collaborative Group Learning," and "Ethical and Legal Problems for Rehabilitation Therapists: Ethical & Legal Responsibilities in Today's Health Care Environment."

Contributing Author

Tina Buettell, MPT is a physical therapist at Town Center Village Outpatient Therapy Clinic in Portland, Oregon. She received her Bachelor of Arts degree in International Studies at Lewis and Clark College, Portland, Oregon, then served as medical coordinator for AFS International Scholarships in New York City, trained as an Iyengar hatha yoga teacher, coordinated nutrition education at Outside-In Medical Clinic in Portland, cofounded and directed an urban-rural community land trust in Oregon, served on the administrative staff at Lewis and Clark College, and taught parent-child creative arts classes.

At age 49, Tina received a Master's degree in Physical Therapy from California State University, Fresno. In addition to her clinical practice, she teaches yoga and dance, cofacilitates wellness programs at a retreat center, and is studying alternative therapies for fibromyalgia. She lives with her husband and teenage son and enjoys "making insurmountable hurdles become just another day's adventure."

Preface

The *PTA Handbook* is a comprehensive guide for physical therapist assistant students as they enter and progress through the educational program and prepare for licensure and transition to clinical practice. As health care providers, we are faced with a multitude of choices every day of our lives.

Many of those choices fundamentally change the nature of our experience from moment to moment. It is much more than the simple perspective of "Is the glass half empty or half full?" We have choices in how to allocate precious resources such as time and energy; whether to choose effective or ineffective strategies; and if, when, and how to take advantage of the opportunities that are available to us. We can choose to nurture the relationships that support us and to learn to say "No" to the challenges that drain our resources.

Students face numerous choices, challenges, opportunities, and obstacles during the professional education process. This book offers an array of strategies for success in physical therapist assistant education and clinical practice. The first few chapters provide both an introduction to physical therapy and a context by describing the current health care environment and the changing roles of physical therapists and physical therapist assistants.

The text then includes a comprehensive path through physical therapist assistant education, including financial considerations, conduct and behavior, performance expectations, requirements, and challenges students face in the educational process. Following this are strategy-based approaches for success that address common issues in learning and skill acquisition, performance anxiety, personal management decisions, ethical challenges, and legal considerations for students. Another component includes special coverage of issues of concern to returning students, students with disabilities, and students challenged with speaking and writing English.

An entire section is devoted to cutting-edge professional issues in physical therapy, including an introduction to evidence-based practice and critical thinking, essentials of information competence, interprofessional collaboration, cultural competence, active participation in conferences, and student roles in the American Physical Therapy Association. The final few chapters address the transition from student life to clinical practice, including preparing for the licensure examination, entering the job market, and common challenges for new graduates including planning for lifelong learning and supervision issues.

This book was written to help entering physical therapist assistant students make healthy choices about entering the field of physical therapy, to assist students to establish sound habits and realistic expectations, and to facilitate success for new graduates in the transition from the academic setting to clinical practice. Clinical and academic faculty may also find these ideas useful in advising students at various stages in the educational process.

The "Putting It Into Practice" exercise at the end of each chapter encourages students to use the resources and tools available to them to make well-informed choices that will facilitate their success.

We welcome your feedback and ideas on how we can make this journey more successful and more fulfilling. The future of physical therapy rests in the hands of the students and new graduates who choose to practice in our current and ever-changing health care environment. We wish you all the best and hope that in some small way this book has made the journey better.

Kathleen Curtis, PT, PhD
Peggy Newman, PT, MHR

PART ONE

The Physical Therapy Profession in the Changing World

CHAPTER 1

The Profession of Physical Therapy

Anita is working in a long-term care facility as a "physical therapy assistant." The Director of Nurses asks her to call the local Community College to see about enrolling in the physical therapy classes. She is surprised to learn that completion of an associate's degree program is required to become a physical therapist assistant.

Can anyone use the title physical therapist? Or physical therapist assistant? What does it take to become licensed? How does a physical therapist assistant fit into the profession of physical therapy?

Misconceptions persist about the academic preparation and role delineation between the physical therapist and physical therapist assistant. Let's take a closer look at the profession of physical therapy and those working in it.

What is Physical Therapy?

Physical therapy is the care and services which are provided under the direction and supervision of a licensed physical therapist. Over 120,000 licensed physical therapists and over 38,000 licensed physical therapist assistants practice in the United States, treating over 1 million people every day.[1,2] The physical therapy profession was founded in the belief that improved physical function makes our lives better.

How Does the Profession Define the Practice of Physical Therapy?

The opening sentence of the *Guide to Physical Therapist Practice* characterizes the physical therapy profession using the following definition:

"Physical therapy is a dynamic profession with an established theoretical base and widespread clinical applications in the preservation, development, and restoration of optimal physical function."[1]

Physical therapists and physical therapist assistants carry out varied roles in many different types of health care, educational, and occupational settings, including hospitals and rehabilitation centers; outpatient clinics; patient's homes; schools; and professional, corporate, athletic, industrial, and community organizations.

The *Model Practice Act* (excerpted in Appendix 1) refers to four distinct areas of physical therapy, including:

1. Examining, evaluating, and testing individuals with mechanical, physiological, and developmental impairments, functional limitations, and disabilities or other health and movement-related conditions

2. Alleviating impairments, functional limitations and disabilities by designing, implementing, and modifying therapeutic interventions

3. Reducing the risk of injury, impairment, functional limitation and disability, including the promotion and maintenance of fitness, health, and wellness

4. Engaging in administration, consultation, education and research[1]

Only physical therapists can provide physical therapy and use the initials "PT" after their names to designate their licensure as a physical therapist. The initials "LPT" and "RPT" were used in the past (and still may be used by some therapists). Physical therapist assistants, under the direction and supervision of the licensed physical therapist, are the only technically educated health care providers who assist in the provision of physical therapy. Only physical therapist assistants may use "PTA" after their names to designate their education and licensure (where applicable) as a physical therapist assistant.

> *Brian reviewed the physical therapy department's personnel list noticing that in addition to the titles "PT" and "PTA" there were "Rehab Tech I," "Rehab Tech II," "ATC," and "Patient Care Associate" listed. "Who can do what in this place?" he wondered.*

Who Works in Physical Therapy?

Physical Therapists

Physical therapists, or PTs, are graduates of physical therapist professional education programs at the college or university level, and are required to be licensed in the state in which they practice. Professional education for physical therapists is at the post-baccalaureate level with the Doctor of Physical Therapy (DPT) being the preferred terminal degree as described in the American Physical Therapy Association's (APTA) Vision 2020 Statement.[3]

Physical therapists perform the five elements of patient/client management—*examination, evaluation, diagnosis, prognosis,* and *intervention*—in order to maximize functional outcomes for people with health problems resulting from injury or disease.[1] They evaluate joint motion, muscle performance, balance and gait, cardiopulmonary function, and performance of activities of daily living among other responsibilities. They provide intervention which may include therapeutic exercise, cardiovascular endurance training, and training in activities of daily living.

They are involved in collaboration with other professionals, consultation in many capacities, education, research, and administration. Physical therapists are responsible for the supervision of physical therapy support personnel, including physical therapist assistants and physical therapy aides.

Physical Therapist Assistants

Physical therapist assistants, or PTAs, are graduates of physical therapist assistant associate degree programs. Many, but not all, states require licensure for physical therapist assistants. Physical therapist assistants provide physical therapy services only under the direction and supervision of physical therapists.

PTAs assist physical therapists with data collection, implement interventions, modify interventions within the PT's established plan of care, participate in discharge planning and document services that they provide. Physical therapist assistants may be involved in educating and interacting with PT and PTA students, aides, volunteers, patient families, and/or caregivers. Some tasks may be performed in conjunction with other health care workers or through supervision of aides.[4] In addition to direct patient care, the PTA often performs functions such as patient transport, maintenance of equipment, and other clinic needs. Specific conditions for supervision of the PTA are outlined in each state's physical therapy practice act.

Physical Therapy Aides

Physical therapy aides are nonlicensed personnel who are usually trained on-the-job under the direction of a physical therapist. The physical therapy aide performs routine tasks either delegated by the physical therapist, or if permitted by state law, by the physical therapist assistant. The aide is permitted to perform specific patient-related duties only with continuous on-site supervision of the physical therapist, or if permitted by state law, the physical therapist assistant. The physical therapist or physical therapist assistant must be in the immediate area to provide continuous on-site supervision.

Other Personnel

Other personnel such as massage therapists, exercise physiologists, or athletic trainers sometimes work with physical therapists in providing care. Depending on state law, these personnel may be licensed or may hold certifications from professional organizations. These personnel should be employed under their appropriate title.

Their roles in patient or client care should be defined by the scope of their education and relevant laws and regulations. The specific physical therapy-related services that are provided by these types of personnel are determined by the physical therapist and must be in compliance with state and federal laws and regulations. In nursing home settings, "rehabilitation aides" continue routine exercise programs as established by the physical therapist. These individuals are not licensed and typically are not formally trained. They are providing nonbillable, routine maintenance exercise/activities which are not considered skilled physical therapy intervention.

Becoming a Part of the "Profession"

Individuals go through a distinct period of role socialization as they acquire specialized knowledge, values, attitudes, and skills while becoming a part of the profession. In addition to knowledge, skills and attitudes, the novice also develops a distinct language. Let's look at the following note, found in a patient's medical record:

> Charlie, a new graduate physical therapist assistant documented patient progress in the patient's medical record by writing: "Pt. amb 40' PWB L c FWW and VC."
>
> The patient's physician is overheard at the nurses' station after reading the chart muttering, "I can never tell whether that's good or bad."

Some sociologists have described professions as social constructs, with their own languages, belief systems, and symbolic lives. The above example shows a message in a language intelligible only to members of the professional culture.

> What does this mean: Pt. amb 40' PWB L c FWW and VC?
>
> Translation: Patient ambulated 40 feet partial weight bearing on the left leg with front-wheeled walker and verbal cueing.

The role socialization period for health professionals extends for a period of as long as 2 years following graduation and entry into the professional field. Research on role socialization within the physical therapy profession shows that clinical role models are likely to be the most powerful determinants of the behaviors and values of novice clinicians.[5,6]

Becoming a Physical Therapist

Physical therapists must complete a postbaccalaureate (masters or doctorate) degree in physical therapy from an accredited education program. At present, there are over 200 colleges and universities nationwide that offer professional education programs in physical therapy. Most of these programs encompass six or more semesters of academic coursework including or followed by a period of extended clinical internship.[7] The Commission on Accreditation in Physical Therapy Education (CAPTE) projects that 72% of all physical therapy education programs will be at the doctoral level by 2010.[8]

After graduation, candidates must successfully pass an examination administered by the Federation of State Boards of Physical Therapy. There are additional requirements for physical therapy practice that vary from state to state by individual state physical therapy practice acts or state regulations that govern the practice of physical therapy.

Becoming a Physical Therapist Assistant

Physical therapist assistants complete a 2-year college education program and receive an associate's degree upon graduation. Eighty-one percent of physical therapist assistant programs are offered at community colleges. The academic program averages 65 semester credit hours over four to six 16-week semesters including general education, applied physical therapy science and technical education and clinical experience.[4] At present, there are over 250 accredited physical therapist assistant education programs in the United States.[8]

Forty-three states/jurisdictions have practice acts that require physical therapist assistants to meet specific educational and examination criteria. In these states physical therapists assistants must be licensed, registered, or certified. Regardless of state licensure, physical therapist assistants may only work under the supervision of physical therapists.[9]

The "Preferred Relationship" Between the PT and PTA

> During an interview for a class project regarding the roles and responsibilities between the PT and PTA, Danielle learns that a physical therapist assistant must effectively work with multiple physical therapists as each PT on staff may delegate to her.

Health care providers must deliver high-quality services with accountability for outcomes that are meaningful to an increasingly savvy consumer. Establishing clearly defined roles and responsibilities, as well as efficient collaboration between the physical therapist and the physical therapist assistant are vital to successfully managing physical therapy practice in this uncertain and challenging environment.

The preferred relationship between the physical therapist and physical therapist assistant is characterized by trust, mutual respect, and an appreciation for individual and cultural differences. The preferred relationship helps to ensure high quality therapy services through effective communication, responsible direction and supervision by the PT, desirable patient outcomes, mechanisms for upholding ethical and legal standards and cost-effective care.[4]

This relationship includes many facets:

* Direction and supervision
* Accepting constructive criticism from each other
* A willingness to become a lifelong learner and seek the contributions of other health care team members; understanding the educational preparation and experiences of each other
* Referencing one another in written and verbal communication
* Demonstrating a mutual appreciation of one another's role(s)[9]

The Evolution of the Physical Therapy Profession

The physical therapy profession had its origins in the post-World War II era rehabilitation needs of returning veterans. In over 75 years, the profession has grown, developed, expanded, and increased its autonomy.

Detailed histories are available both in written and oral forms from the American Physical Therapy Association. The APTA will loan copies of videotapes, audiotapes and transcripts of oral histories by leaders in the profession. See the following site for more information: http://www.apta.org/Research/factsheet_tips/sourcesofinformation/OralHistories

Tables 1-1 and 1-2 indicate some of the key events and persons involved in the early and more recent history of the physical therapy profession.

Vision Statement 2020

The APTA House of Delegates endorsed a vision statement (seen in the sidebar below) which indicates a clear direction for the future of the profession of physical therapy in their June, 2000 meeting.

Vision Statement, APTA House of Delegates, June 2000

"Physical therapy, by 2020, will be provided by physical therapists who are doctors of physical therapy and who may be board-certified specialists. Consumers will have direct access to physical therapists in all environments for patient/client management, prevention, and wellness services. Physical therapists will be practitioners of choice in clients' health networks and will hold all privileges of autonomous practice. Physical therapists may be assisted by physical therapist assistants who are educated and licensed to provide physical therapist-directed and -supervised components of interventions.

"Guided by integrity, life-long learning, and a commitment to comprehensive and accessible health programs for all people, physical therapists and physical therapist assistants will render evidence-based service throughout the continuum of care and improve quality of life for society. They will provide culturally sensitive care distinguished by trust, respect, and an appreciation for individual differences.

"While fully availing themselves of new technologies, as well as basic and clinical research, physical therapists will continue to provide direct care. They will maintain active responsibility for the growth of the physical therapy profession and the health of the people it serves."[3]

Summary

The profession of physical therapy continues to evolve from its origins in the early 20th century. The profession currently faces challenges that will define the future role of the physical therapist and physical therapist assistant in health care delivery. Clearly this profession will continue to play an important role in health care delivery.

References

1. Model Practice Act for Physical Therapy. Alexandria, VA: Federation of State Boards of Physical Therapy; 2002. Available from: http://www.fsbpt.org/pdf/MPA_2002_ Language.pdf. Accessed November 14, 2003.

2. Busse N, ed. *Jurisdictional Licensure Reference Guide, Federation of State Boards of Physical Therapy.* Alexandria, Va: Creative Publishing; 2002.

3. APTA. APTA House of Delegates endorses a vision for the future. Available from: http://www.apta.org/news/visionstatementrelease. Accessed July 28, 2000.

4. APTA. *A Normative Model of Physical Therapist Assistant Education: Version '99.* Alexandria, Va: American Physical Therapy Association; 1999.

5. Jacobson BF. Role-model concepts before and after the formal professional socialization period. *Phys Ther.* 1980;60(2):188-193.

6. Jacobson BF. Characteristics of physical therapy role models. *Phys Ther.* 1978;58(5):560-566.

7. APTA. APTA Background Sheet: The Physical Therapist. A Professional Profile Web page. Available from: http://www.apta.org/Consumer/whoareptsptas/profile. Accessed September 18, 2002.

8. APTA. *Accreditation Update Newsletter. Commission on Accreditation for Physical Therapy Education.* Alexandria, Va: American Physical Therapy Association. 2003;8(1):8

Table 1-1

EARLY EVENTS IN THE EVOLUTION OF THE PROFESSION OF PHYSICAL THERAPY[10-13]

1914, 1916	Widespread polio epidemics occurred during this time. Physical modalities, massage, and corrective exercise were applied by nonphysician personnel, trained in physical education.
1915	Mary McMillan is recognized as the first physical therapist in the United States. She received her training in England and returned to the United States in 1915.
During World War I: (1917-1918)	Reconstruction aides were employed in Army Hospitals. They were women, most from backgrounds in physical education, who participated in 3-month courses during the war to train them in military massage and muscle re-education. They worked in army and veteran's hospitals during the war.
1918	First physical therapy course was organized at Walter Reed Hospital to train Reconstruction aides. Courses were soon established in 14 institutions, the largest of which was Reed College in Eugene Oregon. Standards were administered by the Surgeon General's office.
1921	American Women's Physical Therapeutic Association was founded by Mary McMillan. *PT Review*, a professional journal, began in March, 1921.
1922	Name change from American Women's Physical Therapeutic Association to American Physiotherapy Association (APA)
1928	In the 1920s, a "Council on Physical Therapy" was established in the American Medical Association. By 1928, they had established a standard for schools—a course length of 9 months, with 1200 hours of theory and practice. Entry requirements were graduation from a school of physical education or nursing. From 1936 until 1977, the standards for training and education of physical therapists remained under the purview of the AMA and House of Delegates of the AMA.
1934	The American Registry of Physical Therapy Technicians was established by the American Congress of Physical Therapy (an organization of physicians specializing in use of PT) involved a written examination. Passing the examination allowed one to use the title "Registered Physical Therapist" (RPT), not to be confused by legal licensure allowing one to call themselves RPT. It wasn't until the 1950s that widespread legislation was enacted on a state by state basis.
1935	Standards for Ethics and Discipline were adopted, that addressed the expected behavior in therapeutic intervention and the exclusive responsibilities of the physician for diagnosis, prognosis, and prescription. The physician was considered critical in establishing the legitimacy of the work in physical therapy.
1944	The medical specialty of physical medicine was developed; physicians dropped the name of physical therapist (changed to *physiatrist*) which allowed physical therapist technicians to drop the technician title and use physical therapist as their name.
1940-1945	Rehabilitation concepts introduced in World War II fostered the growth of the physical medicine specialty. In many institutions services of physical therapy were only available via referral to the physiatrist.
1947	Name change of American Physiotherapy Association (APA) in 1947 to American Physical Therapy Association (APTA). By 1946 the organization had over 3000 members.

Table 1-2

RECENT EVENTS IN THE EVOLUTION OF THE PROFESSION OF PHYSICAL THERAPY[10-13]

1960s	Amendments to the Social Security Act necessitated an increase in manpower. The physical therapist assistant was developed based on an APTA Ad Hoc Committee study regarding utilization and training to help meet needs for health care personnel. Fifteen physical therapist assistants graduated from the first two PTA programs in 1969.
	Curriculum changes were instituted to reflect the evolution of the practice of physical therapy. Practitioners needed to not only be skilled in use of PT procedures but also understand the rationale for application. Standards increased breadth and depth of coursework as the foundation of the profession.
1970s	APTA House of Delegates adopted a new document which departed from the course titles, clock hours, and semester hours included in earlier versions. Standards for Accreditation were published in 1978.
	APTA forms Affiliate membership as unique designation for PTA membership.
1980s	APTA adopted a resolution that entry-level education for the physical therapist be that which results in a post-baccalaureate degree.
	APTA adopted the first "Policy Statement on Education & Utilization of the PTA" in 1981.
	Standard of Ethical Conduct for the PTA adopted in 1982.
	APTA became an accrediting agency for PT and PTA education.
	APTA passed a new definition of physical therapy. Physical therapy is (a) treatment by physical means, and (b) the profession which is concerned with health promotion, with prevention of physical disabilities and with rehabilitation of persons disabled by pain, disease or injury; and which is involved with evaluating patients, and with treating through the use of physical therapeutic measures as opposed to medicines, surgery or radiation.
	Clinical Specialization: mechanisms were put into place to recognize therapists with advanced clinical skills. The first clinical specialists were certified in cardiopulmonary physical therapy in 1985.
	APTA Affiliate Assembly Special Interest Group for the PTA is formed in 1989.
1990s	Americans with Disabilities Act signed in 1990, mandating reasonable accommodations to ensure the integration of people with disabilities.
	Number of PTA programs outnumbers PT programs in 1993.
	First entry-level doctorate in physical therapy (DPT) program opened at Creighton University, graduating its first class in 1996.
	Balanced Budget Amendment signed into law in August, 1997, enacting widespread changes in reimbursement for Medicare patients.
	Guide to Physical Therapy Practice, a consensus document outlining patient/client management and scope of physical therapy practice, published in 1997.
	Inaugural National Assembly of PTAs was held in 1999.
2000	Vision statement passed by APTA House of Delegates.

9. APTA. The Future Role of the PTA (RC 40-01); Report to 2002 House of Delegates. (p. 79) Available from: http://www.apta.org/governance/HoD/ 2002HoD/5thHoDPosting/Special Reports. Accessed November 26, 2002.

10. Murphy WB. *Healing the Generations: A History of Physical Therapy & the American Physical Therapy Association*. Alexandria, Va: American Physical Therapy Association; 1995.

11. Pinkston D. Evolution of the practice of physical therapy. In: Scully RM, Barnes MR, eds. *Physical Therapy*. Philadelphia, Pa: JB Lippincott; 1989:2-30.

12. Lippert L. *Physical Therapist Assistant Education: Past, Present & Future*. Presented at: Physical Therapy 2000, American Physical Therapy Association; 2000:11-12

13. Newman P. *History of the Physical Therapist Assistant. Course Materials PTA 2113 Systems/Problems in Physical Therapy*. Oklahoma City, Okla: Oklahoma City Community College; Fall 2002.

PUTTING IT INTO PRACTICE

Consult your textbooks and the American Physical Therapy Association Web site to answer the following questions about the physical therapy profession:

1. What is the APTA's toll-free (1-800) telephone number?

2. Who is the current editor of the journal *Physical Therapy*?

3. During what era did Reconstruction Aides work?

4. Who was the first president of the American Women's Physical Therapeutic Association?

5. What was the name of the first physical therapy professional journal?

6. What organization (outside the physical therapy profession) supervised the development and accreditation of physical therapy programs from their inception in the 1920s until the 1970s?

7. In what year did a bachelor's degree become the **minimum** entry-level educational requirement for physical therapy education?

8. What is the medical specialty name for physicians who specialize in physical medicine and rehabilitation?

9. In what year was clinical specialty certification initiated by the APTA?

10. How many accredited programs exist in your state for the educational preparation of physical therapists?

11. Which of these programs grant a master's degree? A DPT degree?

12. How many accredited programs exist in your state for the educational preparation of physical therapist assistants?

13. When and where will your state chapter conference of the APTA be held this year?

14. Access to physical therapy services without physician referral is currently legal in how many states?

15. Is it legal in your state to provide physical therapy services to a patient without a physician's referral?

16. What is the name of the current president of the APTA?

17. What is the name of the current president of your state chapter of the APTA?

18. What do the initials CSM stand for? (Hint: an annual conference)

19. Which month is National Physical Therapy month?

20. Name one section of the APTA:

21. In what year were standards for utilization of the physical therapist assistant and standards for physical therapist assistant education adopted by the APTA?

22. What disease epidemic created the initial impetus for the physical therapy profession?

23. What degree is currently the minimum entry level educational requirement for physical therapy professional education?

24. What degree will you receive when you complete your educational program? (Be specific as to exact name of the degree-not "associate's degree")

25. What types (program length and requirements) of educational preparation programs are available for physical therapist assistant education?

26. What health care team members can supervise PTAs?

CHAPTER 2

The Changing World and the Future of Physical Therapy

In the past two decades, there have been widespread changes in the health care delivery system in the United States. Managed health care has changed reimbursement mechanisms and mandated widespread cost containment across all levels of care. The roles and practice parameters of the physical therapist and physical therapist assistant continue to evolve in response to these changes.

Cost Containment... Everywhere!

Elaine started her new position as a graduate physical therapist assistant and found that there were five staff members called "Patient Care Associates" who worked side-by-side with the licensed staff members in the department. She talked with one of them who told her that he was trained on the job to perform gait training and therapeutic exercise. She wondered how his training differed from hers.

Changing mechanisms of payment for services have forced health care organizations to develop numerous cost-containment strategies. For example, most physical therapists and physical therapist assistants practice in health care environments which are largely funded by a prospective payment system (PPS). PPS provides payment with a fixed limit or a fixed amount determined by the diagnosis of the patient, rather than by the actual time spent or individual needs of the patient.[1]

Health care providers often experience strict utilization management with increased accountability to third-party payers and health maintenance organizations. This requires an extra burden of paperwork which can be greatly simplified with use of computerized resources.

To manage costs, many health care institutions use on-the-job trained multiskilled workers for physical therapy-related functions and/or reduce the time or number of treatments that patients receive. These workers are sometimes given job titles within an institution of "rehab tech" or "patient care associate."

Physical therapists must therefore be able to prioritize and manage care while delegating and providing supervision for other members of the health care delivery team. State licensure laws vary considerably with regard to specific supervision requirements. Additionally, reimbursement guidelines often determine what services will be covered in the delivery of physical therapy intervention by support personnel.

It is the *physical therapist assistant* who is exclusively qualified and, in most states, licensed to specifically assist the physical therapist in the delivery of physical therapy treatments to patients/clients. Regardless of reimbursement challenges, it is unacceptable to permit unsupervised support personnel to perform entire treatment regimes. It is illegal for support personnel to represent themselves as physical therapists or physical therapist assistants. Furthermore, it is not considered ethical (or in most states legal) for the physical therapist assistant to work under the supervision of anyone besides a licensed physical therapist.

Cost-Effective and Efficient Outcomes

During journal club, Frank wondered why there was so little outcomes research in the physical therapy profession. Both the course instructor and their readings for this assignment had emphasized this point. Their guest speaker presented data which was routinely collected at their facility and indicated that they would like work with other facilities to collect and analyze patient practice patterns.

The focus of physical therapy is to improve physical performance and functional independence that is meaningful to the patient. This may include a person's ability to move about the environment, perform self-care, successfully complete job tasks, and enjoy leisure activities. Third-party payment systems require documentation of functional outcomes of physical therapy treatment, especially in relation to costs. Physical therapists must be able to efficiently and reliably evaluate a person's function and underlying impairments, develop meaningful physical therapy interventions, and objectively measure and document the effectiveness of physical therapy intervention over time.[2]

The *Guide to Physical Therapist Practice* outlines practice patterns which are indicated for various diagnostic groups. *The Guide* also lists objective tests and measurements with references that document the rationale and effectiveness of each procedure.[3] Tests, measurements, and interventions that result in efficient and cost-effective patient outcomes may give physical therapy an advantage in competing for limited health care dollars.

Shift to Prevention and Wellness

> The second-year physical therapist assistant students were assigned a class project to assist the district physical therapy association with preparing an exhibition on computer workstation ergonomics for the PT Month health fair at the mall. The project was approached scientifically, incorporating theories of behavioral change with simple, clear messages about body mechanics, posture, and exercise to prevent repetitive stress disorders.

With diminishing financial resources for treatment of existing illnesses and injuries, attention has been shifted to health promotion, wellness, and prevention of disease and disability. Physical therapists not only provide evaluation and treatment, but also provide services that are aimed at preventing illness and disability. Physical therapists are educated about health behavior and related health promotion strategies. Physical therapist assistants frequently assist with various aspects of the planning and implementation of these activities. More than ever before, excellent communication and patient education skills are critical for both the therapist and assistant.

Integrated Service Delivery

> What do nurses do? What do social workers do? How does occupational therapy differ from physical therapy? When is speech pathology indicated? Do each of these areas utilize licensed assistants? The case study raised all of these questions. What services would be appropriate and the most efficiently delivered to an 85-year-old widow who had just returned home from a 3-week stay in a skilled nursing facility while recovering from a stroke?

As our social service and health care systems increase in complexity and reimbursement dollars shrink, various health care workers must work together closely in order to optimally meet each patient's needs. Interdisciplinary case management has been associated with patients reaching higher levels of function in shorter lengths of time.[4] Integrated service delivery strategies involve interdisciplinary team interaction, interprofessional collaboration, and coordination between providers to deliver skillful services to clients and patients with multiple needs.[5] Physical therapists must be able to foster collaboration and coordination of service delivery, in addition to providing unique and specialized health care services. The physical therapist assistant will inevitably play an instrumental role on this interdisciplinary team.

Shift From Hospitals to Other Levels of Care

> Discharge planning was a word that came up frequently in classroom discussions this semester, including discussion of terms such as social support, prior level of function, mental status, judgment, and current functional level. It seemed that there were so many things to consider.
>
> What determines the level of care that is the most appropriate? Who makes these decisions? What role does the PTA plan in discharge planning?

Over the last several decades, patient length of stay in hospitals and rehabilitation facilities have decreased markedly, with a shift from in-patient services to subacute, outpatient, and home health services.[6] Thus, patients are more likely to receive physical therapy services in a skilled nursing facility, their homes or an outpatient center, rather than in an acute hospital.

Widespread cost containment strategies are changing the rules rapidly in these treatment settings. This requires health care providers to stay informed and work closely with administrators to provide necessary patient documentation and service-related information.

Variation in Supply and Demand for Physical Therapists

When Gina had planned on entering the physical therapy field in high school, physical therapy was forecast as one of the "hottest" professions for the future. Now it seemed like graduates were having difficulty getting full-time positions and were receiving lower salaries than they were several years ago. What happened?

During the late-1980s and into the mid-1990s, there were forecasts of widespread shortages of therapists as a result of the rapidly expanding role of physical therapists and the growing elderly population. In contrast, during the late-1990s, many organizations actually cut or restructured physical therapist and physical therapist positions in response to cost containment initiatives.[6]

Increases in the number of physical therapy and physical therapist assistant graduates combined with organizational staffing cuts led to a surplus of therapists in relation to available positions in some locations for a few years. This resulted in lower salaries, higher case loads, and increased daily patient volume for physical therapists and physical therapist assistants in some areas of the country. While jobs appear to be plentiful once again, the volatile nature of the health care delivery system requires the physical therapist assistant to become savvy about employment trends and develop skills that promote locating and retaining satisfying work.

Key Trends and Statistics That Influence Physical Therapy Practice

Throughout its history, changes in the number and distribution of persons with disabilities or the elderly and the prevalence of the most common public health problems have shaped physical therapy

practice. As mentioned in Table 1-2, widespread outbreaks of poliomyelitis in the 1950s and the Social Security Act of 1965 created an insatiable demand for physical therapy services.

These factors influenced the need for formally educated support personnel. The role of the physical therapist assistant, as an entity within the physical therapy profession, was established in 1967.[7]

Similarly, legislation affecting access to and reimbursement for physical therapy services has played a major role in practice. Let's look at the recent trends and legislation that have influenced the profession of physical therapy.

Disability Statistics

Helena, a first year physical therapist assistant student, who has been hard of hearing since childhood, sat in the first row of the classroom so that she could read the instructor's lips. She listened to the presentation about the Nagi and World Health Organization models of disablement, and wondered if her hearing problems would count as a disability.

Recent US Census estimates reflect that one in five persons in the United States has a disability and one in 10 has a severe disability.[8] Of those with a disability, 8% were between the ages of 5 and 20, and 66% were between the ages of 21 and 64 years old (57% of this age group were employed). The prevalence of disability increases with age; 42% of people over age 65 live with a disability.[9]

This may be a chronic disease process such as heart disease, sickle cell anemia, epilepsy, or cancer; a sensory disability, such as deafness, being hard of hearing, or a visual impairment; a physical disability, such as an amputation, paralysis, or problem with pain or movement; a learning disability, such as dyslexia or attention deficit disorder; a cognitive disability, such as Alzheimer's disease; or a disability related to a mental health condition. Some disabilities are not visible to the casual observer; others are obvious. Some are stable; some are progressive, or intermittent in nature.

What Constitutes a Disability?

For the purposes of identification by the US Census Bureau, a person is considered to have a "disability" if he or she has difficulty performing certain functions (seeing, hearing, talking, walking, climbing stairs, and lifting and carrying), has difficulty performing activities of daily living, or has difficulty with certain social roles (doing school work for children, working at a job and around the house for adults).[8]

A person who is unable to perform one or more activities, or who uses an assistive device to get around, or who needs assistance from another person to perform basic activities is considered to have a severe disability.[8]

See Tables 2-1 and 2-2 for an analysis of conditions causing disability and activity limitations.

Disabilities and Employment

Who has Jobs?

The most recent Survey of Income and Program Participation (SIPP) showed that only....
- 22% of working-age wheelchair users
- 28% of cane, crutch, or walker users
- 26% of people unable to climb stairs
- 23% of those unable to walk three city blocks
- 27% of those unable to lift and carry 10 pounds

...have jobs![10]

For those who do work, the chances that they will earn an equitable wage are slim. People with disabilities are often unemployed and live in poverty. The median monthly income for men with work disabilities averaged $1880 in 1995, according to the SIPP—20% less than the $2356 earned by their counterparts without disabilities. Women with disabilities earned $1511 monthly, or 13% less than the $1737 average for women without disabilities.[11]

Legislative and Economic Aspects of Disability

Before beginning her physical therapist assistant education, Irene worked part-time in the Center for Independent Living. One of the Center clients told her about his recent experience in seeking employment. He had been selected for a position which was matched perfectly with his qualifications. He wondered if he should have mentioned his need for an accessible restroom during the interview. Irene informed him that such accommodation was his right under the provisions of the ADA.

In the past 30 years, we have seen many legislative acts which affect the quality of life of individuals with disabilities. In Table 2-3 are a few examples of the major pieces of legislation that provide the basis for the rights of persons with disabilities in the United States.

Unfortunately, although there is legal protection in many situations, we still have a long way to go in changing public beliefs that it serves *all* people to make entrances to buildings barrier-free, to actively foster opportunities for employment for individuals with disabilities and to provide diagnostic and treatment services to the millions of children and adults with disabilities who live in poverty.

The Aging of America

Jason, home on spring break, visited his elderly grandparents in their retirement community. He was amazed to read their activity calendar. He remarked, "There's more going on here than at my college. Now I see why you're never home!"

Population aging is occurring in the United States and worldwide.

The elderly population in the United States (age 65 and older) increased by 3.7 million (12%) between 1990 and 2000. Seniors now number 35.0 million, about one in eight Americans. This compares to an increase of 13.3% for the under-65 age groups; however, 34% of the group of Americans aged 45 to 64 (the "baby boomers") will reach age 65 over the next twenty years. Since 1900, the percentage of Americans over age 65 has more than tripled from 4.1% in 1900 to 12.4% in 2000.[13]

The oldest segment of the elderly population is growing most rapidly. In 2000, the 65 to 74 age group (18.4 million) was eight times larger than it was in 1900 while the 75-84 group (12.4 million) was 16 times larger and the 85+ group (4.2 million) was 34 times larger.[13] The projected rates of growth of the elderly population are illustrated in Figure 2-1.[14]

Further, population statistics indicate that in the coming decades, the 65+ population will be much more racially and ethnically diverse than it is today. Projections estimate that there will be 80.1 million elderly by the year 2050. It is estimated that about 8.4 million will be African American and 12.5 million will be Hispanic.[13]

New evidence shows that rates of disability and disease may be slowing among older people, suggesting that progress can be made to improve the

---

Table 2-1

CONDITIONS CAUSING DISABILITY BY BROAD ICD AND IMPAIRMENT[12]

ICD Chapter		Number (1000s)	Percent of All Conditions
	ALL CONDITIONS	61,047	100.0
	DISORDERS AND INJURIES	44,721	73.3
13	Diseases of the musculoskeletal system and connective tissue (710-739)	10,530	17.2
7	Diseases of the circulatory system (390-459)	10,170	16.7
8	Diseases of the respiratory system (460-519)	4774	7.8
6	Diseases of the nervous system and sense organs (320-389)	4373	7.2
3	Endocrine, nutritional, and metabolic diseases and immunity disorders (780-779)	3409	5.6
15-16	Certain conditions originating from the perinatal period (760-799), and symptoms, signs, ill-defined conditions (520-579)	2843	4.7
5	Mental disorders (290-316) excluding mental retardation	2035	3.3
9	Diseases of the digestive system (520-579)	1728	2.8
2	Neoplasms (140-239)	1628	2.7
17	Injury and poisoning (800-999), not involving impairment	1205	2.0
10	Diseases of the genitourinary system (580-629)	778	1.3
1	Infectious and parasitic diseases (001-139)	378	0.6
12	Diseases of the skin and subcutaneous tissue (680-709)	362	0.6
14	Congenital abnormalities (740-759)	287	0.5
4	Diseases of the blood and blood-forming organs (280-289)	217	0.4
IMPAIRMENTS		16,326	26.7
Orthopedic impairments		8608	14.1
Learning disability and mental retardation		1575	2.6
Visual impairments		1294	2.1
Hearing impairments		1175	1.9
Paralysis		1071	1.8
Deformities		900	1.5
Absence or loss of limb/other body part		788	1.3
Speech impairments		545	0.9
Other and ill-defined impairments		371	0.6

Note: Conditions in ICD Chapter 11, complications of pregnancy, childbirth, and the puerperium (630-676), are not used.

Adapted from *National Health Interview Survey*. Hyattsville, Md: National Center for Health Statistics; 1992.

Table 2-2 MOST COMMON CONDITIONS CAUSING ACTIVITY LIMITATION[12]		
Rank	Number (1000s)	Percent of All Conditions
ALL CONDITIONS	61 047	100.0
1 Heart disease (390-429)	7932	13.0
2 Deformities, orthopedic impairments and disorders of the spine or back	7672	12.6
3 Osteoarthrosis and allied disorders (715-716)	5048	8.3
4 Orthopedic impairment of lower extremity	2817	4.6
5 Asthma (493)	2592	4.2
6 Diabetes (250)	2569	4.2
7 Mental disorders (290-316), excluding learning disability and mental retardation	2035	3.3
8 Disorders of the eye (360-379)	1577	2.6
9 Learning disability and mental retardation	1575	2.6
10 Cancer (140-208)	1342	2.2
11 Visual impairments	1294	2.1
12 Orthopedic impairment of shoulder and/or upper extremities	1196	2.0
13 Other unknown and unspecified causes	1188	1.9
14 Hearing impairments	1175	1.9
15 Cerebrovascular disease (430-438)	1174	1.9

Adapted from *National Health Interview Survey*. Hyattsville, Md: National Center for Health Statistics; 1992.

health of people age 65+. However, with population aging, living to very advanced age likely will mean disease and disability for increasing numbers of older Americans.[14]

Increasing age heightens the probability of functional limitations. In one survey, over 4.5 million (14.2%) of people between 65 to 80 years reported difficulty with bathing, dressing, and eating, compared with 35% for those age 80 and older. This is much higher than the 2.8% of the 25 to 64 year olds who reported having difficulty with these activities of daily living (ADLs).[15]

Most older people report having at least one chronic condition with many having multiple conditions. The most frequently occurring conditions per 100 elderly in 1996 were: arthritis (49), hypertension (36), hearing impairments (30), heart disease (27), cataracts (17), orthopedic impairments (18), sinusitis (12), and diabetes (10).[12] The link between advancing age and increasing functional problems has enor-

mous implications for long-term care and the need for physical therapy.[14]

National Legislation With a Direct Influence on the Profession of Physical Therapy

Social Security Act of 1965

With the passage of the Social Security Act of 1965, the government began to subsidize two health care plans: the *Medicare* and *Medicaid* programs. This legislation resulted in marked changes in access to health care for the elderly and poor. For example, during the late 1950s less than 15% of the elderly population had any health insurance. The enactment of the Medicare and Medicaid programs helped to provide health insurance to nearly 85% of all Americans by 1966.[16]

Table 2-3
Key Legislative Activity and Disability Issues

Legislation Affecting Persons With Disabilities

Rehabilitation Act of 1973	Mandated no discrimination by federally-funded agencies against workers and students with disabilities and affirmative action requirements for federally funded employers.
Americans with Disabilities Act of 1990	Mandated reasonable accommodations to ensure the integration of people with disabilities in the private sector, including employment, telecommunications, transportation, and public services and accommodations.

Legislation Affecting Children With Disabilities

PL 94-142	Education for All Handicapped Children Act of 1975: mandated a free and appropriate education and the least restrictive environment (ie, mainstreaming). Annual IEP's (Individual Educational Plans) are developed for all children with disabilities.
PL 101-476	Revised provisions of PL 94-142 to include children with autism and brain injury and included training and technology provisions for education of children with disabilities.
IDEA Improvement Act of 1997	Gave parents and school districts more autonomy in determining children's needs for special education services through a mediation process, further defined services available to infants and toddlers, and provided disciplinary sanctions for students who engage in criminal misconduct, unrelated to disability.

Legislation Affecting Older Adults

PL 101-234 – The Omnibus Reconciliation Act (OBRA) of 1987	Major piece of legislation set standards for nursing home personnel; the rights of nursing home residents and set standards for home health agencies.
1990 Nursing Home Reform for Amendments of OBRA	Nursing homes required by law to focus on each resident's highest potential physical, mental, and psychosocial well-being by assessing these abilities and developing individualized care plans. These care plans must be reassessed for any change in function at least quarterly. This created numerous employment opportunities for therapists in the nursing home setting.

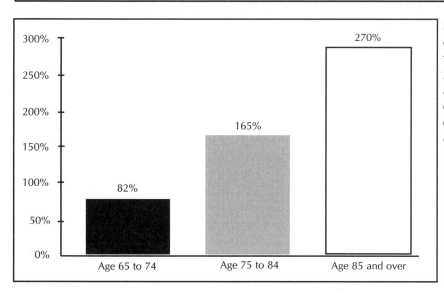

Figure 2-1. Percentage of projected growth in the elderly population by age group from 1990 to 2040. Rapid rates of growth are anticipated for all segments of the elderly population, with the greatest growth occurring in those age 85 and older.[14]

To be eligible for Medicare, an individual must be a citizen or permanent resident of the United States who has worked and contributed to Social Security for at least 10 years and be at least 65 years of age. People under 65 are entitled to Medicare if they have been receiving Social Security benefits for 24 months or have end-stage renal disease. A person can also be eligible if their spouse has met the employment requirement.[16] Medicaid (MediCal in California) is a state-administered program that provides medical assistance to the poor, and is financed through both state and federal taxes. Eligibility is determined by income and other requirements.

Health Care Reform—National Health Insurance Initiative Defeated

In the subsequent decades, as health costs increased logarithmically, it became clear that a significant group of citizens had no medical insurance and were not eligible for either of these public programs. In fact, almost 20% of the US population is currently uninsured. This lead to efforts in the early 1990s to create a system of National Health Insurance. Bitter conflicts erupted between leaders in Congress and the Clinton administration regarding the scope and content of this health care initiative.

In the mid-1990s, following the failure of national health insurance to be adopted by Congress, there was growing concern that the Medicare system would soon have no money, given the aging population demographics and escalating costs of health care. This led to further cost containment in the Medicare system.

The Balanced Budget Amendment of 1997

Perhaps the single piece of modern-day legislation to have the greatest effect on the profession of physical therapy is the Balanced Budget Amendment of 1997. President Clinton signed H.R. 2015, the Balanced Budget Act of 1997 on August 5, 1997.[17]

This legislation, intended to eliminate the federal deficit, created widespread cuts in the Medicare and Medicaid systems, intended to reduce entitlement spending by $115 billion in Medicare over 5 years and $13.6 billion in Medicaid over 5 years. The largest portion of these savings came from reduced Medicare payments to health care providers and hospitals. Hospitals were slated to lose some $40 billion in Medicare (35% of the overall cuts), while payments to managed care plans under Medicare were to be reduced by $22 billion over 5 years. Further reductions in hospital payments, home health services, and skilled nursing facility (SNF) payments also reduced reimbursement for physical therapy services.[18]

Physical therapists were especially hard hit by the provisions of the Balanced Budget Act. The act included a provision that imposed an arbitrary annual cap of $1500 per beneficiary for combined physical therapy and speech therapy services provided by comprehensive outpatient rehabilitation facilities (CORFs), SNFs, and physicians' offices.[17] This extraordinarily low level of reimbursement fell far short of that required to provide necessary services for millions of elderly Americans. The American Physical Therapy Association actively advocated for a moratorium on the $1500 cap until an alternate system could be put into place.

In late 1999, Congress and the White House reached an agreement on a plan to restore more than $12 billion in cuts previously made in Medicare payments. The Balanced Budget Refinement Act eliminated the $1500 caps on Medicare's coverage of physical therapy, occupational therapy, and speech pathology. It also postponed a 15% reduction in payments to home health agencies and increased payments for some patients in skilled nursing facilities.[18]

The Balanced Budget Amendment of 1997 also authorized a prospective payment system (PPS) for skilled nursing facilities. Changes in Medicare reimbursement schedules resulted in widespread decreases in physical therapist staffing of skilled nursing facilities.[18] Further, the Act created a comprehensive assessment of adult home care patients called The Outcome and Assessment Information Set (OASIS) to measure outcomes for the purposes of quality improvement for Medicare-certified home health agencies.[18]

The physical therapy profession, along with other health care providers, vigorously lobbied Congress and the Centers for Medicare and Medicaid Services (CMS) to permanently repeal arbitrary therapy caps and instead contain costs based on the patient/client's condition and past medical history. While gaining support from legislators, Congress adjourned without extending the moratorium on the $1500 therapy caps, thereby allowing the caps to go back into effect in September 2003. Sustained lobbying efforts by health care providers, as well as, increased involvement by elders affected by these caps, led to an amendment within the Medicare Prescription Drug, Improvement, and Modernization Act signed into law by President George W. Bush on December 8, 2003, which immediately restored the moratorium on the Medicare therapy cap extending it through 2005. An appreciation of the effectiveness and efficiency of physical therapy by legislators plays a key role in favorable legislation being passed. All of these changes have had and will continue to have marked implications for the physical therapy profession.[19]

Summary

Changes in the health care delivery system and the changing population demographics have forced a shift in physical therapy practice. Increased accountability, variations in supply and demand for physical therapists and physical therapist assistants, and changing priorities in public health will continue to influence the future of the physical therapy profession.

References

1. Kristy W. Basics of health care financing and reimbursement. In Curtis KA, ed. *The Physical Therapist's Guide to Health Care*. Thorofare, NJ: SLACK Incorporated; 1999:13-47.

2. Chech D, Martin S. *Functional Movement Development Across the Lifespan*. Philadelphia, PA: WB Saunders: 2002:118-119.

3. American Physical Therapy Association. *Guide to Physical Therapy Practice*. 2nd ed. Alexandria Va: American Physical Therapy Association; 2000:s99.

4. Erickson B, Perkins M. Interdisciplinary team approach in the rehabilitation of hip and knee arthroplasties. *Am J Occup Ther*. 1994;48(5):429-441.

5. Hilton RW, Morris DJ, Wright AM. Learning to work in the health care team. *Journal of Interprofessional Care*. 1995;9(3):267-274, 1995.

6. Lopopolo RB. The effect of hospital restructuring on the role of physical therapists in acute care. *Phys Ther*. 1997;77(9):918-32.

7. APTA. The future role of the PTA (RC 40-01), report to 2002 House of Delegates. 2002:78. Available at: http://www.apta.org/governance/HoD/2002Ho/5thHoDPosting/Special Reports. Accessed February 10, 2003.

8. US Department of Commerce, Economics, and Statistics Administration. *Census Brief*. US CBO2-FF11; July 2002.

9. US Census Bureau. CB02-FF.11 12th Anniversary of Americans With Disabilities Act (July 26). Available at: http://www.census.gov/Press-Release/www/2002/cb02ff11.html. Accessed September 24, 2004.

10. Kaye HS. *Disability Watch: The Status of People with Disabilities in the United States*. Volcano, Calif: Disability Rights Advocates, 1997.

11. Kaye HS. The income gap. In: *Disability Watch: The Status of People with Disabilities in the United States*. Volcano, Calif: Disability Rights Advocates, 1997.

12. *National Health Interview Survey*. Hyattsville, MD: National Center for Health Statistics; 1992

13. Administration on Aging. *A Profile of Older Americans: 2002*. Washington DC: National Center for Health Statistics. Available from: http://www.aoa.gov/prof/Statistics/profile/profiles2002.asp. Accessed June 23, 2004.

14. Aging America Poses Unprecedented Challenge, Says New Census, Aging Institute Report [press release]. Washington DC: National Institutes of Health Public Information Office; May 20, 1996. Available from: http://www.nia.nih.gov/news/pr/1996/05%2D20.htm Accessed on June 16, 2000.

15. Administration on Aging. A profile of older Americans: 2002. Available at: http://www.aoa.gov/prof/Statistics/profile/profiles2002.asp. Accessed September 24, 2004.

16. Relman AS. Assessment and accountability: the third revolution in medical care. *NEJM*. 1988;319(18):1220-1222.

17. APTA. The Balanced Budget Act. How it affects physical therapy. Available at: http://www.apta.org/Advocacy/national/National16 Accessed July 30, 2000.

18. APTA. History of medicare therapy caps. Available from: http://www.apta.org/Govt_Affairs/cap_resourcectr/background/history. Accessed January 17, 2003.

19. APTA. 2004 physician fee schedule final rule: summary. Available at: http://www.apta.org/Govt_Affairs/regulatory/Medicare/treatment_settings/privatepractice/2004_feeschedule/2004FeeSchedule-Summary. Accessed September 24, 2004.

1. Interview a person with a disability or a person over the age of 65 about their recent experiences in accessing health care services.

   Briefly describe the person you interviewed:

   What has been this person's experience in finding health care providers to provide services covered by their insurance plan?

   What has been this person's experience in finding health care providers who are able to meet their needs?

   What health care needs are currently unmet?

2. Interview a physical therapist assistant who has been in practice for more than 5 years. What changes has he/she seen in the profession during that time? How has the field differed from his/her expectations before entering the profession? How has practice changed since the implementation of the Balanced Budget Amendment of 1997?

CHAPTER 3

Evolving Roles in Physical Therapy

> Karen had expected to work in an outpatient orthopedic or sports clinic, but found a better paying job closer to home in a skilled nursing facility "Health Center" at a multilevel care, senior residential complex. "You're not going to work in one of those dingy nursing homes, are you?" her older sister had asked, adding, "I couldn't. Those places are so depressing." Karen had done some aide work at a skilled nursing facility and knew her sister was behind the times. Nonetheless, she had some reservations. Her orientation at the facility reassured her. "Wow," she commented. "This place looks like a resort! Beautiful dining room, gardens, fitness room, and skylights to brighten the interior. I'll have to bring my sister to see this."

The Future of Physical Therapy

In this world of constant change, the milieu in which physical therapists (PTs) and physical therapist assistants (PTAs) practice will inevitably change as well. PTs who practice in the next decade will face challenges in service delivery because of the complexity of multiple realities. Sensitivity to these changes is critical for all health care workers. Consider the following forces which shape the practice environment:

* The world's population of those over 65 is growing at an unprecedented rate. The most recent Census Bureau's findings indicate that 13 percent of people in the United States are age 65 or older. In fact, over 9.2 million people living in the United States are 80 years or beyond. The US Census Bureau and the National Institute on Aging (NIA) predict that the global aging phenomenon will continue well into the 21st century.[1] The health care needs of these elders may not be met by a Medicare system that is undergoing constant change and cost containment in an attempt to survive.

* The ethnic diversity of this population is also growing. In some states, combined non-White minorities currently comprise the majority of the population. Language barriers, cultural bias, and socioeconomic challenges influence the delivery of health care services.

* Economic upheaval at the federal and state level have resulted in millions of our citizens living in poverty, lacking access to even basic medical services. Over one-fifth of the population is uninsured by any type of medical insurance program.

* The Balanced Budget Act of 1997 created a downturn in employment opportunities for health care workers, including PTs and PTAs. While in some areas of the country and in some practice settings, the job market tightened, there continued to be maldistribution of physical therapy personnel available to care for those in need of services. Fortuitously, employment opportunities for PTs and PTAs are, once again, plentiful as those needing physical therapy services continue to increase especially in rural and socioeconomically depressed areas.

* Over one-third of disability and disease in this country could be prevented by changing lifestyle habits such as diet and activity. In fact, the Centers for Disease Control has called *obesity* one of the latest epidemics to hit the United States.[2]

* Women's health issues are becoming increasingly important as heart disease, osteoporosis, and related fractures account for significant disability and untimely deaths of elderly women.

* Like most other health professions, physical therapy can no longer rely on reimbursement

from third-party payment systems for their economic security. Other mechanisms of payment and creative modes of service delivery must be explored to address the ever-increasing health care needs of the population.

* Heath care spending is at an all-time high and is projected to continue to rise yearly. It is speculated that by 2011 health care costs will account for 17% of the Gross National Product (GNP).[3] Consumers and third-party payers continue to increase the pressure for cost-effective care. Evidence-based outcomes will continue to be the greatest source of validation for the valuable work that PTs and PTAs provide.

* Internet use has increased exponentially worldwide over the past decade. There are now over 175 million Americans accessing the Internet.[4] Consumers have access to health care information as never before. The value of physical therapy programs and services must be publicized for consumers, businesses, health care providers, and third-party payers to see and understand. Technology use may be the single most important mechanism to publicize the value and availability of physical therapy services.

Consider again, the "Vision Statement" in Chapter 1. Many of the changes noted above must be embraced as the role of the PT is defined within the context of the future health care environment. The roles and responsibilities of the PTA will inevitably be altered as well, yet must remain tied to the basic tenets described by the ethical and practice parameters set by the professional association and various regulatory and licensure bodies.

Key Roles for Physical Therapists ...and What About the Physical Therapist Assistant?

In addition to providing competent intervention, PTs must be skilled in examination, evaluation, diagnosis, prognosis, case management, consultation, delegation of treatment responsibilities to others, patient education, documentation, collaboration, and program development.

The changing health care environment requires practicing clinicians to respond to health care delivery trends and to redesign their organizational responsibilities accordingly.

In keeping with the expanding role and level of responsibility, the profession is moving toward

entry-level PT education at the Doctor of Physical Therapy (DPT) level with a projected 72% of all accredited physical therapy programs offering this as the entry-level degree by 2010.[5]

The challenges confronting the physical therapy profession require critical examination and careful planning to preserve, in fact, *enhance* the image, accessibility, and efficacy of services. Considering the future role and function of the PTA as a partnering stakeholder within these new paradigms is an integral part of this process.

Regardless of the inevitable modifications in where, how long, and who pays for physical therapy services, the caveat remains that the PT is responsible for and directs all services provided, including the determination of the utilization of the PTA in strict accordance with state law, regulatory policies, and ethical standards of practice.[6] Let's examine some of the roles PTs must embrace, as well as the accompanying aspects of the PTA. Be sure to review and keep in mind Table 3-1.

Change Agent

*Linda raised her hand and contributed to the class discussion, "It seems like everything is constantly changing and it's all so complicated. During my clinical rotation last week, I wrote a SOAP note in the patient's chart after we worked with a lady in the hospital but had to use specific forms and **each** box had to be filled in after we worked with the person in the nursing home."*

We have seen significant changes in the physical therapy profession and are likely to see many more in the next few years. PTs and PTAs must remain flexible and informed as the present-day rules may change tomorrow, the next day and even again next week.

But even more importantly than being flexible in the face of change, therapists must assume a proactive role as change agents. Rather than letting external forces dictate constraints on clinical practice, PTs and PTAs must educate others regarding the legal and ethical implications of change as it affects patient care. Therapists must advocate for accessibility and inclusion of physical therapy services as a cost-effective use of health care dollars.

On a larger scale, PTs must take a proactive role in organizational change processes. They must identify and communicate to others the expertise of PTs and determine what can and cannot be compromised in physical therapy service delivery. PTs must be in

---

Table 3-1

THE ROLE OF THE PHYSICAL THERAPIST ASSISTANT[7]

Physical therapist assistants (PTAs) provide physical therapy services under the supervision and direction of the physical therapist (PT).

They:

* Assist with data collection

* Implement patient interventions

* Make appropriate judgments

* Modify interventions within the PT's established plan of care

* Participate in discharge planning and follow-up care; document the care provided

* Educate and interact with PT and PTA students, aides, volunteers, patients, families, and caregivers

* Demonstrate an understanding of the significance and impact of cultural and individual differences

Physical therapist assistants contribute to society and the physical therapy profession through the provision of physical therapy services, teaching and administration. Depending on circumstances, some tasks may be performed cooperatively with other health care personnel or through supervision of aides and volunteers.

Adapted from: APTA. *Normative Model of PTA Education*. Version 99. Alexandria, Va: American Physical Therapy Association; 1999:3.

---

control of changes in their roles and responsibilities rather than letting someone else make those decisions. The PTA plays an important role in communicating the uniqueness of skilled physical therapy intervention to each patient, family member, caregiver, and other health care team members.

The good news is that there are many opportunities to educate others regarding the physical therapy profession in the changing health care environment. PTs and PTAs need to be astutely aware of the past and present history of the profession, as well as, laws, regulations and ethical boundaries governing practice as they secure a place in the future of health care delivery.

Data and Outcome Reporter

Maria, during her final clinical internship, lamented to another intern, "Why do we need to do all this paperwork? Don't they know that we are more valuable actually working with the patients?"

Data. What do we really need to know? And who needs to know it? Documentation. Paper work. Tests & Measurements. Progress Reports. Outcomes.

These processes are the keys to providing evidence of the value of physical therapy services. Organized data collection and systematic analysis and reporting of outcomes are the key to establishing

the efficacy of clinical practices and determining the best methods to deliver physical therapy service.

PTs who can design systems of data collection and analyze and report the results will be able to further establish the value of physical therapy services. Computerized record keeping is an important component of any data collection system as it makes it easier to systematically collect and collate patient outcome data.

It is essential for the PTA to conscientiously document in order to facilitate the collection of meaningful data related to physical therapy care.

Program Developer

Nasir worked for several years on a part-time basis at the local Senior Center prior to entering the physical therapist assistant program. He saw many seniors who were able to maintain an active, healthy lifestyle. He wondered how the lives of seniors might improve even more if physical therapy services could be offered like preventive maintenance on your automobile or periodic dental cleaning by the dentist.

Physical therapy services have traditionally been offered to address problems, after the problem has already occurred. Research has demonstrated that exercise and prevention can minimize, and even prevent, the impairments and functional limitations associated with many disease processes. In addition, conventional service delivery is no longer covered by many insurances. Exploring alternative ways of providing cost effective and meaningful therapy services is and will continue to be a priority for the physical therapy profession.

New program development requires that PTs and PTAs be aware of the needs of a patient population and look at creative ways to meet those needs. It may be through a group class, a community event, a sponsored screening day, a peer network, or a telephone hot line. Innovation in program development is a key to adapting to the changing health care environment.

Collaborator

Oscar sat in his first team meeting around a table with professionals from five other disciplines. He looked over his report and found that several team members who spoke before him had reported conflicting information about the patient's social support network. Perhaps this patient was not able to go home as soon as planned.

We live in a complex world. As educational, social service, and health care systems increase in complexity, members of the health care team must collaborate with one another to provide for the multiple needs of their patients or clients. *Collaboration* means cooperating with each other, joining forces, pooling resources, and working together for the best interest of the patient/client and/or family. There is evidence that outcomes improve and care is provided more efficiently when a collaborative process is used to plan and provide patient or client-centered services. In addition, it is important to include clients, parents, family members, and caregivers in the collaborative process to determine the best plan for each individual client.[8,9]

Interprofessional collaboration involves working together to reach a common goal in a supportive and mutually beneficial relationship with other team members. Collaborative team interactions include voluntary involvement, parity, and shared decision-making power among team members.[9] An awareness of organizational and group dynamics, conflict resolution strategies, leadership, and communication skills characterize effective teamwork.[10]

We are seeing a trend in academic programs to introduce opportunities for students to gain skills in teamwork and interprofessional collaboration.[9-11]

PTs and PTAs become more valuable members of the health care team when they have strong skills in communication and collaboration.

Paula sat in the front row of the classroom. She wondered "Why do we need to spend so much time on patient education? I want to provide hands-on care."

Educator

Education and motivation precede the changes in behavior that lead to prevention of disability and disease. Over one-third of the US population will suffer from disease or disability which can be prevented by diet and exercise. Many of these conditions can be prevented through education and lifestyle change.

To become effective educators, an understanding of the factors that motivate and drive health behavior must be integrated with the patient's specific needs and personality. It is important to utilize available educational technology, develop culturally- and linguistically-appropriate educational materials, and create effective information systems. These practices will maximize the impact on the outcomes that patients can achieve.

Physical therapy intervention must emphasize what patients and their care-givers can do to maximize function, reduce pain and stress, prevent further disability, and return to work. And not to be overlooked, education SAVES money... for consumers, for their employers, and for third party payers.

Roles Exclusive to the Physical Therapist

Patient/Client Management

Roberto decided to write his Capstone paper on Delegation and Supervision in Physical Therapy. He interviewed practicing therapists and read about the history and evolution of support personnel and found that there are many differing beliefs and misinformation in practice about the laws and documents governing this aspect of practice.

Examination, evaluation, diagnosis, prognosis. Each of these terms has specific meanings to the PT. Through laws and core documents that govern phys-

---

Table 3-2

DETERMINING PRIORITIES
FOR PHYSICAL THERAPY SERVICE DELIVERY[12]

1. Which patients need to be seen on a one-on-one basis and whose needs can be met in a group environment?

2. Which patients need daily or twice daily treatment, as opposed to once, twice or three times weekly; and at what level of care?

3. Which patients are changing so rapidly or are so unstable that a professional must constantly reassess the patient responses to treatment before going further?

4. What services can be provided by support personnel?

5. And finally, which patients have needs that are urgent and should begin services immediately and which patients can wait?

Reprinted with permission from Curtis KA. Managing change. In: Curtis KA, ed. *The Physical Therapist's Guide to Health Care.* Thorofare, NJ: SLACK Incorporated; 1999:4.

---

ical therapy practice, the role of the PT has been differentiated as the one uniquely qualified to make decisions to collect and consider evaluative data, to identify the cluster, condition or syndrome(s) present, determine the need for physical therapy intervention, and select the most appropriate intervention strategies (the plan of care). With decreasing resources, it becomes increasingly important that PTs evaluate which patients are most likely to benefit from receiving services. They then must be able to accurately predict the level of anticipated functional outcome, the timing, frequency and duration of the specified plan of care to reach optimal improvements.

PTs today enter practice with specialized skills in screening and triage. PTs need to determine the best use of limited resources. The questions in Table 3-2 are among those used by the PT during the screening process.

Appropriate direction and supervision of support personnel is an important and increasingly complex portion of the PT's responsibility as a clinician.[13,14] Federal and state laws, as well as many insurance companies specifically define whose expertise is required for reimbursement. These laws also protect the safety of the public with regard to the delivery of therapy treatments, also known as interventions. It is the professional and legal responsibility of the PT and PTA to be aware of and follow all federal and state laws and regulations.

In addition, the American Physical Therapy Association publishes its expected practice standards and *Guides for Conduct* of PTs and assistants as part of

the profession's core documents. The *Guide to Physical Therapist Practice* is considered the primary core document for the profession.[5] Updates, including the *Code of Ethics* and *Policies and Position Statements,* are debated and amended as necessary each year by the profession's highest policy making body, the American Physical Therapy Association's House of Delegates.

The profession contends that appropriate supervision requires that PTs provide or direct and supervise the PTA in the provision of physical therapy interventions.[6] Since the core documents of a profession are considered the "gold standard" by external bodies, it is imperative for each physical therapist assistant to be familiar with and uphold the principles as written in The *Guide to Physical Therapist Practice* and the most current policies and positions of the profession. See Appendix 5 for the most recent comprehensive documentation *Direction and Supervision of the Physical Therapist Assistant.*

Case-Manager

Selena heard the clinical instructor say, "This patient will be discharged tomorrow. Where do you think he should go? What level of care is appropriate?" She wondered how this is determined.

To make this decision, PTs consider the patient's needs, the types of treatment environments (acute, subacute, rehabilitation, home health, outpatient), and the roles, skills, and capabilities of various personnel available to meet those needs. The case manager must be a patient advocate, educator, excellent team player and communicator, *and* have the educational preparation and expertise to synthesize all pertinent factors related to the diagnosis, prognosis, and specific plan of care.

The discharge plan is one of the priorities for consideration when beginning a patient's evaluation. Does this patient have what it takes to be successful at the next level of care, whether that will be in an institution, outpatient clinic, or in the home?

PTs who exhibit good delegation and communication skills and use an organized follow-up system can prevent the patient from "slipping through the cracks." While patient/client management is the responsibility of the PT, appropriate utilization of the PTA can maximize service delivery and enhance patient outcomes.

Unfortunately, only some health care consumers are able to survive and navigate in the current health care environment. Most patients require health care providers to be strong advocates to empower them, to educate them, to assist them with access the equipment, services, and referrals they need to appropriately address their health care needs.

Consultant

> The panel discussion at the State Physical Therapy conference had just begun. The first speaker said he was a consultant to a manufacturing plant. I prevent injuries in the workplace. I save my clients thousands of dollars every year. He challenged the audience, "How can physical therapists share their expert knowledge with those who need it most?"

Consultation is a critical role for PTs. Consultation is essentially the process of giving an opinion based on your expertise. This is not a new role for PTs. PTs have been giving their opinions for years, in documenting patient goals and rehabilitation potential, assessments of patient's progress, and discharge recommendations. In the current health care environment, some worry that the complexities of service delivery will be reduced to a series of "cookbook" approaches, critical pathways, and protocols. Sharing one's expertise often makes it clear that a situation is more complex than it may appear on the surface. Identifying "niche markets" that traverse far beyond the traditional clinical setting is becoming a reality for many PTs. For example, more therapists are developing areas of expertise in the area of women's health care. It is quite common to find PTs

practicing alongside gynecologists in women's health clinics.

PTs have many areas of expertise. Some physical therapists possess expert knowledge in the field of movement science and pathokinesiology, others in ergonomics or assistive technology. Still other therapists have received specialist certification in specific clinical domains, such as aquatics, sports, orthopedics, pediatrics, geriatrics, or cardiopulmonary care. Many pursue expertise in health care administration and management.

The role of the consultant is to share one's professional expertise and to educate others. A consultant might provide an explanation of the interrelationships of pathology and functional loss, of impairment and projected outcomes, or organizational change and performance criteria. The consultant often relates known research findings to clinical or environmental problems. Consultants provide critical analysis and advanced clinical decision-making in complex situations.

The PTA certainly may play a role within the consultative venue especially with enhanced skill proficiency through career development activities and mentoring. However, critical analysis and advanced clinical decision-making related to patient care and/or making expert recommendations to others are the responsibilities of the PT.

Summary

Change is constant. PTs and PTAs must be vigilant in monitoring the changing dynamics of the health care environment. Sensitivity to the diverse needs of the changing population, flexibility in choosing the means and methods to meet those needs and accountability in service delivery will be the hallmarks of success in the future.

Thorny issues surrounding the role, responsibilities, supervision, direction, and delegation of the PTA have been debated since the addition of an educated and licensed (in most states) extender of therapy services over 30 years ago. While progress has been made, there is limited consensus and much disparity continues in clinical practice. The utilization of aides and other unlicensed support personnel is a separate but equally as contentious problem.

The onus lies with each and every PT and PTA to be attentive and adhere to the legal and professional expectations of practice.

References

1. National Institutes of Health. World's older population growing by unprecedented 800,000 a month. *US Census and Aging Institute Report.* Available at: http://www.nih.gov/nia/new/press/census.htm. Accessed September 14, 2004.

2. Centers for Disease Control and Prevention. Obesity and genetics: a public health perspective. Available at: http://www.cdc.gov/genomics/info/perspectives/obesity.htm#Public. Accessed September 27, 2004.

3. Sinnott MC. Bifocal vision and the practice of one. *APTA Health Policy & Administration Resource.* 2003; 3(1).

4. Global Internet Statistics. Sources and references. Available at: http://global-reach.biz/globstats/details.html. Accessed September 24, 2004.

5. APTA. *Accreditation Update Newsletter, Commission on Accreditation for Physical Therapy Education.* 2003; 8(1):8.

6. APTA. *Guide to Physical Therapist Practice.* 2nd ed. Alexandria, Va: American Physical Therapy Association; 2001.

7. APTA. *A Normative Model of Physical Therapist Assistant Education, Version 99.* Alexandria, Va: American Physical Therapy Association; 1999.

8. Erickson B, Perkins M. Interdisciplinary team approach in the rehabilitation of hip and knee arthroplasties. *Am J Occup Ther.* 1994; 48(5):429-441.

9. O'Connor B. Challenges of interagency collaboration: Serving a young child with severe disabilities. In: McEwen IR, ed. *Occupational and Physical Therapy in Educational Environments.* Binghamton, NY: Haworth Press; 1995.

10. Hilton RW, Morris DJ, Wright AM. Learning to work in the health care team. *J Interprof Care.* 1995; 9(3):267-274.

11. Richardson J, Edwards M. An undergraduate clinical skills laboratory developing interprofessional skills in physical and occupational therapy. *Gerontol Geriatr Educ.* 1997;17(4): 33-43

12. Curtis KA. Managing change. In: Curtis KA, ed. *The Physical Therapist's Guide to Health Care.* Thorofare, NJ: SLACK Incorporated; 1994:4.

13. Thomas B. Supervising personnel in subacute and long-term care. *Advance for Physical Therapists and Physical Therapist Assistants.* 2003; 14(17):63.

14. Thomas B. Policies on supervision of personnel: Part II. *Advance for Physical Therapists and Physical Therapist Assistants.* 2003; 14(19):65

PUTTING IT INTO PRACTICE

1. Consider your role as a physical therapist assistant and the skills needed to succeed in the role. Think of situations in which you have used these skills in the past. Explore your curriculum and identify opportunities for you to acquire these skills during your educational program. Enter this information in the appropriate boxes below:

Roles	Skills needed to succeed in this role	Situations in which I've used these skills in the past	How to acquire these skills during your education program
Change agent			
Data and outcomes reporter			
Program developer			
Team player			
Educator			
"Delegatee" (subordinate role to the therapist)			
Patient advocate			
Compliance with pertinent laws and core documents			

PART TWO

Becoming a Physical Therapist Assistant

CHAPTER 4

Financing Physical Therapist Assistant Education

Tanya, a single parent, considered enrolling in the physical therapist assistant program when she became disillusioned with her retail sales position. She looked into the expenses of 2 years of education and realized that not only would she have to leave her current position; she would also have to pay for tuition, fees, books, and other related educational expenses. How much would it all cost?

Expenses for Physical Therapist Assistant Education

Depending on whether one chooses to attend a private or public institution, total estimated costs for all educational expenses, excluding living expenses, during physical therapist assistant (PTA) education may range from approximately \$5400 to \$22,000.[1] The estimated cumulative expenses for a student enrolled in PTA education in public and private institutions are shown in Table 4-1.

The majority of PTA education programs are in public institutions.[1] Even so, the costs of attending a five to six semester program in a public institution will be close to \$30,000 including living expenses.

Financial Aid

Uri, a former food service clerk, starting the physical therapist assistant program, waited for the Financial Aid counselor to return from lunch. He worried, "I have taken out so many loans... Is this really worth it? How am I ever going to be able to pay all these loans back?"

Few students can afford to pay for all of the expenses of their education without some form of education financing. There are several forms of financial aid that are available to PTA students. Please check with your local Financial Aid office for forms, deadlines and specifics of the types of financial aid for which you qualify. For example, tuition fee waivers are available at some colleges. This form of financial assistance requires no repayment, however, early application deadlines are quite common.

Loans

A loan is a form of financial aid that must be repaid, with interest. Many students find that they must supplement their savings with government and private loans. Federal education loan programs offer lower interest rates and more flexible repayment plans than most consumer loans, making these loans a feasible way to finance your education[2] (Table 4-2).

Comparing different types of loans can be confusing. There are a number of options including the rate of interest, how interest is calculated and on what schedule interest is accrued. This can make a big difference in the bottom line (ie, the total you will have to pay back, even when borrowing the same principal). Table 4-3 lists some questions which students should be sure to ask when taking out a loan.

Manageable Debt

Educational debt to income ratio is the percentage of your monthly income which is required to pay your loan payment.[2] A ratio of 15% or less is optimal, the lower the better, as most graduates have other expenses as well, such as a car payment, mortgage and other forms of consumer debt. Table 4-4 may help you plan for manageable debt, given an average starting wage of a graduate PTA.

Table 4-1

COST ESTIMATES FOR
PHYSICAL THERAPIST ASSISTANT EDUCATION[1]

	Public Institutions (In-State Rates)	Private Institutions and Out-of-State Tuition Rates
Annual Tuition/fees	$500 to $3000	$6000 to $12,000
Books and supplies	$1000	$1000
Room and board	$5500	$5500
Uniforms and other fees	$100	$100
Personal, transportation, insurance	$2000	$2000
Annual costs*	$9100 to $11,600	$12,600 to $21,600
Cumulative costs* (2 years)	$18,200 to $23,200	$25,200 to $43,200
Cumulative costs* (3 years)	$27,300 to $34,800	$37,800 to $64,800

*includes living expenses

Table 4-2

LOAN PROGRAMS FOR
PHYSICAL THERAPIST ASSISTANT EDUCATION

Student Loans

Some students rely on federal government loans to finance their physical therapist assistant education. These loans have low interest rates and do not require credit checks or collateral. Student loans also offer a variety of deferment options and extended repayment terms. Stafford loans and Perkins loans are two federal programs which are need-based and available for both undergraduate and graduate students.

Parent Loans

The PLUS program (Parent Loan for Undergraduate Students) is available to assist parents to borrow money to support the educational needs of their dependent children which go above and beyond the financial aid package offered by an educational institution. The debt is incurred by the parent, not the student, with these loans. Many adult students are no longer claimed as dependents by their parents and therefore would need to seek their own loan package.

Private Loans

Private Loans, also known as Alternative Loans, help to cover the difference between the actual cost of your education and the limited amount the government allows you to borrow in its programs. Private loans are offered by private lenders who provide different types of private loans, depending on the student's level of study.

Consolidation Loan

This loan allows the borrower to lump all of their loans into one loan for simplified payment.

Table 4-3

CONSIDERATION FOR LOAN COMPARISONS

Questions to Ask When Seeking a Loan

* Is there a loan forgiveness program? (Loan forgiveness programs in which the borrower's loans are paid off in exchange for volunteer work or military service offer an option for easy repayment)

* What will my total debt be? What will my monthly loan payment be?

* How much can I afford to repay each month?

* Is interest capitalized (included in the loan balance) or subsidized (paid by the loan program while you are in school)? What are the additional costs if interest is capitalized?

* What are the terms of loan repayment/deferment? (This is especially important if you are completing a post-graduate internship after receiving your degree)

* How does the total cost of one loan program compare to others?

Table 4-4

PLANNING FOR MANAGEABLE DEBT (A PROFILE OF A PHYSICAL THERAPIST ASSISTANT WITH AN ASSOCIATE'S DEGREE)

	Educational Debt-to-Income Ratio		
	15%	*20%*	*25%*
Gross monthly income*	$2208.33	$2208.33	$2208.33
Maximum *manageable* monthly loan payment (all debts)	$331.00	$442.00	$552.00

*Calculated from a projected annual starting salary of $26,500.

An easy loan calculator is available on-line at http://www.finaid.com/calculators.

Loan Interest Rates

The lower the interest rate, the better. As you can see in the cost comparisons in Table 4-5, a student with $10,000 in total debt will pay *200% more interest* if they are paying interest at credit card rates, which are often as high as 21%.

The message is clear. If a student needs financial assistance to finance an education, there are many relatively low cost loan programs available. The terms of repayment usually accommodate student situations and are far more manageable than credit that is available outside of student loan programs. Do not attempt to finance the costs of your education or your living expenses on credit cards. Borrow the money that you need.

How Long Will it Take to Recover the Costs of My Education?

Typical student loans are for a 10-year term (120 payments); loan payments vary with interest rate and loan principal. You can check typical loan payment amounts in Table 4-5.

Is it Worth It?

Yes!

If you consider that your annual earning potential will increase by $8000 to $10,000 with an Associate's degree, you have covered this payment and gained some. After the first 10 years, you will have devoted 17% of this salary differential to paying off your initial investment (your student loan). But it starts to pay off after that. Over the subsequent 30 years after

Table 4-5

COMPARING LOAN PAYMENTS BY INTEREST RATES*

Loan Interest Rate	8.25%	9.00%	21.00%
Total debt (amount borrowed)	$10,000	$10,000	$10,000
Monthly payment	$123.00	$127.00	$200.00
Total cost of loan (120 months)	$14,718	$15,201	$23,992
Total interest paid on loan	$4718	$5201	$13 992

*Simple interest, 10 year repayment term

Table 4-6

LIFETIME EARNING DIFFERENTIAL COMPARED WITH STUDENT LOAN COSTS

	0 to 10 years	10 to 20 years	20 to 30 years
Student loan costs* (annual total of payments)	$1476	$0	$0
Annual salary *with* Associate's degree	$26,500	$30,000	$35,000
Annual salary *without* Associate's degree	$18,000	$20,000	$22,000
Annual differential in salary with Associate' degree	+$8500	+$10,000	+$13,000
Salary differential less student loan payments	+$7024	+$10,000	+$13,000
Additional lifetime earnings gained with Associate's degree for each 10-year period	+$70 240	+$100,000	+$130,000

*Student loan payments were calculated for a total debt of $10,000 at 8.25% simple interest with repayment over a 10-year period

graduation, with step increases and career progression, this salary difference translates into a cumulative difference in salary of $300,000. So, in 30 years, you will have paid off and gained 30 times over on your initial investment of $10,000 in your education. Look at the value of this investment over time in Table 4-6. Most investors would jump at the chance to have such an investment!

The earlier in your life that you incur these debts, the better. You will have more years of productive earning ahead of you.

Grants and Scholarships

Grants and scholarships are forms of aid that, unlike loans, do not need to be repaid. There are thousands of scholarships available. Scholarships and grant programs usually target students with financial need who have specific educational objec-tives, who have special talents, are members of underrepresented groups or who live in certain areas of the country.

A Web site to help with scholarship searching is available at http://www.fastweb.com/ib/finaid-22f.

For example, in physical therapy, there is a scholarship for members of underrepresented groups (Table 4-7).

The Employment Outlook

Vanessa looked through the classified ads each Sunday for several weeks in the newspaper and saw the same two advertisements for physical therapist assistants. Both offered part-time, temporary positions. She thought "I hope there is more available than that." She wondered when would be the best time to start her job search.

Table 4-7

MINORITY SCHOLARSHIP FUND, AMERICAN PHYSICAL THERAPY ASSOCIATION[3]

Diversity 2000: Physical Therapy Scholarships for a Diverse Future

The Minority Scholarship Fund was created in 1988 to assist minority students in completing their physical therapy education. There is nearly $400,000 in the fund. Since 1988, $365,000 has been awarded to 116 physical therapy students in their final year of physical therapy education and six faculty members pursuing their post-professional doctoral degree. The awards are based upon contributions to minority services and communities, academic achievement, and the potential to contribute to the profession of physical therapy

Reprinted from APTA Department of Minority and International Affairs. Mission statement. Available at: http://eapta.org/advocacy/minorityaffairs/Diversity2000/Diversitybackground, with permission of the American Physical Therapy Association. This material is copyrighted, and any further reproduction or distribution is prohibited.

Over the almost 80-year history of the physical therapy profession, there has been a shortage of qualified physical therapy personnel. In 1997, the Vector Workforce Study, commissioned by the American Physical Therapy Association, shocked the profession by their predictions that there would soon be a surplus of physical therapists and PTAs.[4]

Although the study projected that the need for PTAs would increase overall by 70% between 1995 and 2005, estimates indicated that supply would exceed demand by over 25,000 PTAs by 2005. Since the study was initially published we have seen the demand for physical therapists and PTAs influenced by the growth of the population, by restrictive reimbursement regulations and the spread of the "California model" of managed care.

Simultaneously, educational programs for physical therapists and PTAs rapidly expanded their enrollments and new programs opened during the 1990s.[5] This expansion resulted in an overall increase in the supply of physical therapists and PTAs.

The most recent national surveys (Fall 2001) found that only 3.9% of PTAs who wanted to work were unable to find jobs.[6] This unemployment rate (3.9%) reflects a better picture than the 4.2% reported in Spring 2001 and a substantial improvement from the 6.5% rate reported in Fall 2000. In comparison, the unemployment rate among PTs in Fall 2001 was 1.1%.[6]

Some survey participants reported an involuntary reduction in the number of hours of work, affecting a third of PTAs working in skilled nursing facilities. Many PTAs are working in a combination of part-time employment situations rather than one full-time position. There have also been shifts from skilled nursing facility employment to other practice settings.

The most recent Bureau of Labor Statistics publications indicate that employment of PTAs is expected to *grow much faster than the average* through the year 2010. Federal legislation imposing limits on reimbursement for therapy services is expected to adversely affect the job market for physical therapists and PTAs.

However, over the long run, demand for PTAs is anticipated to continue to rise, with increasing numbers of individuals with disabilities or limited function. This need is driven to a large part by the rapidly growing elderly population and their high rates of chronic disease and disability requiring physical therapy services.[7]

Regional needs for physical therapists and PTAs also vary. Check recent APTA publications for salary figures and local job opportunities.

Summary

There are strong economic factors that support pursuing PTA education. Federal and private loan programs are available which make education accessible to all. In summary, even with a substantial school loan debt, higher education is a good investment for the future.

References

1. APTA. *2002 Fact Sheet Physical Therapist Assistant Education.* Alexandria, Va: American Physical Therapy Association; 2002.
2. FinAid! The SmartStudent Guide to Financial Aid. Loans. Available at: http://www.finaid.com/loans. Accessed September 24, 2004.

3. APTA Department of Minority and International Affairs. Mission statement. Available at: http://apta.org/advocacy/minorityaffairs/Diversity2000/Diversitybackground. Accessed September 22, 2004.

4. APTA. Vector research. Workforce atudy. Available at: http://www.apta.org/Research/survey_stat/workforcestudy. Accessed July 31, 2000.

5. APTA. Program growth. Update on program growth in physical therapy education. Available at: http://www.apta.org/Education/ed_news/ed_news2. Accessed July 31, 2000.

6. APTA. Physical therapist assistant employment survey Fall 2001. Available at: http://www.apta.org/Research/survey_stat/pta_employ_nov01. Accessed November 30, 2002.

7. US Department of Labor, Bureau of Labor Statistics. Physical therapist assistants and aides, 2002-2003. Available at: http://www.bls.gov/oco/ocos167.htm#outlook. Accessed September 22, 2004.

PUTTING IT INTO PRACTICE

1. Complete a budget and project how much financial assistance you will need to complete your education.

Expenses	Monthly	Annually	For Duration of Program
Rent			
Insurance			
Savings			
Other			
Tuition			
Books			
Food and beverages			
Household operations and maintenance			
Child care expenses			
Furnishing and equipment			
Clothing			
Personal allowance			
Transportation			
Medical care			
Recreation, entertainment			
Contributions, donations			
Credit card payments			
TOTAL expenses			
Income			
Salary (after taxes)			
Scholarships			
Loans			
Part-time employment			
TOTAL income			
INCOME LESS EXPENSES			

2. When is the deadline for filing for financial aid applications?

3. When is the next deadline for filing applications for scholarships?

CHAPTER 5

A Primer on Physical Therapist Assistant Education

It had been a busy first day of the second semester. Yolanda looked over the syllabus for the course, Therapeutic Exercise I, and read the paragraph about the practical examination. "Students will differentiate between and demonstrate competent/safe application of: isotonic, isometric, and isokinetic exercise; concentric and eccentric exercise; and open and closed chain exercise to accomplish specific patient goals as set by the physical therapist."

Physical Therapist Assistant Education in the Context of the Physical Therapy Profession

Physical therapy practice today is based on a well-developed body of scientific and clinical knowledge. Physical therapists (PTs) and physical therapists assistants (PTAs) apply knowledge from the basic, behavioral, and social sciences and must demonstrate effective communication skills. Insight and sensitivity to the unique needs of diverse populations are essential to effectively maximize the client or patient's functional potential in society.

Physical therapists are educated at the graduate level. It is projected that more than 70% of all physical therapy programs will be at the doctoral level by 2010.[1] Physical therapists endorse healthy lifestyles and ensure the availability and delivery of effective intervention through the interaction and collaboration of health care team members including support personnel. PTA education exists within the context of the physical therapy profession to prepare competent PTAs who *assist* the PT in achieving established patient-centered functional goals in an effective and cost-efficient manner.[2]

As Zach reviewed the Course Catalogs from the two PTA programs within driving distance from his home, he wondered why one listed all the physical therapist assistant courses during the second year of the program while the other listed them throughout the 2 years along with the general education courses.

PTAs are educated at the 2-year, Associate's degree level with more than 80% of all PTA programs found in community colleges.[3]

PTAs must complete both general education (Math, English, Science) and technical courses (Introduction to PTA, Dynamics of Human Motion). The pattern in which students complete these requirements varies by college program.

The curriculum pattern and sequence of a particular educational program determines how many, and in what order, classes must be taken. For example, basic college classes (such as those that fulfill general education requirements) often must be taken before enrolling in PTA classes.

The number of courses that must be taken simultaneously in one semester and whether required courses are offered during the day, evenings or on-line can influence whether and/or how much a student can work during the program. Students without adequate financial resources, for example, may seek a program that is offered primarily in the evening in order to continue to work while completing their education.

Programs for the preparation of physical therapists and PTAs must meet accreditation standards which are developed and monitored by the Commission on Accreditation in Physical Therapy Education (CAPTE). There are accreditation standards specifically for physical therapy education and another set of accreditation standards unique to PTA education. All developing and existing programs must continuously demonstrate that they meet these standards. Through the accreditation process, the profession assures society that physical therapists

---

Table 5-1

SAMPLE ACCREDITATION STANDARD—PT EDUCATION

The Educational Environment[4]

1. "Professional education programs for the preparation of physical therapists must be conducted in an environment that fosters the intellectual challenge and spirit of inquiry characteristic of the community of scholars and in an environment that supports excellence in professional practice. The institutional environment must be one that ensures the opportunity for physical therapy to thrive as both an academic and professional discipline. In the optimum environment, physical therapy upholds and draws upon a tradition of scientific inquiry while contributing to the profession's body of knowledge."

2. "The program faculty must demonstrate a pattern of activity that reflects a commitment to excel in meeting the expectations of the institution, the students, and the profession."

3. "The academic environment must provide students with opportunities to learn from and be influenced by knowledge outside of, as well as within, physical therapy. In this environment, students become aware of multiple styles of thinking, diverse social concepts, values, and ethical behaviors that will help prepare them for identifying, redefining, and fulfilling their responsibilities to society and the profession. Of major importance is emphasis on critical thinking, ethical practice, and provision of service to meet the changing needs of society. For this environment to be realized, the missions of the institution and the education program must be compatible and mutually supportive."

Adapted from *Evaluative Criteria for Accreditation of Education Programs for the Preparation of Physical Therapists*, Adopted October 30, 1996, Effective January 1, 1998.

---

and PTAs have the required skills to provide high quality health care.

Table 5-1 is a brief excerpt from the *Evaluative Criteria for Accreditation of Education Programs for the Preparation of Physical Therapists* that outlines a few criteria for physical therapy education programs. Table 5-2 is an excerpt from the *Evaluative Criteria for Accreditation of Education Programs for the Preparation of Physical Therapist Assistants* outlining a few criteria for PTA programs.

Let's look at the intended outcomes of PTA education.

Goals of Physical Therapist Assistant Education

Students in PTA education acquire the knowledge and skills to assist the PT with data collection and competently perform delegated interventions in an ethical, legal, safe and effective manner. Upon graduation, the PTA is prepared to effectively communicate with clients/patients, family/caregivers, and other health care team members with recognition of individual, cultural, and economic differences. Graduates are expected to think independently,

problem solve, and participate in life-long learning. PTAs participate with the PT in documenting patient care and in teaching patients, family/caregivers, and other health care providers.[2,4]

There are two major components of the PTA program curriculum: academic and clinical experiences. These two components are interdependent and reinforce one another. The academic setting is designed to provide the information and theory base which is integrated and augmented in the clinical setting. Clinical competence is further developed and validated in the clinical setting through a series of progressive clinical education experiences, called practicums, affiliations or internships.

The curriculum illustrated in Table 5-3 shows a sample of the types of courses that are included in a PTA education program.

Principles of Performance Evaluation

PTA education (like all health provider education programs) is focused around a set of expected outcomes or *competencies*. *Competency-based* education means that learning experiences and evaluation are

---
Table 5-2
SAMPLE ACCREDITATION STANDARD—PTA EDUCATION[5]

1. "Physical therapist assistant education occurs in an institutional environment that supports humanistic principles, inquiry, and dedication to the service of society. The physical therapist assistant education program must be integral to institutional missions and be a logical extension of its education and service programs. The institution, through support for program faculty and policies of the education program, encourages its graduates to practice within the legal, social and ethical context of their careers as physical therapist assistants."

2. "Each academic faculty member is qualified by education and experience to fulfill the assigned responsibilities. She/he hold appropriate credentials where applicable, including licensure, certification or registration. Each academic faculty member maintains activities within the profession consistent with the philosophy of the program and institution."

3. "The physical therapist assistant curriculum includes, or its prerequisites include, elements of general education, including basic sciences that include biological, physical, physiological and anatomical principles, and applied physical therapy science. The course work is designed to prepare the student to think independently, to clarify values, to understand fundamental theory, and to develop critical thinking and communication skills."

Adapted from *Evaluative Criteria For Accreditation Of Education Programs For The Preparation Of Physical Therapist Assistants*. Adopted 11/2000, Effective 1/1/02.

Table 5-3
SAMPLE PTA CURRICULUM[6]
(FRESHMAN YEAR)

Fall Semester	*Spring Semester*	*Summer Session*
PTA 1013 Intro to PT	PTA 1213 Pain & Massage	PTA 1312 Initial Practicum
PTA 1023 Dynamics of Human Motion	PTA 1224 Therapeutic Ex I	
PTA 1113 Pathology for Physical Rehab	PTA 1203 Development, Conditions & Treatment Across the Lifespan	
BIO 1314 Human Anatomy & Physiology I	BIO 1414 Human Anatomy & Physiology II	
Engl 1113 English Composition	HIST 1483 American History To Civil War	
PTA 2014 Electrotherapy & Modalities	or	
PTA 2024 Ther Ex II	HIST 1493 American History From Civil War	
PTA 2113 PTA Systems/Problems & Physiology I	PTA 2034 Practicum I	
	PTA 2134 Practicum II	
PSY 1113 Intro to Psych	PSY 2403 Developmental Psychology	
ENGL 1233 Report Writing	APPM 1313 Math for Health Careers	
	POLSC 113 American Federal Government	

Reprinted with permission from Oklahoma City Community College. *PTA Curriculum*. Available from: http://www.okccc.edu/CourseCatalog/physical_therapist_assist.htm. Accessed 4/4/03.

organized around the major performance behaviors defined by specific criteria that must be exhibited by graduates at entry into the profession. This insures mastery of the concepts, skills and values associated with physical therapy practice.[7,8]

This *criterion-referenced* system differs from a *norm-referenced* approach taken in many prerequisite courses, where student performance is compared to that of other students, not to a set of expected behaviors.[9,10] Most students have had the experience of being "graded on the curve." In a norm-referenced approach, student performance is measured in reference to the group average, which is based on the performance of others. This method does not assure that students meet specific standards of performance, as the group average could be quite low.

Physical therapy education uses a strict standard of performance. Society must have the assurance that health care providers will function at a high standard of care. It *would not be acceptable* for a student to receive a passing grade without mastery of the material. If that were the case, a patient or client's well-being could be in jeopardy. In the physical therapy profession, as in all health professions, each student must demonstrate mastery and meet a predefined level of competency to pass courses and receive credit for clinical education experiences.

A student in a PTA program experiences many forms of performance evaluation, including exams and quizzes, practical or laboratory examinations, papers, projects, presentations, journals, and clinical evaluations. Evaluations may be used as a teaching tool (*formative evaluation*) and or as a certification tool (*summative evaluation*).[11]

For example, during a clinical education experience formative evaluation may occur during daily conferences with a clinical instructor. Summative evaluation occurs when evaluative comments are recorded on the final evaluation form. Student performance is graded based on the accomplishment of specific performance indicators at that point.

Preparing for Mastery

Mastery involves demonstrating **competency**. Competency as defined in the *Normative Model of Physical Therapist Assistant Education: Version '99* is to possess "the requisite knowledge, skills, and behaviors to be a PTA by rendering those aspects of physical therapy care (eg, data collection, components of intervention) as delegated by the physical therapist."[12]

Key elements for mastery to be demonstrated by the student include:

* *Generic Abilities*: There are key behaviors, attributes, and characteristics that must be mastered by PTA students. These generic abilities include such areas as interpersonal communication, responsibility, a commitment to learning and skills in time and stress management.[13] The Generic Abilities are detailed in Chapter 6 in Table 6-3.

* *Clinical Skills*: Students must demonstrate competence in clinical performance skills (assessment, data collection and intervention). For example, a student must be able to determine the type and amount of assistance required to safely and effectively guard a patient during an assisted transfer from a wheelchair to a bed.

* *Integration*: This is the student's ability access interrelated chunks of information. Students must apply general education and applied physical therapy science knowledge to the technical components of the curriculum in order to perform patient care interventions. For example, anatomical principles must be applied in clinical courses and cardiac precautions must be integrated in the intervention of a patient with an orthopaedic disorder.

* *Judgment*: Judgment is reflected in the decisions that the PTA makes, within the clinical environment, that are based on the plan of care established by the physical therapist. This problem-solving approach includes gathering pertinent information through observation, measurement, subjective, objective, and functional findings (data collection); and processing and interpreting the results within the plan of care established by the physical therapist. Students should be aware of and incorporate evidence-based outcomes into this process. For example, a patient's poor response to sitting on the side of the bed can be the result of many factors. The student must understand what is normally expected and make a decision about whether to proceed with treatment or get the patient back to bed immediately.

* *Metacognitive or Self-Regulatory Skills*: Students must be able to monitor their own understanding, develop strategies to properly communicate, assess their own performance, and validate their decisions using sound arguments and rationale. For example, a student must recognize and appropriately respond to a request of an employer which violates ethical guidelines or legal regulations for the practice of a PTA.

Faculty Roles and Responsibilities

Abby sat in the orientation session and listened while the faculty members introduced themselves to the new class. She heard so many interesting things and hoped that she would one day be a faculty member herself.

There are many faculty members involved in providing PTA education. In addition to classroom, laboratory and clinical instruction and student advising, faculty are often engaged in a number of college, professional and service responsibilities which go far beyond their instructional responsibilities. Many academic core faculty members also stay involved in clinical practice.

The faculty in a PTA education program establish acceptable levels of performance within the scope of practice as defined by the profession. They facilitate student achievement of predetermined outcomes and evaluate student performance, providing feedback to the students regarding their performance.

The descriptions in Table 5-4 may be helpful in identifying faculty roles and responsibilities.

Student Responsibilities

Students in a PTA education program have the responsibility for their own learning. This requires that students make choices and accept the consequences of those choices. Students must solicit and provide feedback and participate in the learning experiences that are offered. They must be self-directed and seek help when needed. They must communicate clearly, with respect for themselves and others. There are many similar behaviors that are highly valued in students entering the profession of physical therapy.[13,15]

Qualities of Successful Students

1. Clinical competence
2. Problem solving
3. Self-direction
4. Self-assessment
5. Self-reliance
6. Sensitivity
7. Clear communication
8. Respect for self and others
9. Lifelong learning
10. Self-confidence
11. Creativity
12. Responsibility
13. Accountability
14. Caring
15. Curiosity

Heightened Expectations

Ben read over the examination and could not find an answer that he agreed with for several questions. He went to the front of the room and had a lengthy discussion with the professor who told him to choose, "the best answer." Although the answer was marked wrong, Ben followed up during faculty office hours and eventually received credit because he was able to show references which supported his choice.

One of the greatest challenges for PTA students is to move from the comfort of the "known" and "correct answers" to a place much more consistent with reality. For example, one patient with tennis elbow receives an ice massage and feels instant relief while a second patient with tennis elbow insists he never receive that intervention again! This is an everyday reality in the clinical setting.

The illusion created by years of general education coursework leaves students with the impression that knowledge is stable, irrefutable, and certain. In actuality, very little is certain, absolute fact, especially when a human being is a part of the equation.

This phenomenon alone shakes many students beliefs in the educational process. PTA education requires students to no longer memorize information and then forget it, but integrate a new and complex body of knowledge while monitoring their own progress along the way.

Many students find the volume of work overwhelming, time and financial resources inadequate, and may question, "Why have I chosen to do this?!" The idea that it should be different creates a dynamic that interferes with student progress, creates frustration and dissatisfaction. You may be saying, "So that's why I feel this way!"

Program faculty may inadvertently add to this problem by asking students to demonstrate application of material from other courses or taken in earlier semesters. In order to facilitate student growth, faculty often find themselves in the position of "not giving the answers," but instead pushing students to be accountable for their choices, to find their own

---

Table 5-4

PHYSICAL THERAPIST ASSISTANT EDUCATION PROGRAM FACULTY ROLE DESCRIPTIONS[4,14]

Program Director or Administrator

The core faculty member who is designated and has responsibility for the management of the PTA program. The program director is employed full-time by the institution that houses the PTA program and usually has a faculty appointment. May also be designated the program coordinator or program head.

ACCE (Academic Coordinator of Clinical Education)

The ACCE is a core faculty member who has the primary responsibilities to plan, coordinate, facilitate, administer, and monitor activities on behalf of the academic program and in coordination with academic and clinical faculty. (http://www.apta.org/Education/clinical_edu/model_position)

Core Faculty

Those individuals appointed to and employed primarily by the institution that houses the PTA program. The core faculty is comprised of the program director and ACCE and other appointed faculty members within the program. Members of the core faculty typically have full-time appointments, although some part-time faculty members may be included among the core faculty. The core faculty include physical therapists and physical therapist assistants, and may include others with expertise to meet specific curricular needs. The core faculty have the qualifications and experience necessary to achieve the goals of the program through educational administration, curriculum development, instructional design and delivery, and evaluation of outcomes. The core faculty may hold tenured, tenure track, or nontenure track positions. The primary responsibilities of the core faculty are classroom and laboratory instruction.

Adjunct Faculty

Those individuals who have classroom and/or laboratory teaching responsibilities in the program and who are not employed by the institution, though they may receive honoraria or other forms of compensation. The adjunct faculty may or may not hold faculty appointments. The adjunct faculty may include, but are not limited to, guest lecturers, "contract" faculty, instructors of course modules, tutors, laboratory instructors, and teaching assistants.

Clinical Education Faculty

Those individuals engaged in providing the clinical education components of the program, generally referred to as either Center Coordinators of Clinical Education (CCCEs) or Clinical Instructors (CIs). While these individuals are not usually employed by the educational institution, they do agree to certain standards of behavior through contractual arrangements for their services.

Supporting Faculty

Those individuals with faculty appointments in other units within the institution who teach courses in the technical education portion of the program. Generally not physical therapists or physical therapist assistants.

Table 5-5

STUDENT THOUGHTS ON AMBIGUITY IN PHYSICAL THERAPY EDUCATION

Thoughts on Student Tolerance of Ambiguity, A Learning Experience

Graduate education represents a gateway transition from general, rudimentary knowledge and skills into more specialized, advanced training along a chosen career path. As with any progressive process, the essence of graduate education is developmental change, like learning to walk; and, as in learning to walk, zealous as it may be, there is risk, frustration, and uncertainty.

Uncertainty of meaning, significance, or attitude that may result in intellectual or emotional tension between two or more logically incompatible points of view is called ambiguity, from the French, "ambigere," to wander about, waiver, or dispute. It is mystery arising from a vague knowledge or understanding that has multiple interpretations.

Ambiguity often involves doubt, confusion, inconsistency, unpredictability, as well as change. The challenge of ambiguity in graduate education is reflected in the many choices, conflicting opinions, double entendres, unstable definitions, understatements, oversights, and general absences of clarity that confront students daily. The goal is growth and insight; the hazard is feeling confused, overwhelmed, and out of control.

Tolerance of ambiguity implies coping with choice and uncertainty. It employs strategies that help maintain psycho-emotional equilibrium and includes cognitive techniques that bring thinking and action in line with reality, counteracting irrational beliefs and assumptions that may have no basis in truth.

Why tolerate ambiguity? Why put up with the confusion and tension of multiple conflicting interpretations rather than demand to know what the hell is going on, and why, and how to deal with it? Sometimes it's reasonable not to passively accept sloppy communication or double meanings, but by considering a broader, perhaps more rational view of what it's all about, the student begins to accept (if not comprehend) not only undefined external events, perplexing people, and unfamiliar pressures, but inner personal truths and strengths as well as hurts, fears, and hang-ups triggered by stress and change.

"Real-world" integration of self and other involves letting go of ultimate control. Ambiguity negates control; there is no direct control possible in an ambiguous situation. Expectations become irrelevant. New, more sophisticated ways of thinking must replace dualistic—right vs wrong—thought. Anxiety about uncertainty is unproductive, stressful, and symptomatic of grappling for control.

Tolerating ambiguity, on the other hand, facilitates learning, adapting, seeing both sides, getting along, and getting the job done. It is integral to stress management, to becoming a professional and to the process of graduate education, itself.

Many irrational beliefs may occur to you as a student. Beware: Habitual patterns of thinking often conflict with a world view conducive to change and to adaptation to graduate education.

Tina Buettell
1997

---

answers and to apply classroom material to clinical problems. Again, this can be frustrating for students who are more accustomed to faculty members who assume roles of authority and pass on their truths to students who are only too happy to write them down.

Table 5-5 is the contribution of a student in an entry-level PT education program experiencing such conflicts. She wrote these words to try to confront many of the beliefs that were interfering with her participation in the physical therapy program. Her words have helped many students to examine their beliefs and experiences.[16]

Table 5-6

STUDENT EXPECTATIONS[17]

Responsibilities of the Student

1. Come to class: You cannot learn about physical therapy from a book. This is a hands-on profession. Classes require your participation. Your ultimate obligation to your patients requires that you learn as much as you can. Capitalize on the expertise that your professors and clinical instructors' have to offer.

2. Dress appropriately: Proper attire is required when involved with patients, clinical sites and/or guest speakers. Your self-presentation is critical to your reception by patients, faculty and colleagues.

3. Prepare for and participate in class: Read the material assigned. Your instructors will assume that you have completed the material and may not cover it in class. Remember that your questions help your classmates as much as they do you, but also remember that you need to direct questions towards areas of confusion, rather than a general lack of knowledge.

4. Keep up: Budget your time for studying so that you do not fall behind. Prioritize your commitments and realize how much time/energy each requires. Organize your class and assignment schedule on a calendar you carry with you.

5. Be active: Participate in meetings, special events, committees. Be willing to volunteer and work with members of the program on fundraisers, community service opportunities and professional association opportunities.

6. Give feedback: Give your opinions, compliments, and criticisms in a responsible way. You may make individual appointments with faculty to make your views known.

7. Communicate: Leave phone messages with faculty if you will miss class. If you are having personal or family difficulties, communicate this BEFORE it causes you to miss class or assignments. Also develop good communication with classmates, friends, and family.

8. Be prompt: Arrive at class, meetings, clinical sites on time. This is not only common courtesy, but also required of a physical therapist assistant.

9. Stay healthy and take care of yourself: Watch your diet, sleep, and exercise. Practice stress management techniques. Identify and use your support system.

10. Be courteous: Even under times of stress, treat others as you wish to be treated.

11. Be responsible for yourself: You are an adult and expected to manage your own life. Handle your problems in a responsible manner.

Adapted from Newman PD. *Student responsibilities. PTA Program Handbook.* Oklahoma City, Okla: Oklahoma City Community College; 2003.

More on Physical Therapist Assistant Education

Having accepted a position within a PTA program, you assume an increased level of commitment and responsibility to your classmates and program faculty. Although the majority of PTA students juggle multiple responsibilities, including family/childrearing and work obligations, program faculty assume you have chosen to apply and are serious about joining the physical therapy profession. Some of the key differences between the expectations of general education and a PTA program are listed below: Take a look at the guidelines in Table 5-6 which further indicate student responsibilities.

Student Responsibility, Self-Direction

PTA students are expected to be self-directed and take responsibility for their actions. Students are responsible for informing faculty members when and if they will not be in class. The student is responsible for making any special arrangements for missed classes, exams or late papers. It is essential to realize that some assignments/exams may not be made up at all. Absence may result in failure in that experiential learning (discussions, patient simulations, lab practice with faculty input) cannot be recreated.

Table 5-7

INTERACTION WITH FACULTY IN PHYSICAL THERAPIST ASSISTANT EDUCATION

Establishing good working relationships with faculty.

1. Some physical therapist assistant programs are more formal than others. It is wise to ask how a faculty member would like to be addressed before assuming it is fine to call them by their first name.

2. Schedule appointments with both academic and clinical faculty. Leave voice or e-mail messages and give faculty an opportunity to call you back. Don't expect immediate attention at times that are convenient for you to drop by. Observe academic faculty office hours and realize that you may also have access to faculty by appointment at other times.

3. Both academic and clinical faculty members are busy people with multiple other responsibilities. Give the faculty member the opportunity to hear your concern, interest, or problem with the time and attention that it deserves. Don't put off talking about a problem; small concerns often mushroom and escalate in a short period of time.

4. Communicate directly with faculty, not through another faculty member, staff member, or student. Faculty members may not get the message. They also may not disclose key information to other students or faculty in respect for your privacy and confidentiality.

Adapted from Newman PD. Establishing good working relationships with faculty. *PTA Program Handbook*. Oklahoma City, Okla: Oklahoma City Community College; 2003.

Autonomy and Choice

PTA students are assumed to be adult learners. The student is expected to work with autonomy and independence, asking for feedback and help as needed. Academic honesty is held in the highest regard since cheating of any kind translates into short-changing a patient or client in the future.

Responsibility for Self in All Situations With Colleagues, Patients, Families

In addition to being a responsible student, the student in PTA education is also likely to be responsible for the well-being of others during clinical learning experiences. It is critical that students practice in compliance with all laws, regulations, and ethical guidelines, understanding that their actions reflect not only themselves, but also the academic program, the clinical institution, and the profession of physical therapy. Accurate self-assessment concerning competencies, strengths, and weaknesses is critical.

Relationships With Academic and Clinical Faculty

Both academic and clinical faculty play a key role in student development. Get to know the faculty. Establish good working relationships with both aca-

demic and clinical faculty members. Seek their guidance and assistance as needed.

Recognize that faculty roles in PTA education make it inadvisable to have social relationships with students. This is especially important in clinical education, where you may be working closely with a clinical instructor for 40 to 50 hours per week. Table 5-7 addresses some typical questions that students have in working with faculty.

Computer Competence

College graduates are expected to be computer-literate and have the ability to use technology competently. The resources of the Internet, government agencies, medical data bases, and even your college library are available without leaving home. An increasing number of assignments and educational experiences are available on-line. Check with your institution regarding their requirements for technological literacy. The licensure examination for physical therapists and PTAs is computer-based.

Information Competence

What used to be "going to the library" has become a navigational task by computer. Knowing where to look and how to search are critical skills that will determine your success in researching papers and projects throughout your education and your career (see Chapter 17 on Information Competence).

Grades

Acceptance into many PTA programs is at least partially based upon academic achievement—grade point average (GPA). For many students accustomed to being at the top of their high school and general education classes, PTA education often involves the added stress of being in classes with an entire class of students who have been at the top of the class. Although competition is discouraged in most programs, sometimes old habits are hard to break. Although typically a "C" or better is required to continue on in the program, many students put additional pressure on themselves to "be the best." This causes extra stress. Student effort is better directed in supporting and receiving support from colleagues in study groups and communication with professors.

Clinical Education

Clinical education is a critical component of PTA education. Most educational programs include 16 to 18 weeks of clinical education experience during the educational process.[2] These experiences are courses within the curriculum, for which students enroll, pay tuition, and receive academic credit. Clinical faculty members provide direct supervision of students during clinical education experiences. Clinical faculty are usually employees of the facilities to which the students are assigned. The academic institution makes the clinical assignment of students to learning experiences, provides the administration of the clinical education course and assigns the final grade. It is a joint responsibility of clinical and academic faculty to insure that clinical learning experiences are high quality and effective learning experiences for the student.

The *Academic Coordinator of Clinical Education* (ACCE) is the person on the academic faculty who arranges clinical education assignments. There are many factors that enter into the assignment of students to clinical learning experiences including availability during a given time period, type of facility, past experience of the student, interests of the student, level of the student, and geographical location. In most cases, students have input into the choice, but few students get their first choice in all cases. Students should check with the ACCE regarding policies and procedures for selecting and assigning clinical education sites.

In general, students cannot arrange their own clinical learning experiences. There are many considerations in selecting a clinical learning site. Clinical facilities are evaluated by a number of criteria before becoming involved in the clinical training of student physical therapists. Academic institutions contract with the clinical institution or organization to provide clinical training of student physical therapists. These are legal agreements that cover issues such as liability and malpractice, in addition to outlining the responsibilities of the academic institution, the student, and the clinical facility before, during, and after the clinical learning experience. Months of paperwork and negotiations often go into establishing an agreement between an academic institution and a clinical learning facility.

Clinical performance is measured on a specific instrument. Many programs for PTA education are using the *Clinical Performance Instrument* (CPI). The CPI is defines 20 key behaviors such as "Conducts self in a responsible manner." and then gives sample behaviors that illustrate the key behavior. Each educational program establishes the level of performance required on clinical performance during each clinical learning experience. Clinical experiences may be graded on a Credit/No Credit, Pass/Fail, or letter grade basis. See Chapter 7 for more information on clinical performance evaluation.

Capstone Classes/Comprehensive Practical Examinations

PTA education requires a way to measure that you have comprehensive mastery of the material presented during your educational experience. Every program has either a comprehensive written and/or practical examination, an extensive project or a summary course (often called a "capstone") demonstrating mastery of the content of your education. Check with your program for specific requirements.

Summary

PTA education presents challenges that differ from the educational experience with which most students have familiarity. PTA education requires demonstration of mastery of content and demonstration of acceptable clinical performance. Every program has slightly different requirements; acquaint yourself with the specifics of your program.

References

1. APTA. *CAPTE Accreditation Update*. Department of Accreditation. Alexandria, Va: American Physical Therapy Association; January, 2003:8.

2. APTA. *Normative Model of Physical Therapist Assistant Education: Version 99*. Alexandria, Va: American Physical Therapy Association; 1999:3-9.

3. APTA. *The Future Role of the PTA (RC 40-01) Report to the 2002 House of Delegates*. Alexandria, Va: American Physical Therapy Association; 2002. Available from: http://www.apta.org/governance/HOD/2002HOD/5thposting/specialreports. Accessed November 26, 2002.

4. APTA. Evaluative criteria for accreditation of education programs for the preparation of physical therapists. Available at: http://apta.org/Education/accreditation/eval_criteria_menu. Accessed September 22, 2004.

5. APTA. *Evaluative Criteria for Accreditation of Education Programs for the Preparation of Physical Therapist Assistants*. Alexandria, Va: American Physical Therapy Association; 2002.

6. *PTA Curriculum, Oklahoma City Community College; 2003*. Available from: http://www.okccc.edu/CourseCatalog/physical_therapist_assist.htm Accessed April 4, 2003.

7. Davis CM, Anderson MJ, Jagger D. Competency: the what, why, and how of it. *Phys Ther*. 1979; 59(9):1088-94.

8. May BJ. Competency based education: general concepts. *J Allied Health*. 1979;8(3):166-71.

9. May BJ. Competency based evaluation of student performance. *J Allied Health*. 1978;7(3):232-7.

10. May BJ. Evaluation in a competency-based educational system. *Phys Ther*. 1977;57(1):28-33.

11. Bloom BS, Hastings ST, Madeus AF. *Handbook of Formative and Summative Evaluation of Student Learning*. New York, NY: McGraw-Hill Inc, 1971.

12. APTA. *A Normative Model of Physical Therapist Assistant Education: Version 99*. Alexandria, Va: American Physical Therapy Association; 1999: 190.

13. May WW, Morgan BJ, Lemke JC, et al. Model for ability-based assessment in physical therapy education. *J Phys Ther Educ*. 1995;9(1):3-6.

14. APTA. Model position description for the academic coordinator/director of clinical education. Available at: http://apta.org/Education/educatorinfo/model_position. Accessed September 22, 2004.

15. Hayes KW, Huber G, Rogers J, Sanders B. Behaviors that cause clinical instructors to question the clinical competence of physical therapist students. *Phys Ther*. 1999;79:653-671.

16. Buettell C. *Thoughts on Student Tolerance of Ambiguity, a learning experience* [unpublished manuscript]. California State University, Fresno; 1997.

17. Newman PD. *Student Responsibilities. PTA Program Handbook*. Oklahoma City, Okla: Oklahoma City Community College; 2003.

PUTTING IT INTO PRACTICE

1. What is the name, title, and credentials of the person who directs or oversees your physical therapist assistant education program? Who serves as your advisor?

2. What is the name, credentials, and area of clinical expertise of the Academic Coordinator of Clinical Education in your education program?

3. What comprehensive examinations/projects are required in your program to demonstrate mastery? At what point in your course of study will you complete these requirements?

4. How many weeks of clinical education are included during your professional education program? During which quarters or semesters? Is any of this part-time?

5. How are clinical affiliation assignments determined? Do students have input? When are assignments made for each affiliation?

6. What are the minimal performance standards you must meet to successfully complete the program?

7. Outline the names and course numbers of the courses you will take each semester of the program, starting with the current semester:

CHAPTER 6

Standards of Behavior and Conduct

> *Carmen arrived for the laboratory orientation session early. She waited in the second row for the professor to enter the room. Professor Landau started the lecture by handing out a paper outlining standards of expected conduct in the lab.*

Standards of Conduct

What are standards of conduct? Perhaps one of the first places that many students are overtly exposed to standards of conduct is in the laboratory, where safety, ethical, and liability issues demand that specific rules be established and followed. Both legal and ethical issues govern the handling of human anatomical materials.

Consider the Guidelines in Table 6-1, which are excerpted from an anatomy course syllabus. These guidelines provide clear expectations of student conduct in relation to conduct in and around the anatomy laboratory.

Behavior and Conduct in Physical Therapy

Standards of conduct commonly address such attributes as dependability, appearance and presentation, initiative, empathy, cooperation and conflict resolution, verbal and written communication.

Many physical therapist assistant (PTA) programs incorporate the 10 *generic abilities* for students within the curriculum. These generic abilities are defined in Table 6-2.

Codes of Student Behavior

Acceptable behavior is defined for students in similar ways by many professions and disciplines. Academic institutions publish student codes of conduct. The underlying principles are usually similar. (Table 6-3)

Students who join professional associations may also be bound by the codes of conduct of the professional organization. The American Physical Therapy Association defines guidelines for professional conduct of its members by the Code of Ethics and guides for conduct exhibited in Appendices 2 and 3. The student code of conduct in Table 6-4 refers to and includes the *Code of Ethics and Guide for Professional Conduct*.

Appearance and Dress

> *It had been a rough morning. Dawn forgot that today was dress code day—a guest speaker was coming in her Orthopedics class. She was the only student in class in cut-off jeans and sandals. Should she stay for the lecture or go home and change? She felt embarrassed as she tried to hide in the far corner of the classroom.*

You have only a few seconds to make a first impression. The way that you appear may determine whether patients and clients trust you, feel that they will be safe with you, disclose confidential information, or even consent to receiving services. Even though it seems unfair, it even influences whether other professionals will respect your opinion. It may influence whether you land a job or get a raise.

Although the standard "daily uniform" may be jeans with an old T-shirt or sweatshirt, professional dress requires attention not only to what you wear, but personal hygiene, hair, nails, and identification. Take a look at the sample dress code in Table 6-5.

Table 6-1

SAMPLE GUIDELINES FOR STUDENT CONDUCT[1]

Standards of Student Conduct—Anatomy Laboratory

Students will observe the following standards of conduct while in the laboratory:

1. Any student not wearing a laboratory coat or jacket will not be allowed to remain in the dissecting room.
2. Students registered for the course and authorized persons are the only people allowed in the dissecting room. Relatives, spouses, and friends are absolutely not allowed access to the dissecting room.
3. The dissecting room will be open during the scheduled laboratory periods, and at various other times to be arranged. Other times may be arranged upon the approval of the instructors.
4. There is to be no smoking or eating in the laboratory at any time. No food or drinks are allowed in the anatomy laboratory or in the adjacent hallway. No smoking is permitted in these areas. Do not store food in the lockers in the lab.
5. Models, specimens, etc. are not to be removed from the laboratory.
6. The outside doors to the laboratory must remain closed at all times.
7. Handle scalpels and other sharp instruments with care! Do not use them to point and put them down when you are not actually dissecting with them.

Adapted from Jamali M. Course Syllabus. PT 3514 Laboratory for Gross Anatomy. Arkansas State University, College of Nursing & Health Professions. Available at: http://www.clt.astate.edu/mjamali/pt3514.htm. Accessed 6/25/2000.

Table 6-2

GENERIC ABILITIES IMPORTANT TO PHYSICAL THERAPY[2]

Generic Ability	*Definition*
1. Commitment to learning	The ability to self-assess, self-correct, and self-direct; to identify needs and sources of learning; and to continually seek out new knowledge and understanding.
2. Interpersonal skills	The ability to interact effectively with patients, families, colleagues, other health care professionals, and the community and to deal effectively with cultural and ethnic diversity issues.
3. Communication skills	The ability to communicate effectively (ie, speaking, body language, reading, writing, listening) for varied audiences and purposes.
4. Effective use of time	The ability to obtain the maximum benefit from a minimum investment of time and resources.
5. Use of constructive criticism	The ability to identify sources of and seek out feedback and to effectively use and provide feedback for improving personal interaction.
6. Problem solving	The ability to recognize and define problems, analyze data, develop and implement solutions, and evaluate outcomes.
7. Professionalism	The ability to exhibit appropriate professional conduct and to represent the profession effectively.
8. Responsibility	The ability to fulfill commitments and to be accountable for actions and outcomes.
9. Critical thinking	The ability to question logically; to identify, generate, and evaluate elements of logical argument; to recognize and differentiate facts, illusions, assumptions, and hidden assumptions; and to distinguish the relevant from the irrelevant.
10. Stress management	The ability to identify sources of stress and to develop effective coping behaviors.

Reprinted with permission from May WW, Morgan BJ, Lemke JC, et al. Model for ability-based assessment in physical therapy education. *J Phys Ther Educ*. 1995;9(1):3-6.

Table 6-3

SAMPLE ELEMENTS OF STUDENT BEHAVIOR STANDARDS

Student Behavior and Conduct

1. Respect for the rights of all individuals without regard to regard to position, race, age, gender, handicap, national origin, religion, or sexual orientation, including compliance with laws prohibiting activities such as sexual harassment such as the Title IV of the Civil Rights Act of 1964 and by Title IX of the Education Amendments of 1972.

2. Appropriate handling of information, records, or examination materials.

3. Respect for patients' confidentiality, privacy, modesty, and safety.

4. Proper appearance and conduct (professional appearance, speech, and behavior), including wearing identification badges, appropriate dress for professional activities, and exemplary personal hygiene.

5. Compliance with all existing laws, policies, and regulations.

6. Respect for property and instructional material.

Table 6-4

SAMPLE OF PHYSICAL THERAPIST ASSISTANT STUDENT CODE OF CONDUCT

Students will conduct themselves in a manner that is consistent with their future aspirations in the physical therapy field. To that end, the following expectations reflect qualities such as appropriate appearance and presentation, collegial respect, and accountability to [the institution's] codes of student conduct; the *American Physical Therapy Association Standards of Ethical Conduct for the Physical Therapist Assistant*, the *Guide for Conduct of the Physical Therapist Assistant*; and applicable local, state and federal laws in all interactions with academic and clinical faculty, academic or clinical staff, colleagues, patients, family, and research subjects.

1. Students will observe published codes of dress and appearance as requested by academic or clinical faculty and staff, including proper clothing to permit practice of evaluation and treatment techniques in laboratory sessions. Students should assume required dress requirements for any engagement, laboratory or clinical experience off campus, and for any class which involves patients or outside speakers.

2. Students will arrive on-time or early to scheduled classes, laboratories, or clinical assignments and will not interrupt classes or treatments in session. It is the student's responsibility to make up material missed due to absence and to notify academic and/or clinical faculty members regardless of the reason for the absence.

3. Students will notify the designated academic or clinical faculty or staff member regarding their anticipated late arrival or absence prior to the scheduled session.

4. Students will not bring guests into the classroom or clinical setting unless previously cleared with the designated faculty member.

5. Students will not bring children or pets into a university classroom or clinical setting.

6. Students will use appropriate, courteous, and respectful communication whether by e-mail, (individually and on department-sponsored list-serves), by letter, voice-mail, telephone, or in face-to-face communication with academic and clinical faculty, academic or clinical staff, colleagues, patients, family, and research subjects.

continued

> ──────── Table 6-4 (continued) ────────
>
> ## SAMPLE OF PHYSICAL THERAPIST ASSISTANT STUDENT CODE OF CONDUCT
>
> 7. Students will observe appropriate codes of conduct per the American Physical Therapy Association *Standards of Ethical Conduct for the Physical Therapist Assistant, the Guide for Conduct of the Physical Therapist Assistant* and Physical Therapy Practice Act, (California Business and Professions Code, Chapter 5.7 Physical Therapy) and Regulations of the Physical Therapy Examining Committee (California Code of Regulations, Title 16, Division 13.2. Physical Therapy Examining Committee of the Board of Medical Quality Assurance) in all interactions with academic and clinical faculty, staff, students, employers, patients, and families. This expectation will also include conduct in off-campus personal or employment situations in which the student may potentially be in violation of these codes of conduct.
>
> 8. Students will observe the Codes Governing Student Conduct (Sections 41301 to 41303, inclusive in Article 1, Subchapter 3, Chapter 5, Title 5, California Administrative Code; Education Code Sections 66017, 69810 through 69813 inclusive; and Penal Code Sections 626 through 626.4 inclusive), which establish grounds for expulsion, suspension and probation of students.
>
> Adapted from Professional behavior policy: Student code of conduct. In: *Student Manual, Department of Physical Therapy.* Fresno, Calif: California State University, Fresno; 2000.

Language and Conversations

> *The student PTA list-serv had been up and running for a few months. Eddie posted an ethnic joke poking fun at a common accent. May (a fellow student) was irate. She wrote on the list-serv, "I don't think that joke is funny, nor do I think it belongs on a list-serv that represents our future profession." What do you think? Is May over-reacting?*

Although Eddie's intention was not to offend May or behave in an irresponsible way, his communication does not show sensitivity to others. The ensuing discussion after this event certainly created ample opportunity to explore cultural biases and establish proper conduct for internet use.

The language we use is another example of expected behavior. Whether speaking or writing, make an effort to use appropriate language and use judgement as to whether a topic of conversation, joke or random thought is appropriate for the context.

Also, be careful of what you write. A patient's medical record is a legal document. Your documentation must be clear and reflect the physical therapy care provided.

Confidentiality

> *The instructor gave an example of a problem employee, without using the employee's name or making any reference to a facility or point in time. Frances thought the situation sounded vaguely familiar and she knew that the instructor was a district supervisor of the same company for which she worked. She went to work the next afternoon and asked her fellow employees at the clinic about the case the instructor used. They gossiped about the details of why a former colleague was fired. Who has breached confidentiality here?*

Student PTAs frequently have access to confidential information about clients and patients. They may also have access to confidential information about colleagues, supervisees, students, and faculty. Using good judgment requires thinking about the reasons why someone would need to know information.

In the situation above, even if Frances could identify the employee and situation with certainty, it serves no legitimate purpose for her to discuss the case with her colleagues. Avoid the temptation to enter into discussions of a colleague's situation or a patient's diagnosis, personal life, or other details, even in private.

Table 6-5

SAMPLE STUDENT DRESS CODE[4]

Purpose

To provide guidelines for proper attire, while placing responsibility on the student to dress appropriately at all times.

General Appearance

Clothing

- Dress should be neat, clean, practical, safe, avoiding extremes of fashion, and appropriate to staff duties and work area.
- No blue jeans, faded denim of any color, or sweat pants.
- Shirts should have appropriate neckline (ie, not too low), be plain or simple, and in conservative colours.
- Shorts, if worn, should be no shorter than 4 inches above the knee.

Footwear

- Socks (or pantyhose) should be worn with shoes.
- Shoes to be well maintained and closed toe—casual shoes may be worn.
- Athletic shoes can be worn if in good condition.
- No sandals or clogs.

Accessories

- Jewelry should be minimal: smooth surface rings, watches, and small earrings.
- Conservative make-up.

Miscellaneous

- Hair: Clean, long hair appropriately tied back.
- Nails: To be clipped and cleaned; brightly colored nail polish not recommended.
- Hygiene: All students should be clean with no discernable body odor. The use of fragrances and colognes is prohibited.

NAME TAGS TO BE WORN AT ALL TIMES!

** Students will be expected to adhere to the dress code policy of the facility/agency to which they are assigned for placement if it is different than the student dress code policy.

Adapted from University of Manitoba School of Medical Rehabilitation, Division of Physical Therapy. Available at: http://www.umanitoba.ca/faculties/medicine/units/medrehab/pt. Accessed on August 18, 2004.

Patients have rights to privacy and confidentiality. Under the Health Insurance Portability and Accountability Act of 1996 (HIPAA), the only communication about patients that is necessary to provide, manage, and coordinate care is permitted.[5]

Avoid casual conversations about individual patients with clinical instructors and colleagues. Never engage in communication about individual patients in public places or with individuals not involved in providing care for that patient.

Keep in mind that PTA students may have access to privileged information during their clinical coursework. Respect that privilege and do not abuse it.

Personal Space, Privacy, and Modesty

Grant spoke with his elderly female patient's family about his mother's seeming lack of "motivation" to begin walking after her hip fracture. She bitterly complained about her physical therapy appointments. Her daughter-in-law talked with her for a few minutes and returned to tell Grant that she was embarrassed to be lifted and touched by a young man.

Be aware that our concept of personal space is *culture-specific*. We may feel uncomfortable being touched on certain body parts or having people stand too close. This applies to working with both fellow students and patients.

With Other Students

Limits of personal space and modesty may vary widely among your classmates. There are many situations in the PTA program where you will be well within the personal space of another student. Show sensitivity to issues of privacy and modesty. Your colleagues must give their permission for you to touch them. It is not your right. Be sure that you ask your colleague first and inform him/her about what to expect, just as you would a client or patient.

Allow instructors, students, and colleagues an opportunity to assist you in performing laboratory exercises that make you feel uncomfortable. If you have objections to others touching or practicing on you, inform the instructor or laboratory assistant. There are solutions that will meet everyone's needs.

With Patients and Clients

Physical therapy procedures often involve touching and treating body parts which go beyond normal social boundaries. You are allowed past these boundaries in your role as a PTA. It is only in that role you are accorded these privileges. Keep in mind that you also have responsibilities to preserve patient dignity and privacy.

Be sure to observe draping guidelines and expose only those areas necessary for treatment. Be sure to inform patients and clients as to what you intend to do and the purpose of the procedure. Obtain consent before beginning. If you feel uncomfortable, ask another staff member to stay in the treatment area with you.

Sexual Harassment

Hannah finished the ultrasound treatment to the patients upper thigh area. As she turned to put away the machine, the patient grabbed her hand and pressed it to his crotch and said, "Now that's more like it."

What should Hannah do or say?

The best approach is to be direct, simple and clear. A statement such as "Let go of my hand right now. Don't do that again. Is that clear?" would indicate the unacceptable behavior. She should request a change in staff if she continues to feel uncomfortable working with this patient.

Sexual harassment, unwanted sexual attention, comments, or overt sexual behavior is never appropriate, yet it is fairly common in physical therapy.[6-8]

Whether the source of sexual harassment is patients or clients, other students, faculty or clinical staff, deal with it directly. Indicate that it is unwanted and inappropriate. Do not keep it to yourself. Take action. Talk with a faculty member, supervisor or clinical director about the proper channels for action.

Remain calm. Define unacceptable behavior clearly. Document the incident in writing through whatever procedures are appropriate at your college or clinical facility.

Summary

Standards of conduct and behavior commonly address dependability, appearance and presentation, initiative, empathy, cooperation, conflict resolution, and verbal and written communication. Published codes of conduct define limits and boundaries of PTA behavior.

Students must be especially aware of standards for behavior and conduct in clinical activities, including presentation and attire, language, confidentiality, and modesty. All students who are members of the American Physical Therapy Association must observe the standards of conduct described in the *Guidelines for Conduct of the Physical Therapist Assistant*. Students should check institutional policies for other regulations that govern student conduct.

References

1. Jamali M. Course Syllabus. PT 3514 Laboratory for Gross Anatomy. Arkansas State University, College of Nursing & Health Professions. Available from: http://www.clt.astate.edu/mjamali/pt3514.htm. Accessed 6/25/2000.

2. May WW, Morgan BJ, Lemke JC, et al. Model for ability-based assessment in physical therapy education. *J Phys Ther Educ.* 1995;9(1) 3-6.

3. Professional behavior policy: student code of conduct. In: *Student Manual, Department of Physical Therapy.* Fresno Calif: California State University, Fresno; 2000.

4. University of Manitoba School of Medical Rehabilitation. Physical therapy dress code. Available at: http://www.umanitoba.ca/faculties/medicine/units/medrehab/pt. Accessed August 18, 2004.

5. Centers for Medicare and Medicaid Services. Health Insurance Portability and Accountability Act of 1996 (HIPAA, Title II) Part 160—General Administrative Requirements. Available from: www.cms.hhs.gov/hipaa/hipaa2/regulations/transactions/finalrule/txfin01.asp. Accessed August 18, 2004.

6. O'Sullivan V, Weerakoon P. Inappropriate sexual behaviours of patients towards practising physio-therapists: A study using qualitative methods. *Physiother Res Int.* 1999;4(1):28-42.

7. deMayo RA. Patient sexual behaviors and sexual harassment: A national survey of physical therapists. *Phys Ther.* 1997;77(7):739-44.

8. McComas J, Hebert C, Giacomin C, Kaplan D, Dulberg C. Experiences of student and practicing physical therapists with inappropriate patient sexual behavior. *Phys Ther.* 1993;73(11):762-9; discussion 769-70.

PUTTING IT INTO PRACTICE

1. Locate and make a copy of the pages of your student handbook or catalog which refer to student conduct. What aspects of conduct are covered by these policies? What are the consequences for failure to observe these standards of conduct?

   How are students in your PTA education program expected to dress for:

   Daily classroom activities?

   Guest speakers?

   Laboratories?

   Clinical experiences?

2. Suppose you find out that one of your classmates has been working as a physical therapy aide, often unsupervised in a local physical therapy practice. You are aware that this practice is a violation of both state law and the APTA Code of Ethics. How would you handle the situation?

3. Why is it important that student PTAs observe standards of behavior and conduct? What are the ramifications of violations of these standards?
   For the student?

   For his/her classmates?

   For the program academic or clinical faculty?

   For the educational program?

   For the physical therapy profession?

CHAPTER 7

Student Performance Evaluation

Evaluation Within the Curriculum

> Irene waited outside the classroom for her first practical examination. She wondered, "Am I really ready for this?" She had practiced for hours the night before on her roommate but still she worried about this new experience. The door opened. A classmate left the room and didn't look upset. She thought, "OK, I'm going to be fine."

Most evaluations within the physical therapist assistant (PTA) curriculum are tied into a general purpose, explained in Chapter 5, to insure that students demonstrate mastery of specific knowledge, attitudes, and skills and meet predefined standards of performance.

There are several types of performance evaluations during the PTA education experience including written and practical examinations, writing evaluations, presentation ratings, and clinical performance evaluations.

Written Examinations

Most students are experienced with written examinations through their academic experiences in primary school. There are many strategies that are valuable for succeeding on written examinations.

Forced-choice questions on written examinations are most commonly of three types:
1. Multiple choice
2. True-false
3. Matching

Constructed answers include three common types as well:
4. Fill in the blank
5. Short-answer
6. Essay

Multiple-Choice Examinations

A multiple-choice question has a stem and multiple *options*. Successful test-takers pay attention to some specific characteristics in these two components of the question that may provide clues that increase the examinee's chances of selecting the correct answer. It may also help to eliminate potential poor choices.

Example
A skin graft in the left axilla, makes palpation of this muscle difficult in the posterior fold:
A. Pectoralis minor
B. Rhomboids
C. Latissimus dorsi
D. Coracobrachialis

To answer this question, we need to know surface anatomy and which muscle groups are palpable in the posterior axillary fold. Since A and D are both in the anterior thorax, and B does not cross the axilla, we can eliminate all choices *except* C, which is the correct answer.

Unless there is a penalty for guessing, always guess. Even if there is a penalty for guessing, it is to your advantage to guess if you can reduce your choices from 4 to 2, by a process of eliminating implausible options. Table 7-1 gives some tips for success on multiple choice exams.

True-False Questions

Because there are only two options, you have a 50% chance of being correct on a true-false question. Unless there is a penalty for guessing, it is always to your advantage to guess.

Read carefully. Watch for specific determiners (always, never, only) and the direction of the statement (not, unable). These words will often exclude an answer or be overlooked by a test-taker in a hurry.

Example

T   F   The only people not at risk for HIV infection are married men and women.

Matching Questions

With matching questions, it is always important to read directions carefully. Know where you will place the correct answer and find out how many times an option can be selected. Eliminate the incorrect responses first, then work with the rest.

Place the number of the correct term in Column B that represents each abbreviation in Column A. You may use each item only once. Consider the context and the likelihood that one of two possibilities is incorrect.

Example

__a. LOL	1. Taking care of business
__b. TCB	2. Two geese in the forest
__c. TGIF	3. Little old lady
__d. PI	4. Postal inspector
	5. Totally courageous boss
	6. Thank goodness it's Friday
	7. Principal Investigator
	8. Lots of luck

Fill in the Blank

Be careful to read the question carefully and to match your answer to the question that is asked. Be sure that your answer fits grammatically (the part of speech: neurological vs. neurology) and the same level of complexity or classification of terms.

Example

In a multiple-choice question, there is a stem and multiple _____.

First by reading the sentence, we know that this should be a noun and it should be plural. So, then we can narrow down the response to answers? or choices? Or, if we recall the specific terminology used earlier in this chapter, we would of course respond "options."

Short-Answer

Short-answer questions allow a two to three-sentence response to a directed question. Read the question carefully. Respond directly in line with the question asked. Be specific, clear and concise. Number the responses if appropriate. If asked, give a simple rationale for your answer.

Example

Give three characteristics of a lower motor neuron lesion.

Response: Three characteristics of lower motor neuron lesions are:

1. *Flaccid muscle paralysis*
2. *Absent deep tendon reflexes*
3. *Hypotonicity in response to passive movement*

Essay

Essays are longer samples of timed writing which indicate your ability to organize your thoughts and respond to a more complex issue. Be sure to read the question carefully.

Essay questions often ask for responses that compare key features of one phenomenon with another. They may ask for arguments in favor or arguments against a particular stance. They sometimes ask for a response and then a rationale for that response.

Help the reader understand your answer. Organize your responses to the question in the same order as the question is asked. Use subtitles to organize your response where appropriate. See the example of an essay question on page 64 .

Writing Assignments

Types of writing assignments and styles are covered in Chapter 8. Writing is evaluated and graded in the context of the purpose of the assignment. There are some desirable characteristics of all types of writ-

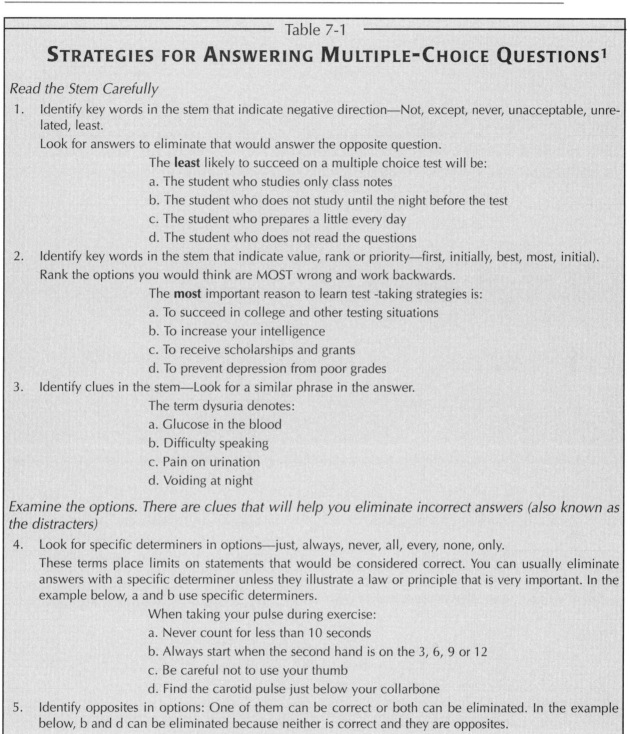

--- Table 7-1 ---

STRATEGIES FOR ANSWERING MULTIPLE-CHOICE QUESTIONS[1]

Read the Stem Carefully

1. Identify key words in the stem that indicate negative direction—Not, except, never, unacceptable, unrelated, least.

    Look for answers to eliminate that would answer the opposite question.

    > The **least** likely to succeed on a multiple choice test will be:
    > a. The student who studies only class notes
    > b. The student who does not study until the night before the test
    > c. The student who prepares a little every day
    > d. The student who does not read the questions

2. Identify key words in the stem that indicate value, rank or priority—first, initially, best, most, initial).

    Rank the options you would think are MOST wrong and work backwards.

    > The **most** important reason to learn test -taking strategies is:
    > a. To succeed in college and other testing situations
    > b. To increase your intelligence
    > c. To receive scholarships and grants
    > d. To prevent depression from poor grades

3. Identify clues in the stem—Look for a similar phrase in the answer.

    > The term dysuria denotes:
    > a. Glucose in the blood
    > b. Difficulty speaking
    > c. Pain on urination
    > d. Voiding at night

Examine the options. There are clues that will help you eliminate incorrect answers (also known as the distracters)

4. Look for specific determiners in options—just, always, never, all, every, none, only.

    These terms place limits on statements that would be considered correct. You can usually eliminate answers with a specific determiner unless they illustrate a law or principle that is very important. In the example below, a and b use specific determiners.

    > When taking your pulse during exercise:
    > a. Never count for less than 10 seconds
    > b. Always start when the second hand is on the 3, 6, 9 or 12
    > c. Be careful not to use your thumb
    > d. Find the carotid pulse just below your collarbone

5. Identify opposites in options: One of them can be correct or both can be eliminated. In the example below, b and d can be eliminated because neither is correct and they are opposites.

    > In relation to the average child, a hyperactive child is:
    > a. Easily taught in a large class
    > b. Nonviolent except when provoked
    > c. Difficult to focus on a task
    > d. Often abusive to other children

continued

Table 7-1 (continued)

STRATEGIES FOR ANSWERING MULTIPLE-CHOICE QUESTIONS[1]

6. Identify equally plausible/unique options.

    If there are two items which are no better or worse than the other option, you can usually eliminate both. In the example below a and c are similar and thus neither are correct.

    > If your computer screen does not illuminate when you turn on the computer, the first thing you should do is:
    >
    > a. Turn the power off and on again quickly
    >
    > b. Check the brightness controls of the monitor
    >
    > c. Shut it off; wait 30 seconds, then turn on again
    >
    > d. Hit the monitor gently on the side

7. Identify duplicate facts in options.

    When an option contains 2 or more facts that are identical and you can identify one part as being correct, you can usually eliminate two options that are distracters. In the example below the only two answers with a "typical college student" age group are a and c. Therefore b and d can be eliminated.

    > The most common age groups on campus (including all students, faculty and staff) are:
    >
    > a. 21 to 25 and 45 to 50
    >
    > b. 16 to 20 and 31 to 35
    >
    > c. 21 to 25 and 56 to 60
    >
    > d. 36 to 40 and 51 to 55

Adapted from Curtis KA. *Test-taking, UNIV 001: University Orientation*. Fresno, Calif: California State University; 1999.

Example Essay

Instructions

Answer the following questions. Organize your response. (You may use scrap paper to do this) Be clear and concise. Be sure you answer all parts of the question. Write legibly and in the available space. Illegible answers cannot be graded.

Question

In the managed care era, several trends have occurred which affect the delivery of physical therapy services. Indicators forecast further downsizing of health care institutions and a shift to prospective payment systems.

*Why is evidence-based practice an attractive alternative in this changing health care environment? Describe three problems that the physical therapy profession may face in using this practice model. **Your response?***

First re-read the question. Outline your response. There are two questions asked in the above question. This essay is asking you to consider evidence-based practice within a defined context.

A well-written essay would start with an introductory paragraph defining evidence-based practice, then answer the first question. The responses to the first question must be in reference to the described trend of downsizing of health care institutions and shift to prospective payment systems. Why is evidence-based practice especially important under these conditions?

Then the responses to the second question could consist of three paragraphs to describe three problems that may arise as physical therapists and PTAs attempt to use evidence-based practice. The final paragraph should be a summary statement addressing the value of evidence-based practice.

Use subtitles such as Evidence-Based Practice, Problems, and Summary to organize your response and make it easier for the reader to identify your responses to various parts of the question. Use words like first, further, and finally to help the reader define where your points begin and end.

ing, including clarity, topic development and correct grammar and spelling.

It is often helpful for students to assess their own writing and that of their peers prior to turning in assignments. The scoring criteria used in Table 7-2 may be beneficial in reviewing your work.

Presentation

Strategies for preparing projects and presentations are covered in Chapter 8. Performance during a class presentation is often graded. Students are usually graded on content, style, quality of presentation and evidence of having met the objectives of the assigned project. Look at the sample assignment and evaluation form in Table 7-2 for evaluating a presentation.

Peer evaluation is also very important. Here is an example of a peer evaluation form that can be completed by the audience during a class presentation.

Practical Examinations or Performance Assessments

Example

Presentation Feedback Form   Date:_____

Subject: _____

Speaker(s): _____

1. What was most helpful or most interesting about this presentation?

2. What would you like to know more about this subject?

3. What suggestions would you make regarding this presentation?

4. What new ideas or insights have you gained from this presentation?

Practical examinations are commonly used in courses that cover physical therapy tests and measures and/or interventions. They are usually case-based and require the student to read a case and then simulate performance with another classmate or standardized patient.

A *standardized patient* is a paid volunteer who plays the role of the patient for the purpose of examining students. Standardized patients are usually trained and may have real diagnostic findings which students must accurately measure and treat per the simulated physical therapist's evaluation and plan of care.

During a practical examination, students are given the opportunity to interact with a "patient" and provide test/measures and treatment procedures following completion of this content within the curriculum. Additionally, many programs require a comprehensive practical examination as an important means for the academic faculty to confirm student competence as a prerequisite to participating in full-time clinical internships.

The following example is typical of a case study you might be given during a practical examination.

Grading of a practical examination is done by observation of student performance. Student performance and choices during the examination reflect problem solving and safe judgment, as well as, understanding and competent application of course content. Communication skills come into play as stu-

Case Study[3]

This is a 62 y.o. hispanic female with hx of severe DJD right knee who underwent TKA x 1 day. Pt lives in one story home alone with adult children living in town. PMH includes HTN, LBP and DM. She has received P.T. previously for her LBP. Has never used an assistive device. Received orders this A.M. for transfer/gait training WBAT R.

The P.T. performed eval and initial treatment this A.M. and has put this patient on your schedule for this afternoon. This A.M. the pt. transferred supine to sit with mod asst x 1; sat on the edge of bed x 5 mins while performing deep breathing exs; stood at bedside with a standard walker x 5 mins requiring min to mod assist x 2 working on erect posture and accepting weight on R; took 3 steps requiring verbal/tactile cues and mod assist x 1 when became nauseated and requested to go back to bed. Vitals remained stable. The "P" from the initial note includes: transfer training, gait training with assistive device WBAT R, ther ex and pt/family education.

In your Rx work towards achieving the following goals:
Pt. will:

1. Transfer I supine to sit to stand in 2 Rxs.

2. Ambulate with walker to bathroom with min assist x 1 & no verbal cues for safety or walker management in 3 Rxs.

3. Demonstrate R knee AROM -5 – 90 degrees flexion in 3 Rxs.

4. Demonstrate LE strengthening ex program satisfactorily prior to DC.

Table 7-2

SAMPLE ORAL/WRITTEN PRESENTATION WITH GRADING CRITERIA FOR *PTA SYSTEMS/PROBLEMS IN PHYSICAL THERAPY*[2]

Oral/Written Presentation

1. The student will select three choices of an orthopedic or neurological condition involving a child or adult client.

2. The student will have one of the three conditions selected assigned to them. *NO DUPLICATIONS OF TOPICS WILL OCCUR*

    If in the assignment process, there are limited choices due to duplication of the conditions turned in by students, RANDOM ASSIGNMENTS WILL BE MADE.

3. Out of class time will be required to research and prepare for this project.

4. The student will prepare a 5 to 7 page typewritten report including the required outline topics. Please use 12-point font.

5. The student will contact one physical therapist (or assistant) colleague who works with clientele with this condition in order to complete this project. Failure to complete this aspect of this assignment will result in a zero.

6. The student will observe this colleague evaluating and/or treating a person with this neurological condition in the clinic.

7. The written report will include at least two (2) references from a peer-reviewed journal to support information in the written/oral report. Referencing must be done according to the publication manual of the American Psychological Association.

8. The student will present a 15-minute oral presentation to the class including a BRIEF demonstration of one treatment strategy that is commonly used with this type of client by a physical therapist and/or assistant. Be able to discuss the underlying rationale for this treatment approach. Failure to arrive for your scheduled presentation time and participate during classmate's presentations may result in a zero.

9. The student will provide each classmate with a copy of the written report (with references) at time of oral presentation.

10. The student will use client-centered, non-discriminatory language.

Oral/Written Presentation Grading Criteria

NAME: _____   DATE: _____

Oral Presentation

___/20	Speaking skills
___/05	Eye contact/clarity/volume/body language
___/05	Conciseness/vocabulary
___/05	Audio-visual material informative and clear
___/05	Report copies distributed to classmates
___/10	Sequential/organization
___/10	All required components addressed/physical therapy management presented
___/10	Therapy treatment technique clinically sound and appropriately demonstrated
___/70	Oral presentation subtotal

Written Report

___/50	Includes all outline topics and appropriate length
___/10	References with abstracts included
___/50	Clinically sound therapy management and most of report focuses on therapy management.
___/20	Uses appropriate spelling/grammar / medical terminology / punctuation
___/20	Organization
___/150	Written report subtotal

TOTAL: ___/220

Adapted from Newman PD. *Oral/Written Presentation, PTA 2113 Systems/Problems in Physical Therapy*. Oklahoma City, Okla: Oklahoma City Community College; 2003.

Table 7-3

SAMPLE PERFORMANCE EVALUATION CRITERIA (COMPREHENSIVE CHECK OUT)

Evaluation Form

Student Therapist: _____ Problem #____

Patient: _____ Date:_____

Please rate the student therapist assistant using the following rating scale:

Completes skill competently entirely without assistance = 3

Completes skill competently with minimal assistance = 2

(Requires 2 or less verbal cues from evaluator)

Completes skill competently with assistance = 1

(Requires more than 2 verbal cues from evaluator)

Unable to complete/safely complete skill or omits this skill component = Needs Improvement (NI)

1. Introduces self appropriately.   _____
2. Dressed appropriately.   _____
3. Communicates (verbally/nonverbally)appropriately.   _____
4. Explains treatment/answers questions.   _____
5. Performs re-evaluation tests & measures. List specifically: ie, MMT, goniometry, gauges amount of assistance, palpation.

   _____   _____
   _____   _____
   _____   _____
   _____   _____

6. Chooses appropriate treatment/interventions within PT's plan of care:

   _____   _____
   _____   _____
   _____   _____
   _____   _____

7. Monitors safety/comfort/modesty of patient.   _____
8. Chooses appropriate exercises/instructs correctly.   _____
9. Issues home exercises/instructions correctly.   _____
10. Provides safe/effective treatment session.   _____
11. Demonstrates problem solving/proper judgment.   _____

Comments:

Evaluator: _____ Pass: _____ Redo: _____

*The student must re-do if they receive one (1) NI or more than two (2) #1's.

Adapted from Newman PD. *Comprehensive Skills Evaluation Form*. Oklahoma City Community College; 2003.

---

dents must question the patient, give instructions and listen to what the patient says. Performance also includes a psychomotor component in that students must position themselves and the patient appropriately and demonstrate effective and safe handling skills. Take a look at the practical examination performance evaluation criteria in Table 7-3.

Assessment Center

An assessment center (also called an objective, structured clinical examination [OSCE]) involves the evaluation of various components of clinical competence which are measured in a series of stations.[5,6] The student progresses from station to station carry-

---

Table 7-4

PHYSICAL THERAPY STUDENT ASSESSMENT CENTER[7]

Assessment Center	*Stations Activity*
Station One: Chart Review	Perform chart review of basic medical and social history information.
Station Two: Interview	Perform a 5-minute interview with the "patient" role-played by a faculty member.
Station Three: Evaluation Planning	Design and prioritize evaluation procedures. Complete a written questionnaire, answering questions about the functional limitations, diagnosis and important medical problems, contraindications, and precautions for the patient. List evaluative priorities and give the rationale for choices.
Station Four: Evaluation Performance	Perform several evaluation procedures on the patient. Procedures include surface palpation, goniometric assessment, manual muscle testing, and reflex and sensory testing. Students rated on organization, safety, accuracy, and effectiveness in performing each evaluative procedure. Write a short note documenting evaluative findings.
Station Five: Treatment Planning	After reviewing the physical therapy evaluative findings, establish functional goals and a treatment plan directed toward meeting those goals. Identify contraindications or precautions considered in the treatment planning process.
Station Six: Treatment Performance	Present treatment plan and explain rationale. Perform a selected part of the treatment plan on the patient. The students are rated on their ability to explain and demonstrate their instructions to the patient, to adjust equipment, to prepare the treatment area, to exhibit proper body mechanics, to take appropriate precautions for patient safety and to apply treatment skills.

Adapted from Curtis KA, Haston L. *Basic Physical Therapy Skills Assessment Center: Evaluation Alternative for Entry-Level Physical Therapy Students.* Miami, Fla: University of Miami, 1994.

---

ing out specified activities in a limited time frame. Student performance is graded with specific outcome measurements. It generally involves a number of different components which simulate decision-making and skills needed for clinical practice.

An example of a Physical Therapy Assessment Center and the types of activities students might perform are listed in Table 7-4.

Clinical Performance Evaluation.

The *Physical Therapist Assistant Clinical Performance Instrument* (CPI) is a clinical rating instrument in wide use in PTA clinical education. It was developed to evaluate knowledge, skills and attitudes in 20 clinical performance criteria. Each of the 20 performance criteria is accompanied by a list of sample behaviors that serve as examples of the item (Table 7-5).

The instrument uses a 10-cm rating visual analog scale, on a continuum from "novice clinical performance" at the low end to "entry-level performance" at the high end to rate each of the 20 indicators. Both instructors and students are able to rate progress on this line. Instructors must also record narrative comments on each page of the 23-page instrument. Compare these two definitions in Table 7-6.

Summary

Student performance is evaluated at many points and through many different processes during the educational process. Students who understand the criteria on which they are being graded and practice in ways that simulate exam conditions should fare well. Sound preparation and effective use of test-taking strategies are keys to success not only during the

---
Table 7-5

EXAMPLE OF PERFORMANCE CRITERIA AND SAMPLE BEHAVIORS FROM CLINICAL PERFORMANCE (CPI)[8]

Physical Therapist Assistant Clinical Performance Instrument: Performance Criteria and Sample Behaviors

9. Participates in patient status judgments within the clinical environment based on the plan of care established by the physical therapist.

    Sample Behaviors

a. Explains rationale for judgments.

b. Makes judgments within the context of ethical issues, informed consent, and safety considerations.

c. Utilizes information from multiple data sources to make judgments.

d. Uses a clinical problem-solving process that includes considering decision rules (eg codes, protocols), thinking, data collection, and interpretive processes.

Adapted from APTA. *Physical Therapist Assistant Clinical Performance Instrument.* Alexandria, Va: American Physical Therapy Association. 1998;9.

Table 7-6

DESCRIPTIONS OF NOVICE AND ENTRY-LEVEL PERFORMANCE[8]

Clinical Performance Instrument Performance Definitions

Novice clinical performance:	A PTA student who provides quality care only with uncomplicated patients and a high degree of supervision. Without close supervision, the student's performance and judgement are inconsistent and require constant monitoring and feedback. This is typically a student who is inexperienced in clinical practice or who performs as though he or she has had limited or no opportunity to apply academic knowledge or clinical skills.
Entry-level performance:	A PTA clinician performing at entry-level consistently and efficiently provides quality care with simple or complex patients in a variety of clinical environments under the supervision of a physical therapist. Usually needs no guidance or supervision except when addressing new or complex problems.

Adapted from APTA. *Physical Therapist Assistant Clinical Performance Instrument.* Alexandria, Va: American Physical Therapy Association; 1998; v-vi.

---

academic program but in successfully obtaining licensure as well. Performance evaluation serves a critical role in determining clinical competence and identifying student needs.

References

1. Curtis KA. *Test-taking, UNIV 001: University Orientation.* Fresno, Calif: California State University; 1999.

2. Newman PD. *Oral/Written Presentation, PTA 2113 Systems/Problems in Physical Therapy.* Oklahoma City, Okla: Oklahoma City Community College; 2003.

3. Newman PD. *Comprehensive Skills Check/Tutorial.* Oklahoma City, Okla: Oklahoma City Community College; 2003.

4. Newman PD. *Comprehensive Skills Check/Tutorial Evaluation Form.* Oklahoma City, Okla: Oklahoma City Community College; 2003.

5. Harden RM, Gleeson FA. Assessment of clinical competence using an objective structured clinical examination (OSCE). *Med Educ.* 1979;13:41-54.

6. Deusinger SS, Sindelar B, Stritter FT. Assessment center: a model for professional development and education. *Phys Ther.* 1986;66:1119-1123.

7. Curtis KA, Haston L. *Basic Physical Therapy Skills Assessment Center: Evaluation Alternative for Entry-Level Physical Therapy Students.* Miami, Fla: University of Miami; 1994.

8. APTA. *Physical Therapist Assistant Clinical Performance Instrument.* Alexandria, Va: American Physical Therapy Association. 1998; 9:S v-vi.

PUTTING IT INTO PRACTICE

1. Survey your course syllabi for the current semester. Write the dates of all quizzes, written examinations, practical examinations, and assignments due on your daily planning calendar.

2. On what dates do you have multiple examinations or assignments due?

3. Record the results of any tests or assignments you have completed thus far on your syllabus.

4. What clinical performance rating system is used in your curriculum?

5. If you were given the choice of an examination or a project as a means to evaluate your performance, which would you choose? Why?

6. Most successful students are fairly accurate in their self-assessment of their skills and knowledge.

   What opportunities in the past have you had to evaluate your own performance?

   What opportunities do you or will you have in the professional education program to perform self-assessment?

CHAPTER 8

Presentations, Papers, and Projects

Oral Presentations

Jolene noticed on the course outline that a group case presentation was required during the 12th week of the class. She worried, "I've never been a good public speaker, but even worse, what if I end up in a group with someone who doesn't do the work?

Presentations, papers, and projects are common requirements during the educational process. Within the health care professions, they form the basis for communication between disciplines, for starting new programs or research projects and for contributing to the base of scientific knowledge. Knowing how to effectively communicate your ideas, information, and research findings is an important skill.

Types of Presentations

There are many opportunities to present information to colleagues, professors, clinical instructors, and others. Each type of presentation may have a different purpose and therefore have different requirements.

In-Class

Students in college classes often must do an individual or group presentation as part of the requirements of a course. These presentations are usually focused on a specific topic, issue, or content related to the course. These presentations are usually short (15 to 30 minutes) and focused with specific objectives and expected outcomes. The audience is usually fellow classmates and the course instructor. These types of presentations are usually graded using specific criteria.

In-Service (Clinical)

Students are frequently requested to do in-service presentations as part of their clinical education experience. The focus of these presentations is often left to the student's choice, with input from the clinical instructor. Usually the purpose is to provide a review of the latest literature and demonstrate an understanding and application of clinical information. In-service presentations tend to be scheduled in 30 to 60 minute periods, often during a lunch or staff meeting time. The audience is usually the clinical staff, other students and clinical instructors.

Examinations

Presentations are also done for the purpose of a clinical or academic examination. A student might be required to present a case study, literature review, or research findings. A student in these cases is often required to meet specific criteria, address certain issues or questions and respond appropriately to questions. The audience may be one or more faculty members (academic and/or clinical) either with or without fellow students.

Research

Research presentations are done for several purposes, depending on the location and audience. These types of presentations might be done to demonstrate successful completion of a project to an academic review committee, to share research findings with other investigators and colleagues at a scientific meeting and to add to the body of evidence-based knowledge underlying the profession of physical therapy.

Designing a Presentation

In designing a presentation, it will be helpful for you to consider the following issues:

Purpose and Objectives

State the purpose and intended outcomes of your presentation. For example, your purpose might be to present your research findings in a simple, understandable way.

Objectives are what you hope that your audience will know, feel, or be able to do following your presentations. These intended outcomes give your presentation a direction and help you to measure whether you have achieved your intended outcome. If your objectives are specific and measurable, it will be easier to tell if you have achieved them than if they are more general and vague. Compare these two objectives:

> *Participants will understand and appreciate the causes and results of the inflammatory process.*
>
> *Participants will be able to define inflammation, infection, edema, and induration and differentiate the etiology and tissue pathology of each of these four processes.*

Which is more measurable, more clear? Which describes an outcome? Objectives are as much for the presenter as they are for the audience. They keep you on track and help define the content you will present and path you will take.

Audience

Who is your audience? Are they colleagues or consumers? Do they have the same background or do they differ in levels of education and specific previous exposure to the subject matter? What are their needs with respect to the subject matter? What vocabulary do they use? Should your presentation be in lay language or use medical terminology?

Needs Assessment

A needs assessment determines your audience's background and present level of knowledge. This might be accomplished by an informal questionnaire to a few representative members of the group, brief interviews, or more extensive surveys. Don't fall into the trap of assuming that all members of the audi-

ence have the same background or that this background is similar to that of the presenter. Remember that in preparing to do a presentation, you are probably becoming far more knowledgeable than your audience.

Subject Content

The subject content that is presented should be related to the intended outcomes of the presentation. The subject content should be organized in an outline or list form as you develop the presentation. Try to simplify, condense and summarize material for your audience.

Define terms before using complicated or technical terminology. Be sure to introduce sections of your presentation and make it clear when you are moving from one section to the next. Use simple subtitles, advanced organizers, and other techniques that will keep your audience with you.

Presentation Activities

Select an appropriate presentation technique and/or learning activity. The descriptions in Tables 8-1, 8-2, and 8-3 should help you to differentiate what presentation techniques may be most appropriate. Consider the value of lecture, question and answer, demonstration, discussion, and experiential techniques to present the material. Although lecture is frequently the mode chosen, other activities may actually be far more effective in presenting material and accomplishing your objectives.

Reinforce and supplement your presentation with visual aides and written handout materials. Make your materials compliment but not duplicate your presentation. Never read your written materials verbatim to the audience.

Instructional Media

Do not overlook the importance of media in adding to your presentation. An electronic slide presentation, a short video, and/or photographs or diagrams may help markedly to improve understanding and keep your audience's attention. See Tables 8-4 and 8-5 which describe types of media and guidelines for presentation.

Also think in advance about reading materials you can recommend which might compliment or augment your presentation.

Table 8-1

SIMPLE PRESENTATION TECHNIQUES[1]

Lecture

We have all experienced lecture in our formal education. It is most useful when the leader wants to transmit information that the participants do not have. Lectures are best when they are:

- SHORT (less than 5 minutes of monologue at a time!)
- SIMPLE (building on what participants know)
- VISUALLY INTERESTING (so participants can see concepts and ideas)
- PARTICIPATIVE (involving participants via questions)

A mini-lecture is helpful to introduce the topic and provide a brief description of the problem and important background material. Participants should be INVOLVED as soon as possible to maintain their interest and attention.

Questions

The leader can insert questions in the lecture to stimulate and involve the participants. Asking for agreement/disagreement or for common experiences of participants is an easy way to begin. ("How many of you have experienced this?" or "Does this sound familiar? I see a few of you nodding your heads.")

Demonstration

Lecture can often be enhanced with demonstration of skills or techniques. Demonstration is best followed by practice and a return demonstration. When demonstrating the leader should be sure that participants can see the demonstration. The leader should take care to illustrate and identify the key points of the demonstrated skill.

Adapted from Curtis KA. *Training Programs for Clinical Instructors*. Los Angeles, Calif: Health Directions; 1988.

Table 8-2

DISCUSSION TECHNIQUES[1]

Purpose and Types of Discussion

Discussion provides for participant sharing of knowledge, experience and skills on the subject. Holding a discussion helps the leader to take advantage of the combined background that the group brings. Discussion is a valuable method to generate ideas and give participants new approaches to a common problem.

Discussion Techniques

Brainstorming

Brainstorming is a useful technique to generate many ideas in a short period of time. A question is asked and participant responses are recorded on a flip chart or board for all to see. It is important the leader record responses and refrain from evaluation of responses until the group runs out of ideas.

Question and Answer

This technique is useful to involve participants and diverge from straight lecture. The instructor asks a question and then calls on an individual participant to answer the question. The leader should have a predetermined list of questions and follow-up questions to ask, which are tied into the lecture material.

continued

Table 8-2 (continued)
DISCUSSION TECHNIQUES[1]

Case Study

This provides a means for participants to analyze a case and apply the techniques and principles of the learning experience to it. The case provides a situation to be discussed. The leader should have a list of discussion questions prepared in advance. Participants should be encouraged to share experiences which help in making the jump from the case to their own experiences.

Fish Bowl Discussion

A small group of four or five representatives are chosen to sit in front of, or in the center of the larger group. This is particularly valuable to focus the group on their reaction to a particular exercise or experience. At the end of the fish-bowl discussion, all participants have had the same experience, either directly or vicariously.

Panel Discussion

The panel discussion takes place in front of a larger group, with questions directed to the panelists initially by the leader or facilitator. Panelists typically represent different points of view or may come from different occupational groups or specialty areas.

Adapted from Curtis KA. *Training Programs for Clinical Instructors*. Los Angeles, Calif: Health Directions, 1988.

Table 8-3
EXPERIENTIAL PRESENTATION TECHNIQUES[1]

This term applies to a variety of techniques that allow the participant to *experience* what you want to teach, rather than just studying or talking about it. Learning occurs via the reactions and emotions participants experience while they participate in the exercise. The leader has a key role in helping participants to analyze their experience and relate it to the objectives of the learning experience.

Role Playing

Role playing is helpful to provide an opportunity to practice a new process or skill and illustrate different perspectives which one takes on in a "role." It is not "play-acting," as it is intended to simulate reality. Role-playing provides a realistic, look at the participant's behavior, emotions, and experience in a "real" situation.

Role playing is most successful when participants are given a loosely defined situation, a role to play and attitude or position to take. The role play should be followed up with discussion by participants and observer(s). This discussion should help to relate the experience to the skills, concepts, or ideas that it was intended to illustrate and support.

Games and Simulations

Games and simulations are carefully structured learning activities which assist participants to explore their group working relationships and responses to a variety of situations. The value of using simulations is that if a mistake is made, no one is hurt. Games and simulations must have contingencies built-in for the decisions and actions that participants take. For instance, if a participant makes a decision to proceed with a particular action, there must be feedback which indicates the consequence of that choice. Therefore, the rules and results must be carefully defined.

Videotaping

This is time-consuming but quite valuable as an experiential learning tool. When videotape is used, it is essential that participants have sufficient time to observe and analyze their performance, with instructor feedback.

Adapted from Curtis KA. *Training Programs for Clinical Instructors*. Los Angeles, Calif: Health Directions; 1988.

Table 8-4

INSTRUCTIONAL MEDIA CHOICES

Types of Instructional Media

Overhead projector transparencies:	Useful to project words, charts, graphs, cartoons. Can be easily made on photocopy machine; lights stay on. Instructor can write or draw on transparency.
Electronic Slides/LCD projector:	Can be used to present computer-generated materials and video onto a large screen. Special effects can be incorporated into computer program. Photographs, charts, graphs, videos, sounds, words, different colors are all possible. Lights must be off. Easy to control and advance. However, be careful of technical difficulties and incompatible versions of software, operating systems, and media.
Videotape/DVD/CD:	Able to demonstrate complex interactions, movement with both visual images and sound. Often must be edited and cued for effective presentation.
Audio tape/CD:	Excellent for instruction or review with accompanying written materials.

Table 8-5

GENERAL GUIDELINES FOR USING INSTRUCTIONAL MEDIA[2]

Strategies for Successful Media Use

1. Keep it simple. For word slides, or overhead transparencies, use no more than seven lines of text.
2. Make sure that the projected image is visible from all areas of the room.
3. If you can't see it well, don't use it. (Do not use tiny figures on charts) If showing a table, use no more than three rows and columns of figures. Fewer will be more understandable.
4. Use media to enhance your presentation, but be sure to explain adequately also.
5. Allow the audience to see and read before you talk. Pause slightly before speaking.
6. Use titles. A title on a slide or transparency helps the audience to absorb and organize the material.
7. Insure that volume and visibility are adequate for a video tape presentation. You may want to darken the room.
8. Be prepared! Check out all equipment and your media BEFORE beginning your presentation.

Adapted from Curtis KA. *PH TH231 Seminar in Health Care Issues Course syllabus*. Fresno, Calif: California State University, Fresno; 1997.

Equipment and Facilities

Reserve the equipment you will need. Double check on the availability of equipment and support personnel at the presentation site. Arrive early to test your presentation on the actual equipment you will use. Some of the following equipment may be helpful to your presentation:

* Overhead projector (for overhead transparencies)
* LCD projector and laptop computer (for electronic slides)
* Video cassette player
* Microphone
* Laser pointer

Evaluation

Evaluations are done for many purposes. They serve as a form of feedback for the presenter and as validation of learning or achievement for the participants.

Speakers should seek involvement of the audience to assess whether their objectives have been met and

---

Table 8-6

EVALUATION TECHNIQUES FOR EVALUATING A PRESENTATION

1.   Paper and pencil test, survey, or reaction.
2.   Performance evaluation of participants.
3.   Behavioral observations of participants.
4.   Participant self-evaluation.

---

to review the effectiveness of each phase of the presentation. Evaluations can take many forms. Consider the list in Table 8-6 and consider what evaluation techniques you might choose. Some sample evaluation forms are shown in Chapter 7.

Papers and Writing Assignments

There are various writing assignments which you will be involved with in the course of your education. It is important that you understand the purpose, guidelines, and parameters of each assignment. Some of the more common types of papers follow:

Review of the Literature

A review of the literature is a systematic and thorough compilation and summary of published research on a particular topic. It is important when writing this type of paper to narrow the topic enough to allow for thorough and relevant coverage of published sources. This type of paper may serve as the basis for an introduction to a research proposal or may be publishable as a review article on a particular subject.

Case Report

A case report or case study is an in-depth report of an example of a phenomenon. Usually case reports involve the application of theoretical or research-based information to clinical or administrative examples. For example, one might write a case report to present the unique management of a patient or development of a new administrative structure to address transdisciplinary care. A case report usually presents a chronological series of events and often describes the effect of an intervention or change over time.

Research Abstract

Research abstracts are short summaries of a larger article. They typically include the key elements of purpose, subjects, instruments, methods, results, and conclusions. Most articles have abstracts which are written preceding the article. Abstracts are indexed in databases such as the Cumulative Index to Nursing and Allied Health Literature (CINAHL) and serve as a preview to help you determine if the article meets your needs.

Research Critique

Critiques are discussions of the strengths and limitations of published research articles. Critiques require that the writer has a background in both the subject matter, previous research in the area and in research methodologies. A critique generally follows a prescribed format, commenting on issues such as the relevance and importance of the study, the sampling technique, the validity and reliability of instrumentation, the variables measured, the statistical analyses chosen, and the generalizability of the findings reported. Some journals (such as *Physical Therapy*) often publish a peer-reviewed "discussion" following a research article.

Position Paper

A position paper is often focused around a controversial issue. This type of paper requires that the writer succinctly summarize the issue, provide relevant arguments from several positions, and then choose a particular stance. It is important that this type of writing focus on the establishment of an argument and position, using sound rationale and acknowledging consideration of alternative points of view.

Reaction Paper

A reaction paper is a more personal account of an event or experience than any of the previous types of writing. The writer should use the first person voice, "I found…." when describing the experience. A reaction paper usually involves the application of theoretical or research-based findings to a real-life experience. For example, students might write a reaction paper after visiting a hospice facility and discuss their observations and feelings about the experience in relation to assigned readings.

Patient-Related Documentation

There are numerous opportunities during the physical therapist assistant (PTA) education program to practice writing patient-related documentation including daily progress notes. Be clear, concise, and use professional terminology where appropriate. Be careful not to use excessive or non-standard abbreviations and avoid professional jargon. Consider who will be reading this documentation and keep in mind that insurance claims reviewers and even physicians often do not understand abbreviations like TTG (toe-touch gait), VC (verbal cueing), or SBA (stand-by assist).

The Writing Process

Drafts and Revisions

Good writers always go through numerous drafts while developing their ideas, the structure of the paper and the proper grammar, spelling and syntax. It often helps to have a colleague read and review your work. Be sure to use computer-based spell checking and grammar assists. Avoidable errors detract from your work and make it appear that you have not invested much effort.

What is the Point?

Understanding the purpose of writing is important in determining what you write. Be sure to identify the focus and theme of each paragraph and check to make sure that you are communicating your ideas effectively.

Avoid Common Writing Errors

Take a look at Table 8-7 for common writing errors. Have you made some of these common errors?

Professional Language

Kelly and Al both prepared reviews of the same article they had read. Al took a casual, friendly approach and concluded her review as follows: "This was a totally cool article that I think everybody ought to read. I learned lots of neat stuff about how to get patients to do their exercises and I really liked all the pictures of people working out, and that kind of thing." Kelly took a more professional approach: "This article presents relevant new research that clinicians may find useful for their orthopedic patients. The authors conclude that social support is a necessary component of patient adherence.

Be aware that you must choose the language style that is appropriate for the type of writing and reader. As a rule of thumb, most professional writing requires professional language. Be critical of your writing and watch the terminology you use.

Terminology and Definitions

It is a good idea to start every technical writing piece with basic definitions of the terminology you are using. A few introductory sentences should suffice as you introduce each new topic in your paper.

Plagiarism and Copyright Infringement

Plagiarism involves misrepresenting the work of another, whether published or unpublished as one's own work. This can be as simple as using phrases of other authors without proper citation. To avoid plagiarism, always cite your sources.

Be sure that you are citing the original source. The *original source* is that of the author(s) whose work is being described. Do not cite the article or book in which you read about another study. Look at the reference list at the end of the piece and find the original source. Find the original paper and read it for yourself. Your citation should always be the original source, not another author who has cited this source in his or her work.

Copyright infringement involves copying published material, whether text, illustrations or photographs without permission. Be careful…. even copying a photograph from an internet site into an electronic slide presentation is a copyright infringement. Always ask permission from the copyright owner before incorporating someone else's work into your writing or presentation. (Copyright infringement applies even if the sources are properly referenced.)

Review the laws regarding plagiarism and copyright infringement in Chapter 12.

Referencing Styles

Instructions for a paper or other writing assignment should designate which referencing style to use. Common styles for professional writing in the health fields include American Medical Association (AMA) and American Psychological Association (APA) styles. Your library should have references available which detail these reference styles.

The journal, *Physical Therapy*, uses AMA style. Table 8-8 shows a sample of how references are done for journal articles, books, book chapters, and online journals and Web sites using AMA style.

Table 8-7
COMMON WRITING ERRORS[3]

Goal	Incorrect	Correct
Make sure that subjects and verbs agree.	Mary is more capable than he is at suctioning.	Mary is more capable than him at suctioning.
Avoid using nouns as verbs.	This change will impact the way we do things.	The impact of this change will be significant.
Make pronouns and subject agree. Watch out for the word they/them when referring to one person.	The patient called to complain that I could not see them this afternoon.	The patient called to complain that I could not see (him or her) this afternoon.
Only use apostrophes to indicate possession or a contraction, NOT a plural (except for the word it).	Charles's voice is very loud. The CD's and disks were very expensive. I have found it's cord under the bed.	Charles' voice is very loud. The CDs and disks were very expensive. I have found its cord under the bed.
Don't confuse "affect" and "effect."	The affect is not known. How can I effect this outcome?	The effect is not known. How can I affect this outcome?
Don't split infinitives.	He lifted the patient to slightly move the sheet.	He lifted the patient to move the sheet slightly.
Start sentences with words other than "hopefully" or "basically."	Hopefully, I will hear about the scholarship this week.	I hope to hear about the scholarship this week.
Use people-first language	Disabled people need more job opportunities.	People with disabilities need more job opportunities.
Use the active voice wherever possible.	John was selected for the job.	The Search Committee selected John for the job.

Adapted from So You Wanna.Com. So you wanna avoid common writing errors? Available at: http://www.soyouwanna.com/site/syws/wrerros/wrerrors.html. Accessed August 24, 2004.

Peer Review

Peer review is a process that occurs throughout professional writing. It involves a subject matter expert or colleague reviewing your submitted writing. Following peer review, authors then have the option to revise their work. Table 8-9 shows a very simple peer review form which students can use to review the work of their colleagues.

Although it may not always be easy to hear criticism of your writing, peer review is a valuable process. Through this process, writers benefit from having someone else with a similar background critically read their work. Reviewers often become better writers as well.

In general, peer-reviewed professional writing receives the highest credibility and distinction in publication. Peer-reviewed journals serve as the original sources of scientific knowledge and serve as a vehicle for communicating new knowledge.

Projects

Class Projects

Projects take many forms. Courses within the PTA curriculum will require individual or group projects that encourage students to apply course material into a meaningful learning experience. This might be through a service learning project, such as doing volunteer work at a community center. It might involve researching a clinical topic or doing an in-depth case study of a patient or client.

Collaborative Projects

Group projects allow students to collaborate to complete a project. This model is, in reality, how most work in the real world is done. Students may have an opportunity to work with other student PTAs or with students from other disciplines.

Table 8-8

REFERENCING USING AMA STYLE[4,5]

Follow AMA style (eg, *Journal of the American Medical Association*; *Physical Therapy*). Double-space citations in your list of references. References should be numbered in the order of their citation in the text. When citing references in the text, the numerals appear outside periods and commas, inside colons and semicolons. When more than two references are cited at a given place in the text, use hyphens to join the first and last numbers of a closed series; use commas without space to separate other parts of a multiple citation (for example: As reported previously,[1,3-8,19]). Some common examples follow:

1. *Journal articles (up to 6 authors)*:

    Doe JF, Roe JP III, Coe RT Jr, Loe JT Sr, Poe EA, Voe AE. How to write a research proposal. *JAMA*. 1981; 244:76-97.

2. *In the case of more than 6 authors*:

    Doe JF, Roe JP III, Coe RT, et al. How to write a research proposal. *JAMA*. 1981;244:76-97.

3. *In the case of a journal article that does not have consecutive pages throughout volume: (The month or the day of the issue is preferable to the issue number)*:

    Doe JF, Roe JP III, Coe RT Jr, Loe JT Sr, Poe EA, Voe AE. How to write a research proposal. *Sci Am*. November 1981;244:76-97.

4. *In the case of a journal article published in a supplement*:

    Gordon AS. Standards for cardiopulmonary resuscitation (CPR) and emergency cardiac care (ECC). *JAMA*. 1974;277(suppl):833-868.

5. *In the case of abstracts*:

    Pailard M, Resnick N. Natural history of nosocomial urinary incontinence. *Gerontologist*. 1981;24:212. Abstract.

6. *Books*:

    Spencer H. *Pathology of the Lung*. 3rd ed. Elmsford, NY: Pergamon Press; 1976:46-51.

7. *Books with an editor*:

    Gray H; Goss CM, ed. *Gray's Anatomy of the Human Body*. 29th ed. Philadelphia, Pa: Lea and Febiger; 1973:1206. (Note Gray is author and Goss is editor)

8. *Chapter or sections of books*:

    Schulman JL. Immunology of influenza. In: Kilbourne RD, ed. *The Influenza Viruses and Influenza..* Orlando, Fla: Academic Press; 1975:373-393.

10. *Online journals*:

    Roach KE, Ally D, Finnerty B, et al. The relationship between duration of physical therapy services in the acute care setting and change in functional status in patients with lower-extremity orthopedic problems. *Phys Ther*. [serial on-line] 1998;78:19-24. Available from: American Physical Therapy Association, Alexandria, Va. Accessed July 3, 2003.

11. *Online Web site*:

    Health Sciences Libraries University of Washington. The AMA Style Guide page. Available from: http://healthlinks.washington.edu/hsl/styleguides/ama.html. Accessed July 2, 2003.

Note: the title of the journal, title of book, or Web site should be in italics, however if this is unavailable you may substitute it with underline.

Adapted from Iverson C, Flanagin A, Fontanarosa PB, eds. *American Medical Association Manual of Style: A Guide for Authors and Editors*. 9th ed. Philadelphia: Lippincott, Williams and Wilkins; 1997.

Table 8-9
SAMPLE OF SIMPLE CRITERIA
FOR STUDENT PEER REVIEWED WRITING[7]

Follows stated instructions for content of paper:

Rating Criteria

_____   not done, major areas of content missing

_____   done to a limited extent, could be improved in quality or quantity of content.

_____   exceptionally well done, organized, and complete

Writer takes a position and develops that position:

Rating Criteria

_____   not done, superficial and limited in development of position

_____   done to a limited extent, some examples given but writer's position is not clearly explained or supported in all areas

_____   exceptionally well developed, complete, good examples which illustrate the points made

Expression is clear, concise and language is appropriate:

Rating Criteria

_____   not done, uses terminology incorrectly or uses broad generalizations.

_____   done to a limited extent, possible alternatives in terminology or sentence structure, some generalizations

_____   exceptionally well done, uses first person voice where appropriate, wide range of appropriate terminology, meaning is clear.

Paper is without typographical and grammatical errors:

Rating Criteria

_____   >5 errors

_____   3 to 5 errors

_____   zero errors

Adapted from Curtis KA. *PH TH 142 Concepts in Patient Compliance: Course Syllabus.* Fresno, Calif: California State University, Fresno; 1998

Collaborative projects are excellent learning experiences for the real world. How does one create a collaborative project? The organization of group members for completion of a project can be simplified by breaking down the steps of the project and then assigning responsibilities and timelines for completion. The worksheet in Table 8-10 provides a sample of a project management worksheet for student research.

Summary

Presentations, papers and projects are required throughout the educational process. Students can learn and implement effective strategies to complete these requirements. The skills acquired in the preparation of presentations, papers and collaborative projects are essential for future practice as a health care team member.

Table 8-10

SAMPLE STUDENT PROJECT MANAGEMENT WORKSHEET[8]

Project Management Worksheet Student Research		Personnel Names				
	Timeline	1	2	3	4	5
1. Literature search						
Library search						
Organization of references						
Procurement of references						
Assignment of reading						
Storage and organization						
2. Writing Proposal						
Preliminary Drafts						
Final draft and all forms, figures, and appendices						
3. Obtaining necessary approvals						
Faculty consulted as needed						
4. Logistics						
Data collection						
Schedule group meetings						
5. Design of presentation/audiovisuals						
Development of materials						
Revisions						
6. Writing final paper						
Preliminary drafts						
Final paper, tables, figures, references						
7. Preparing Presentation						
Audiovisual materials						
Handouts						
Organization of presentation						
Prepare rationale & anticipate questions						
8. Presentation						
Platform presentation						
A-V materials						
Delivery						

Adapted from Curtis KA. Project worksheet. *Student Research Manual*. Fresno, Calif: California State University, Fresno; 1999.

References

1. Curtis KA. *Training Programs for Clinical Instructors.* Los Angeles, Calif: Health Directions; 1988.

2. Curtis KA. *PH TH231 Seminar in Health Care Issues Course syllabus.* Fresno, Calif: California State University, Fresno; 1997.

3. So You Wanna.com. So you wanna avoid common writing errors? Available from: http://www.soyouwanna.com/site/syws/wrerrors/wrerrors.html. Accessed August 24, 2004.

4. Iverson C, ed; Flanagin A, Fontanarosa PB. *American Medical Association Manual of Style: A Guide for Authors and Editors.* 9th ed. Philadelphia, Pa: Lippincott, Williams and Wilkins; 1997.

5. Health Sciences Libraries University of Washington. The AMA style guide. Available from: http://healthlinks.washington.edu/hsl/styleguides/ama.html. Accessed August 23, 2004.

6. Crane LD, Kroll P, Curtis KA, et al. More support for student research. *Phys Ther.* 1992;72(8):608-9.

7. Curtis KA. Peer-reviewed grading form. *PH TH 142 Concepts in Patient Compliance: Course Syllabus.* Fresno, Calif: California State University, Fresno; 1998.

8. Curtis KA. Project worksheet. *Student Research Manual.* Fresno, Calif: California State University, Fresno; 1999.

PUTTING IT INTO PRACTICE

1. Trade papers with a colleague prior to turning in a writing assignment. Use the rating criteria below to give each other feedback on your papers.

Follows stated instructions for content of paper:

Rating Criteria

_____   not done, major areas of content missing

_____   done to a limited extent, could be improved in quality or quantity of content.

_____   exceptionally well done, organized, and complete

Writer takes a position and develops that position:

Rating Criteria

_____   not done, superficial and limited in development of position

_____   done to a limited extent, some examples given but writer's position is not clearly explained or supported in all areas

_____   exceptionally well developed, complete, good examples which illustrate the points made

Expression is clear, concise and language is appropriate:

Rating Criteria

_____   not done, uses terminology incorrectly or uses broad generalizations.

_____   done to a limited extent, possible alternatives in terminology or sentence structure, some generalizations

_____   exceptionally well done, uses first person voice where appropriate, wide range of appropriate terminology; meaning is clear.

Paper is without typographical and grammatical errors:

Rating Criteria

_____   >5 errors

_____   3 to 5 errors

_____   zero errors

2. Observe an instructional presentation. This could be an observation of one of your classes or a speaker at a professional conference. How would you describe the purpose, audience, needs assessment, subject content, and presentation activities involved? What instructional media was used? How was the effectiveness of the session evaluated?

Purpose

Audience

Needs Assessment

Subject Content

Presentation Activities

Media

Evaluation

PART THREE

Essentials for Success for Physical Therapist Assistant Students

CHAPTER 9

Managing the Learning Process

Improving Classroom Retention and Comprehension

> *Liza was overwhelmed. She realized during her pathology test that she had not studied the right material. Rather than the anatomical features of the cardiopulmonary system she had memorized, the test focused on the relationships between cardiac output and oxygen transport with cardiac dysfunction.*

Information Processing

Information processing is a cognitive science that deals with the brain's ability to sort and make sense of information. Research indicates that we can best increase our ability to use and retain information when we consider the relationship and relevance of that information. We need to consider how it relates (in similar or different ways) to past information and clarify how we will use this information.[1]

Concept Formation

We form *concepts* as we process information. A concept is the set of rules used to define the categories by which we group similar events, ideas or objects.[1,2] We are aided in concept formation by the following strategies.

USE ADVANCED ORGANIZERS

It helps when we label and define the concept to be learned. Categorize new information and define the attributes of the concept. For example, write titles and subtitles (eg, Pathology, Signs, Symptoms) fre-

quently in your notes and in the margins of your texts. It is important to actively process, categorize, and classify the information as you read.

Using a highlighter while you read is a *passive* technique that does not enhance comprehension or learning. Writing key notes in the margin or on another sheet of paper with a pencil is an active technique that enhances retention.

GIVE EXAMPLES AND NONEXAMPLES OF THE CONCEPT

Think of examples that would be either true or false. This may be a useful way to prepare for examinations as well. (For example, cardiac myopathy results in decreased cardiac output which negatively affects oxygenated blood delivery versus increased cardiac output.)

APPLY THE INFORMATION

Practice application of inductive reasoning by using examples and experiences to reach a conclusion. Make up cases and see if you can reach a diagnosis. Consider the following:

> *A 54-year-old woman, status-post 2 days total hip arthroplasty is complaining of severe calf pain as you enter her room for this morning's therapy session. Her calf appears reddened, hot, and swollen. What may likely be suspected given this clinical picture?*

Also practice deductive reasoning by using the diagnosis to predict the findings. Consider a diagnosis and see if you can define the characteristics of a typical clinical presentation.

Consider the following:

> One of the patient's you will treat for a therapist who is ill today is being seen for "wrist pain." You learn that this patient works full time as a computer programmer and hobbies include playing interactive video games with buddies that live in various parts of the country. What may be contributing to this person's wrist pain?

As you can see from the above example, deductive reasoning involves recalling definitions and descriptions, where inductive reasoning involves reaching a conclusion. It may be more difficult to do inductive reasoning as there is always the possibility that one will reach an incorrect conclusion.

Improving Memory and Retention

There are many study processes which can be used to aid memory and retention of information:[1,2]

PAY ATTENTION

* Attend all classes and pay close attention; hearing the same concepts repeatedly will assist you to establish ways of conceptualizing new information.
* Sit in a classroom location where you can easily see and hear, away from distractions which may decrease your ability to pay attention.
* Study for short periods of time and use your time productively.
* Look for indicators from the instructor about what information is important.

USE WHAT YOU'VE LEARNED IN THE PAST

* Skim reading assignments prior to class.
* Look at figures, charts, and photographs in the text which may further illustrate this information.
* Discuss previously covered content prior to the next class.
* Record and listen to lectures while driving, folding clothes or doing other "chores."

LOOK FOR WAYS TO IDENTIFY IMPORTANT INFORMATION

* Identify concepts that are repeated in handouts, during lectures on the board or in transparencies.
* Highlight and organize your further reading and review around these concepts.

ORGANIZE THE INFORMATION

Even if the classroom presentation is not in an order that makes sense for you, try your best to impose an order in your mind and your notes. This can be done in several ways:

* Show a logical sequence from one step to another for a procedure.
* Go from simple to complex, easy to more difficult.
* Arrange historical events in chronological order.
* Cross-reference notes by source and subject matter; identify differences and similarities.
* Explain your understanding to others, especially those who are learning the same material. Listen to what others explain to you and discuss differences in your understanding. Consult the instructor for clarification if necessary.

CATEGORIZE (CHUNK) RELATED INFORMATION

* Develop lists to compare and contrast information. For example, create a table that lists treatment indications, contraindications, and precautions across the top and diagnostic categories down the side. See if you can fill in all the boxes from your lecture and reading material.
* Think "across" courses. How will the information you are learning be important when it comes to guarding a patient to insure safety? Look back at your notes and rediscover the relationship of information covered in past courses to your present learning.

RECOGNIZE AND USE OPPORTUNITIES FOR REPETITION OF LEARNING

You will have many opportunities to do this from the academic to the clinical learning situation.

* Apply the same information or principle in different situations.
* Schedule periodic reviews of previously learned concepts and skills and see if you can apply them to new situations.
* Jog your memory using drills and other memory techniques.

ANCHOR NEW INFORMATION TO SOMETHING YOU ALREADY KNOW

* Think about how this applies to clinical situations you have experienced. How does this information change what you would think about or do in a similar situation?

* Use all your senses to experience the new information. What details did you notice that enhance or change your technique? How did it feel? What feedback did you receive?

WORK WITH A STUDY GROUP

Study groups are the single most effective way that students can improve their performance. Collaboration and group learning are very effective processes which are relevant to future practice.[2]

* Be accountable. Students stay more focused when they have partners or a group that is depending on their participation.

* Check your understanding. Information processing and retention is greatly enhanced by verbally summarizing learning in writing or in discussion.

* Share your thoughts and listen. In addition to aiding in retention, you may pick up a great idea, a new perspective, or a time-saving strategy by working with others.

Psychomotor Learning

Many skills that physical therapist assistant (PTA) students must learn involve *psychomotor learning*, requiring physical movement, as well as a cognitive component. Most physical therapy skills do involve both cognitive and physical components such as operating machines, lifting a patient, using a computer or re-measuring a patient. Howard Gardner's theory of multiple intelligences suggests that different abilities can be separately developed and that there may not be such a close link between different types of abilities, such as kinesthetic and verbal abilities.[3]

Basics of Skill Learning

An understanding of the following principles will aid in psychomotor learning:

* *Avoid trial and error learning*: Once learned, a skill is not "unlearned;" it is only replaced by the learning of another skill. Therefore it is important to avoid trial and error learning, which may create bad habits that later have to be corrected. Concentrate on what you are learning, solicit feedback and correct your performance. This will prevent your having to relearn later.

* *Perfect practice makes perfect performance*: Practice is required for skill acquisition. It is important that the practice be guided: Practice only makes perfect if what is being practiced is correct.[4] Learning incorrect methods can interfere with progress. Effective practice provides for knowl-

edge of results which reinforces and motivates future action.

* *Be patient*: Fatigue and complexity of material to be learned interfere with the speed of learning. Be patient and use all of your senses (vision, hearing, feeling) to process, learn, and practice. Schedule frequent, short practice sessions and stop when you feel fatigued. Work with different partners and be open to honest feedback from your "patient" as to how it feels to have you moving them/performing that intervention.

* *Think, first*: Be careful when transferring learning from one situation to another. Different patient positioning or different physical environments may create a need to perform differently. Think before you act.

We all feel awkward at times. Seasoned physical therapists and PTAs may become particularly gifted at various aspects of performing interventions, but students must be able to learn how to competently perform all skills required for successful entry-level practice. The steps in Table 9-1 may aid your psychomotor learning.

Facilitating Clinical Learning

Morgan reviewed her mid-term CPI evaluation and read her clinical instructor's comments, "Morgan seems to have difficulty with identifying important changes in the patient's performance." The clinical instructor later explained that she would like to explore what is happening that prevents Morgan from focusing on these changes.

First, we must acknowledge that clinical information processing uses a monumental amount of information. Students must read and digest pertinent components of the patient's medical record including the physical therapist's initial evaluation with plan of care, participate in data collection, observe physical signs and symptoms, and select from long-term memory the appropriate clinically relevant information needed to adjust or withhold treatment based on patient status and responses to intervention.[5] The environment is full of information that must be filtered and processed. How can we most effectively accomplish this task? What do we know about clinical information processing?

Novices and Experts

It may be useful to look at what differentiates novice from expert performance. Novice and expert performance tends to follow certain patterns. There

---

Table 9-1

LEARNING STRATEGIES[2,4]

Useful steps for learning and practicing skills:

✳ Write down what should be done, why, and how. How should it feel? To what should I pay attention?

✳ Verbalize all the necessary steps in the correct sequence as you perform them.

✳ Rely on all your senses for feedback. Concentrate on how it feels to perform the activity smoothly and without hesitation. Maximize your chances for success in early skill practice. When you know that you are performing correctly give yourself a chance to experience successful completion of the task.

✳ Break down a sequence of a complex activity into parts and perform each part of the sequence or pattern of activity well. Anticipate the next part of the sequence and prepare yourself to be in the right position and insure that the required conditions exist for the next step. For example, it is important to maximize lifting safety by positioning the load close to the body prior to initiating the lift.

✳ Introduce variety to the performance of a skill. Now that you have mastered the skill on the right side of the patient, are you equally as comfortable working on the left side? Can you plan for the differences required?

---

is quite a bit of evidence that these types of behaviors occur across professions and/or subject matter.[6-9] Think of an area in which you have developed expertise, such as computer use or playing the game of chess. See if these descriptions sound familiar to you.

NOVICE PERFORMANCE

The novice focuses primarily on objective findings, observable signs, and rules to use to make decisions. The novice's performance is governed by these rules and may lack flexibility. The novice tends to be concerned with details and may not have the experience base to be able to prioritize which information is critical and which is not. Novices tend to use systematic approaches to try to control the huge amounts of information which bombard them. Detailed forms, lists of checklists, and protocols are very comforting for a novice.

EXPERT PERFORMANCE

The expert, on the other hand, uses a largely intuitive process, looking at the whole picture, modifying his or her approach in response to deviations from expectations. Expert performance is characterized by its fluid and flexible nature. The expert is able to simultaneously carry on a conversation and make observations. Much of this process goes on "in the expert's head" and is often not verbalized. An expert often unconsciously and automatically processes a great deal of information and arrives at a conclusion often without a systematic or organized

approach to arriving at a decision. Most importantly, the expert processes information *within a context*, with a view that recognizes cues and vital information which change from situation to situation.[10]

Where novices tend to use more of an "rule-oriented" process, the expert tends to have a more holistic view. Let's look at some evidence that further defines the process.

Pattern Recognition

There is evidence that experts retain information by organizing the information in familiar patterns. Research conducted on physicians and medical students showed that physicians differed from medical students in their recall of critical information in a written text. Physicians showed significantly greater recall of critical cues and made more accurate diagnoses than did the medical students, when the information was presented in a pattern which they were used to seeing (medical history-physical exam-lab findings). The recall of physicians decreased to approach the level of the medical students when the same information was presented in random order.[11]

The expert is different from the novice by his or her ability to *recognize and interpret* critical cues in *patterns of information*. Students need support in developing their thought processes to see these patterns. There are some specific steps that students can take to identify and organize the information in the environment.

Steps to Better Information Processing

Cognitive psychologists have identified that each of the following steps aids in our information processing abilities. Students and their instructors can systematically approach the task of decision making by using some of the following guidelines.[12]

Identify the Key Cues

A *cue* is something that grabs your attention. It might be a note written in a chart, an observation of a sign or symptom or a key question that you ask the patient. Ask yourself the following questions:

* What are the key cues I am seeing, hearing, or feeling?
* Do they differ from my instructor's view? Identify those differences.
* What cues are most critical?
* Think of the intensive care unit with monitors beeping, phones ringing and many conversations going on simultaneously. To what must I pay attention to know that the patient is okay?
* How do I know that a patient receiving gait training will be safe to walk by himself to the bathroom?

Organize and Prioritize the Cues

The next step is to organize the cues into logical units of information. This involves prioritizing information and organizing it in a way that one is able to identify patterns. (For example, a PTA identifies that a patient has difficulty with sitting balance on the edge of the bed. There are many other activities that involve sitting, some supported, some unsupported. This patient may have difficulty in all sitting positions, such as in a wheelchair or on a toilet. These cues have implications for safety precautions for all activities of daily living.)

We can systematically collect and sort various pieces of information into categories such as subjective information from the patient, family, or caregiver; objective data-collection measurements and observations about patient performance and reactions; judgments regarding patient status and progress towards goals established by the physical therapist; and treatment planning within the plan of care established by the physical therapist (PT).

The following questions may help to organize the cues:

* What subjective information have I elicited that is of greatest concern?

* Does the patient have significant past medical history as I consider the patient's current status?
* What are the positive findings of the tests and measurements? Are there any red flags?
* What medications may interfere with performance?
* What findings indicate the need for further follow-up?
* What information may change the approach I take? (Such as how the patient responds, patient preferences or occupational demands.)

Reviewing the Pattern

The *Guide to Physical Therapist Practice* has established practice patterns for many diagnostic groups. As an initial step, it may be helpful to consider what pattern applies to the patient based on the physical therapist's examination and diagnosis. This will help to guide your thinking, jog your memory, and make a well-reasoned decision regarding the interventions you may choose within the therapist's established plan of care. The following questions may be helpful:

* What patterns of signs and symptoms do you expect with certain diagnosis? For example, hyperactive deep tendon reflexes and paralysis are consistent with an upper motor neuron lesion.
* What time frame do you have to work with the patient before the physical therapist's goals are expected to be reached?
* What is your reasoning in using specific critical pieces of information to monitor this patient's progress?

Identify Deviations From the Pattern

This step of the process is the most difficult as it requires constant attention to the cues in the environment and reconsideration of assumptions which you may have made. Initial impressions may lead to false conclusions unless you take this essential step. Consider this case:

> *Mr. Atkins has experienced worsening back pain since his last therapy visit on Friday. You learn that he began to feel worse while gardening over the weekend. He can hardly walk into therapy on Monday due to intense pain and numbness in the left leg. You notify the physical therapist, who comes right over to examine Mr. Atkins. The PT calls the patient's physician while the patient waits. The physician requested that the patient be sent right over to be examined.*

This PTA's action led to an immediate trip to his physician. The patient was soon diagnosed with a prolapsed disk and was scheduled for decompressive laminectomy later that week. Deviations from the pattern are important because they change the expected course of action. They may indicate problems, precautions or referrals that physical therapists must make. These questions may assist you to start this process:

* What critical pieces of information are not fitting the expected pattern?
* How does this patient's signs and symptoms deviate from what I typically see?
* Are there complications, contraindications or precautions that may result from these deviations?
* Do I need to contact the PT now or have the PT see the patient on the next visit?

Synthesize and Draw Conclusions, Integrate Information Into a Plan

The key question here is "So what?" What difference does it make that I know this information? You may reach any of the following conclusions.

* Knowing this, I might choose one approach over another.
* Knowing this, I will have to involve the patient's care-givers in my plan.
* Knowing this, the patient may not be able to participate in the indicated duration or frequency for optimal treatment.
* Having identified symptoms that don't fit in the expected pattern, I am going to contact the PT to discuss my concerns and have the patient re-examined.

After developing a diagnosis and prognosis, the PT designs an intervention, including a plan of care which is intended to result in expected changes in the condition. It is within the intervention component of practice that the PTA makes the clinical judgments necessary to adjust/withhold intervention, weigh alternatives and select appropriate responses within the plan of care established by the physical therapist.

Metacognition and Reflection

Metacognition, or an ability to monitor and alter one's process of thinking, assists in helping to refine the process of problem-solving. The multidimensional and complex nature of the clinical environment requires constant processing of clinical information. "Thinking about one's thinking" provides insight into attention, pattern recognition, and clinical reasoning processes.

Recent research supports the value of *reflection* during the learning process.[10,13,14] Reflection allows us to consider the meaning of information and the thoughts we had in response to this information. Reflection includes both consideration of the procedure and interaction involved.

Research has shown that PT reasoning occurs in context, with cues and patterns of information developing different meanings in varying conditions. The knowledge base of expert physical therapists develops through reflection.[10] With increased experience and engagement in reflective processes, physical therapists are able to develop reasoning processes that incorporate multiple perspectives.[14]

Life-Long, Self-Directed Learning

Both physical therapists and PTAs assume responsibility for their own career development, long after the formal educational program ends. Reflection provides a key tool to identify, select, and critique appropriate learning needs, tasks, and resources, and formulate new knowledge to address these needs.

Maintaining an active learning environment promotes independent thinking and an atmosphere where learners have responsibility for learning. It is beneficial for students to seek answers to their questions on their own, rather than always relying on faculty to provide answers. Such self-directed learning helps learners to improve their self-assessment skills and develop self-reliance. Students who develop a pattern of independent learning while in school will find these skills invaluable for life-long learning and continuing career development. See Chapter 25 for more strategies for life-long learning.

Summary

There is ample evidence to support a systematic approach to information processing to facilitate student learning. Researchers have found that methods of clinical reasoning differ in novices and experts in predictable ways.

Principles of information processing can be applied to clinical learning to enhance clinical problem solving. Further, an active consideration of these thought processes and reflection on our experiences facilitate development of a rich base of knowledge.

References

1. Curtis KA, Haston LM. *Teaching Accountable Clinical Decision Making in Physical Therapy: Integration of Entry-level Clinical Evaluation and Treatment Skills Courses.* Miami, Fla: University of Miami; 1994.

2. Graham CL. Conceptual learning processes in physical therapy students. *Phys Ther.* 1996;76:856-865.

3. Gardner H. *Frames of Mind: The Theory of Multiple Intelligences.* 10th ed. Basic Books; 1993.

4. Hunter M. *Mastery Teaching.* Thousand Oaks, Calif: Corwin; 1994.

5. APTA. *A Normative Model of PTA Education: Version '99.* Alexandria, Va: American Physical Therapy Association; 1999;13:50.

6. Benner P. *From Novice to Expert: Excellence and Power in Clinical Nursing Practice.* Menlo Park, Calif: Addison Wesley; 1984.

7. Shepard KF, Hack LM, Gwyer J, Jensen GM. Describing expert practice in physical therapy. *Qual Health Res.* 1999;9(6):746-58.

8. Jensen GM, Shepard KF, Gwyer J, Hack LM. Attribute dimensions that distinguish master and novice physical therapy clinicians in orthopedic settings. *Phys Ther.* 1992;72(10):711-22.

9. Jensen GM, Shepard KF, Hack LM. The novice versus the experienced clinician: insights into the work of the physical therapist. *Phys Ther.* 1990;70(5):314-23.

10. Jensen GM, Gwyer J, Shepard KF. Expert practice in physical therapy. *Phys Ther.* 2000;80(1):28-43.

11. Coughlin LD, Patel VL Processing of critical information by physicians and medical students. *J Med Educ.* 1987;62:818-828.

12. Curtis KA. Facilitating critical thinking in clinical education. Presented at: San Joaquin Valley District Meeting, American Physical Therapy Association. May 13, 1997; San Joaquin, Calif.

13. Cross V. Introducing physiotherapy students to the idea of "reflective practice." *Med Teach.* 1993;15(4):293-307.

14. Dahlgren MA. Learning physiotherapy: students' ways of experiencing the patient encounter. *Physiother Res Int.* 1998;3(4):257-73.

PUTTING IT INTO PRACTICE

1. Select your class notes from one class period in a course you are currently taking. Reference the material to your books and reading assignments by writing notes in the margins. Note any discrepancies by asterisk. Make an appointment to talk with your instructor about any discrepancies you find or questions which arise during this activity.

2. Identify a new motor skill which you are learning. This might be performing a transfer, guarding a patient during gait training, or doing a "wheelie" in a wheelchair.

   Write down what should be done, why and how.

   How should it feel? To what should you pay attention?

   Write down all the necessary steps in the correct sequence of performance.

3. Choose a class session to analyze. Reflect on what drew your attention during this class.

   What were the cues to which you responded?

   What was most important in the material covered or skills learned?

   Reflect on how you might apply this information. Why is it important to know?

CHAPTER 10

Will I Do Well Enough?

Nicole looked over her first pathology exam as it was discussed in class. This was the first exam of the physical therapist assistant program. She winced as she saw the grade, "68" in bold letters at the top of the exam. "How could this have happened?" she questioned inwardly. "I have never had a D before. I have always made straight A's."

Performance Anxiety

Performance anxiety is a manifestation of stress, occurring when worry and fear interferes with performance and causes distress for the performer. This can occur for musicians doing a performance, for speakers giving a presentation, or for students taking tests or practical examinations.[1]

The symptoms of performance anxiety are varied and can range from simple "butterflies" and mild excitement to totally debilitating panic attacks. Physical symptoms might include heart palpitations, extreme perspiration, dry mouth, shaky knees and hands, trembling voice, shortness of breath, dizziness, nausea, urinary frequency, diarrhea, and/or a sense of dread. Emotional symptoms include feeling frightened, sad, frustrated, angry, or a combination of these. Intellectually, there may be difficulty in paying attention, concentrating and remembering. Take a look at Table 10-1 and see if you have experienced any of these symptoms.

The person experiencing performance anxiety may withdraw, feel more isolated, have a low sense of personal effectiveness, or feel guilty or ashamed regarding the current situation. Coping strategies are often ineffective, resulting in reaction and worry, rather than more effective preventative action.

Worry and Decreasing Performance

Research shows that anxiety resulting in worry and self-doubt interferes with information processing and memory.[1-6] Performance tests show that worry tends to divert attention and valuable cognitive processing time just when you need it most.

So, in addition, to not knowing what is on the text, if a student worries about it while trying to succeed on the examination, performance is likely to be even worse!

Just as the physiological, emotional, and intellectual manifestations of anxiety are varied in the moment that we feel stressed, our longer-term responses to stress can also vary.

Illness

Research shows that student susceptibility to illness increases during examination periods, resulting in far greater incidence of viral and upper respiratory infections during these periods of stress.[7-10] Similarly, persons under extreme physical stresses, such as marathon runners, show increased vulnerability to illness post-marathon.[11] There is evidence that physical exhaustion, anxiety, stress, and worry are related to compromised immune function and higher incidence of illness.

Fatigue

Overwhelming fatigue and excessive sleepiness is a common response when chronically faced with situations in which there is little sense of control over the outcome. Fatigue is a common symptom of depression as well. Fatigue interferes with attention and focus; its effects on performance are dramatic and far-reaching.

Substance Abuse

Substance abuse involves the use of external chemicals or drugs, such as alcohol, legal and illegal drugs, caffeine, or tobacco. Substances are often used

---
Table 10-1
RESPONSES TO ANXIETY[1]

Physical Symptoms

Racing pulse

Perspiration (can be extreme)

Dry mouth

Shaky knees and hands

Trembling voice

Shortness of breath

Dizziness

Nausea

Bladder and rectal pressure

Emotional Symptoms

Fear

Sadness

Frustration

Anger

Dread

Intellectual symptoms

Difficulty paying attention

Problems with concentration

Poor memory

---

to numb the pain of anxiety or depression.[12-14] The performance impairment and serious health risks that accompany the abuse of these substances are undesirable for anyone.

Depression and Suicide

Clinical depression can be a serious problem for students. Be aware of the symptoms and problems listed in Tables 10-2 and 10-3. Suggest that any student or colleague experiencing these symptoms seek professional help.

Identifying the Source of the Problem

Olivia had always succeeded in the past with minimal effort. What was the problem now? As she read over the test questions, she felt like she had studied for a different test. She had a sinking feeling and felt her palms begin to sweat.

Olivia's story is common among high ability students who have been successful in the past and face difficulties with the intensive demands of the physical therapist assistant program. There are a number of common problems that lead to performance difficulties on examinations.

Effort

Many students have a history of past success with less than maximal effort. In both physical therapist and physical therapist assistant education, the complexity of the material presented and the sheer volume of information one faces require different strategies to improve performance.

STUDY TIME

Take a look at your study time. It is reasonable to expect that you will be spending 2 to 3 hours studying for each in-class hour. If you are spending this amount of time and not seeing positive results, you are may be choosing the wrong information to study or using ineffective learning strategies. See Chapter 9 to review some more effective learning strategies.

READING PRIORITIES

The volume of reading required may at times exceed your capability to read it. You must become good at skimming, reading abstracts, conclusions, looking for key words, definitions and other critical information. You may not be able to read all assigned reading for full comprehension and retention, yet you will be responsible for these facts.

Talk with your professor about what information is most important to study. Use your class notes as a guideline. Watch for key phrases and repetitive information in your notes and books.

USE LEARNING STRATEGIES

Chapter 9 presents many strategies enhancing for information processing, comprehension and mastery of material. Put these techniques into place to assist you.

FIND AND USE A SUPPORT SYSTEM

Identify what academic support services are available on campus. These may include tutoring, mentoring, advising, and extra help or study sessions. Meet with a study group to help maximize your efforts.

REDUCE DISTRACTIONS AND DIVERSIONS

Explore ways to reduce the distractions in the environment in which you study. Find a place in a quiet corner of the library or designated place in

---

Table 10-2

SYMPTOMS OF DEPRESSION*

- Persistent sad or "empty" mood.
- Feeling hopeless, helpless, worthless, pessimistic and or guilty.
- Substance abuse.
- Fatigue or loss of interest in ordinary activities, including sex.
- Disturbances in eating and sleeping patterns.
- Irritability, increased crying, anxiety and panic attacks.
- Difficulty concentrating, remembering or making decisions.
- Thoughts of suicide; suicide plans or attempts.
- Persistent physical symptoms or pains that do not respond to treatment.

Not all people with depression will have all these symptoms or have them to the same degree. If a person has four or more of these symptoms, if nothing can make them go away, and if they last more than two weeks, a doctor or psychiatrist should be consulted.

Adapted from SA/VE—Suicide Awareness/Voices of Education. P.O. Box 24507. Minneapolis, Minn 55424-0507. Phone: (612) 946-7998. http://www.save.org. E-mail address: save@winternet.com.

Table 10-3

SUICIDAL SYMPTOMS*

- Talking about suicide.
- Statements about hopelessness, helplessness, or worthlessness.
- Preoccupation with death.
- Suddenly happier, calmer.
- Loss of interest in things one cares about.
- Visiting or calling people one cares about.
- Making arrangements; setting one's affairs in order.
- Giving things away.

A suicidal person urgently needs to see a doctor or psychiatrist.

Adapted from SA/VE—Suicide Awareness/Voices of Education. P.O. Box 24507. Minneapolis, Minn 55424-0507. Phone: (612) 946-7998. http://www.save.org. E-mail address: save@winternet.com.

---

your home where you won't be disturbed. Change seats if you are distracted by a person sitting next to you. Commit to and keep a regular study schedule in an environment that will support, not interfere, with your efforts.

Time Management

Do you have conflicting obligations, such as work, child care or family responsibilities? Are you using your time efficiently? Are you procrastinating? Review Chapter 11 for time management techniques.

Limited Clinical Background

Sometimes students who have had minimal contact with patients and clinical exposure lack a context in which to apply the information they are learning. This may interfere with being able to identify the most important information. Pay attention to the specific examples given in class. These examples will help you understand and use this material.

Unable to See "The Big Picture"

Are you excessively concerned with details? Many courses emphasize details and few courses pull together "the big picture." Many students find themselves studying compartments of facts and information for tests and lack opportunities to think about how this information applies to a patient's problems or physical therapy practice.

Actively ask yourself, "How am I going to use this information?" or "Why is this important for me to learn?" If you or your classmates are unable to answer these questions, seek assistance from the faculty. Learning information in context will assist with retention and future application. (Review Chapter 9 for the details.)

Career Doubts

Sometimes problems with performance lead students to question whether they are well-suited for a career as a physical therapist assistant. Consider what attracted you to the physical therapy field. If these reasons are still valid, you may want to explore what strategies you can employ to facilitate your future success.

Your future success is dependent on your satisfaction and happiness doing this work. If you are having doubts, talk with an advisor, trusted faculty member, or clinical mentor. Do not brood alone with your doubts.

You are not alone, nor are you abnormal to question your choices. Questioning allows you to consider and reaffirm your choice. Even if you choose not to continue your studies to become a physical therapist assistant, the reflection involved in reaching this decision is a valuable growth process.

Take Action!

Let's first consider the basics of a healthy lifestyle. Are you getting sufficient rest, eating a healthy diet and participating in regular exercise? Many students would answer no, no, and no! Examine these areas and make needed changes. Despite multiple demands and responsibilities, you must make caring for yourself a priority.

Lifestyle Habits

REST

Be sure that you are getting enough sleep. Fatigue interferes with both information processing and memory. Reduce caffeine intake. Don't sleep during the day, especially if you are waking up at night. If anxiety is keeping you awake, take action to address it.

NUTRITION

Be sure that you consume a healthy diet that is going to give you sufficient energy for the work you are doing and prevent long-term health problems. Don't let the time pressures of your educational program reduce the quality of the diet you consume. There are many alternatives to eating campus "fast-foods."

Many college students gain weight. In addition to high-calorie, high-fat convenience eating, insufficient exercise may also be a consideration. Don't let this add to your worries.

EXERCISE

Regular aerobic exercise such as walking, swimming, or biking and resistive exercise such as lifting weights is critical to prevent (and improve) many health problems associated with a sedentary lifestyle. Further, regular exercise habits now may protect you from common work-related injuries later. And as an added bonus, there is a growing body of work that supports the connection of exercise and movement to enhanced information processing, mood elevation, and stress reduction.

Study Habits

STUDY GROUPS

Working in a group is effective! Organize a group if you are not already in one. Group work allows you to organize your study time, focus on specific class requirements and questions and to process essential information with others.

WORK HARDER/INCREASE STUDY TIME

Are conflicting interests reducing your study time? Consider the following strategies to increase your effectiveness in studying:

* Can you study at home or would studying in the library increase your efficiency and concentration?
* Do you need to reduce work or personal commitments?
* Can you maximize commuting time with listening to tapes of lectures or reviewing your notes?

SEEK ALTERNATIVE MEANS OF ENHANCING YOUR KNOWLEDGE BASE

Are you just not getting it? Seek alternative sources. There may be computer-based resources,

Internet sites, videos and other self-directed resources that are available to augment and supplement the course material. Check with faculty, library staff, professional networks, and student resource guides.

STUDYING MORE EFFECTIVELY

Review the tips in Chapter 9 on learning and information processing research. Specifically look for the following problems in your studying strategies:

Are You Having Difficulty?

* *Prioritizing and selecting what to study?*
* *Identifying relationships between bits of information?*
* *Reading everything and not remembering anything?*
* *Not finding the information you need?*
* *Applying information?*

Remember that cognitive processing research shows us that comprehension and memory of newly acquired information is *greatest* if YOU make sense of the information, talk about it, summarize it, write it in your own words, establish a context for the new information and apply it to real-life situation.

Reading a textbook with a highlighter in hand is a waste of your valuable time. You must do something active with what you are reading which will enable you to relate it to something else, apply it, categorize it, or put it into context.

MONITOR YOUR THOUGHTS

Petra lay awake in her bed worrying about the exam she took earlier that day. She discussed her answers later with her classmates and realized she had made many mistakes. She could not stop thinking about the questions she read incorrectly and worried. "What if I flunk out of school? What would I tell my parents? I've worked so hard for this."

The thoughts that we have, especially after an unexpected failure, are related to underlying beliefs about ourselves, may increase anxiety and reduce our future expectations of success.[15] These thoughts may ruin our enjoyment of the challenges and learning experiences ahead. They may dampen feelings of success and take the fun out of sharing achievements and accomplishments with colleagues.

Chapter 9 introduces the concepts of *metacognition* and *reflection*. Take a few minutes to think about the thoughts that you frequently have. Are you guilty of

"making mountains out of molehills?" Everyone has probably had one or two nights laying awake and thinking about the "worst things that could happen." You can change the negative thought patterns that interfere with your performance. The first step is to be aware of them.

Check Table 10-4 for common habitual negative thought patterns that interfere with performance and some suggested ways of coping with these bad habits.

Use Your Resources

FACULTY INVOLVEMENT

Use faculty resources early and often! Ask for help as soon as you note a problem. Use faculty office hours, teaching assistants, and extra review times that are available. Be specific about your questions. Here are some good questions to start:

---

* *What information is most important to study?*
* *What relationships between facts are most critical?*
* *Can you explain discrepancies between the reading and lecture notes? (Have specifics in mind)*
* *What additional resources may help my understanding?*

TUTORING

Are there tutoring services available? If you need help, investigate college or program resources that might provide a tutor. Is there another student that could spend several hours a week with you?

FOCUS ON CLINICAL APPLICATIONS

It may help to see a clinical application of the information. There are several strategies which may be effective:

* Study with classmates who have more diverse clinical experience. Ask them to relate their experiences and apply this information.
* Seek opportunities to spend a few hours a week with a faculty member in practice.
* Use your vacations and down-time to gain some clinical experience.

COUNSELING SERVICES

Investigate free counseling services through your student health center. Student concerns are their specialty. Don't let a problem get out of hand. Take action to address issues such as performance anxiety, stress, personal conflicts, and depression early and effectively.

Table 10-4

COMMON NEGATIVE THOUGHT PATTERNS[15]

Pattern of Thinking	Characteristics of This Thought Pattern	A Better Way to Think	What to Say to Yourself and Others
Filtering	Magnifying the negative details, while filtering out the positive aspects of a situation.	Shift your focus. Think of strategies to cope with the problem rather than the problem itself. Focus on the positive aspects of the situation, your personal qualities, past successes and positive events. Be realistic about the situation. If it is a one-time occurrence or a temporary problem think of it that way.	"I am usually a very capable student; I misunderstood the instructions on this part of the exam."
Polarized thinking	All things are good or bad, perfect or a failure. There is no middle ground.	Realize that every situation is more complex than simply good or bad. There is a continuum that reflects reality. Think in terms of percentages.	"I am able to do this well 95% of the time."
Overgeneralization	Coming to a general conclusion, based on a single incident or piece of evidence. Expecting bad things to happen over and over.	Quantify, rather than using words that are qualitative (terrible, horrendous, awful). How many times has this happened? Examine how much evidence you really have for your conclusion and evidence that would be against your conclusion. Throw out the conclusion until you have consistent evidence to support it. Avoid statements using words like "every, all, always, none, never, everybody, and nobody." Use words, instead like "sometimes" and "often."	"Some of my classmates did very well on the first exam. I am succeeding in this course, even though my performance on the first exam didn't really reflect how much I know."
Mind-reading	Thinking that you know how other people feel about you and why they act the way they do, without their telling you.	Check out your perceptions. Ask people what they think or feel. Be direct. Look at the evidence you have to support your conclusion and the evidence which would be against your conclusion. What are some other logical explanations?	"I'm worried because it seems like you are angry with me. Is there any truth to what I'm saying?"

continued

Table 10-4 continued

COMMON NEGATIVE THOUGHT PATTERNS[15]

Pattern of Thinking	Characteristics of This Thought Pattern	A Better Way to Think	What to Say to Yourself and Others
Catastrophizing	Expecting disaster. "What if... I fail this exam? What if... I don't have enough money to pay my tuition next semester?"	Make an honest assessment in terms of odds or percent of probability of the event happening. Realistically look at the chances of this happening. Take constructive steps with tasks within your control to prevent future problems, instead of worrying about them.	"I have had only two "C's" all the time I've been in college. There is a very low likelihood that I will fail now, because I'm more interested and involved in my studies than I have ever been." "I can apply for a loan. Even though I don't want to be in debt, it will allow me to finish my education without the added stress of compromising my studies by working too much."
Shoulds	Working from a list of strict rules about how you and other people should act. People who break the rules make you angry and you feel guilty if you break the rules.	Question any rules or expectations that include the words "should, ought, or must." Realize that ALL action comes from personal choice. Also, there is no prescribed way to feel about a particular situation. Think of exceptions to these rules that seem to run your life. Realize what are YOUR values and opinions and what CHOICES you are making in your life and don't impose them on others.	"I'm choosing to spend this Sunday afternoon with my friends, rather than studying."
Being right	You must be right and prove that your actions are correct. Being wrong is not acceptable to you and you will go to any length to demonstrate your correctness.	Actively listen to what others have to say. what you think you've heard to verify your understanding. Defuse the immediate situation. Agree to disagree with another person. Focus on what you can learn from the other person's perspective.	"I understand your point of view. I look at the situation differently."

continued

Table 10-4 continued

COMMON NEGATIVE THOUGHT PATTERNS[15]

Pattern of Thinking	Characteristics of This Thought Pattern	A Better Way to Think	What to Say to Yourself and Others
Doubting yourself	Having constant self-doubts and fears of failure. You assume that you are the only one with these feelings.	Realize that success in every situation may not be possible. However, the choices you make are under your control. Think about how you define success and what steps you can take to insure that you'll be successful the next time.	"I can make choices that will help me to be successful."
Blaming	Holding others responsible for your problems. Or turning blame inwards as an indicator of failure.	No one can be at fault for the actions and choices you have made, as a responsible adult. Identify the choices you have made that have created the situation you are now in. Look at the options you now have for coping with it.	"I chose to focus on other work during the first few weeks of the semester, which has allowed me to fall behind in my reading. I will focus the next few days on catching up."

Adapted from McKay M, Davis M, Fanning P. *Thoughts and Feelings: Taking Control of Your Moods and Your Life.* Oakland, Calif: New Harbinger Publications Inc, 1997.

SUPPORT GROUPS

There may be organized support groups for students, such as those run by a women's resource center, a re-entry center, a students with disabilities center, or related to specific health or mental health concerns. Support is a key factor in your success. Don't overlook the value of emotional support in improving your performance. Sometimes just knowing that others share your feelings and anxieties allows you to then focus on the tasks at hand.

HELP LINES AND HOT LINES

Ask for help when you need it. Anonymous help lines and hotlines are available in every city across the country. They often also serve as referral centers to other resources in your university and community.

Train Your Relaxation Response

Some of the most effective ways to reduce anxiety involve altering your physical responses like breathing and muscle tension.[16] Try some of the following to train your relaxation response.

DEEP BREATHING

You are more likely to take shallow breaths when anxious. If you change your focus to breathing deeply and slowly you can begin to relax. Place your hand on your abdomen and inhale in a way that makes your abdomen expand. As you exhale, your abdomen should move inward. Practice by taking 10 to 15 slow deep breaths, two or three times per day. Then, during a stressful situation, focus on taking 2 to 3 deep breaths, and you will feel more relaxed.

SELECTIVE MUSCLE RELAXATION

Muscle tension also increases with anxiety. You can consciously relax your muscles to reduce muscle tension. Focus on a particular muscle group during deep breathing, such as your neck or shoulders, and tense and then relax the muscle. Focus on releasing the tension in the muscle, repeating "relax" to yourself. You can add selective muscle relaxation to deep breathing in a stressful situation.

DEVELOP A RITUAL

Rituals are behaviors we use to give us a sense of familiarity, achieve a focus and reduce anxiety. Think about the basketball player who bounces the ball three times before shooting a free-throw. Develop a simple ritual that will help you to relax. This might involve arriving early to choose a preferred seat, bringing a bottle of water with you or using a particular pen that makes you feel comfortable. It could involve privately saying a phrase that affirms your ability or a spiritual belief.

Rituals work when they lower anxiety. Avoid choosing rituals that are likely to increase anxiety, such as when you forget that "lucky rabbit's foot!"

Summary

Performance anxiety and related stress is a frequent concern for students. Changes in lifestyle and study habits may direct and focus your efforts more effectively. Examining and monitoring negative thought patterns can be helpful to reduce anxiety. Taking control of the choices you make will help to focus your efforts on strategies to lower anxiety and facilitate success. Outside resources such as academic and emotional support services are often helpful to students experiencing worry and anxiety. Although this is an intense and demanding time, it will pass quickly and you will soon be working in your desired career.

References

1. Barnes RG. Test anxiety in master's students: a comparative study. *J Nurs Educ.* 1987;26(1):12-9.

2. Garcia-Otero M, Teddlie C. The effect of knowledge of learning styles on anxiety and clinical performance of nurse anesthesiology students. *AANA J.* 1992; 60(3):257-60.

3. Gasper K, Clore GL. The persistent use of negative affect by anxious individuals to estimate risk. *J Pers Soc Psychol.* 1998;74:1350–1363.

4. Ikeda M, Iwanaga M, Seiwa H. Test anxiety and working memory system. *Percept Mot Skills.* 1996;82:1223-31.

5. Onwuegbuzie AJ, Snyder CR. Relations between hope and graduate students' coping strategies for studying and examination-taking. *Psychol Rep.* 2000;86:803-6.

6. Youseff FA, Goodrich N. Accelerated versus traditional nursing students: a comparison of stress, critical thinking ability and performance. *Int J Nurs Stud.* 1996;33(1):76-82.

7. File SE. Recent developments in anxiety, stress, and depression. *Pharmacol Biochem Behav.* 1996;54(1):3-12.

8. Leonard BE, Song C. Stress and the immune system in the etiology of anxiety and depression. *Pharmacol Biochem Behav.* 1996;54(1):299-303.

9. Stahl SM, Hauger RL. Stress: an overview of the literature with emphasis on job-related strain and intervention. *Adv Ther.* 1994;11(3):110-9.

10. Stein M, Keller SE, Schleifer SJ. Immune system. Relationship to anxiety disorders. *Psychiatr Clin North Am.* 1988;11(2):349-60.

11. Peters EM. Exercise, immunology and upper respiratory tract infections. *Int J Sports Med.* 1997;18(Suppl) 1:S69-77.

12. Kushner MG, Abrams K, Borchardt C. The relationship between anxiety disorders and alcohol use disorders: a review of major perspectives and findings. *Clin Psychol Rev.* 2000;20(2):149-71.

13. Roth SM. Anxiety disorders and the use and abuse of drugs. *Clin Psychiatry.* 1989;50(Suppl):30-5.

14. Pohorecky LA. The interaction of alcohol and stress. A review. *Neurosci Biobehav Rev.* 1981;5(2):209-29.

15. McKay M, Davis M, Fanning P. *Thoughts and Feelings: Taking Control of Your Moods and Your Life.* Oakland, Calif: New Harbinger Publications Inc; 1997:32..

16. Mann W, Lash, J. Some facts psychologists know about test and performance anxiety. Available at: http://www.psc.uc.edu/sh/SH_Test_Anxiety.htm. Accessed July 13, 2003.

PUTTING IT INTO PRACTICE

1. Automatic thoughts.

   Think of your experiences in the past week. Make a notation of several times that you can recall that you have experienced an unpleasant emotion, self-doubt, or negative thought.

   Record the thoughts that you had at the time in the second column. Refer to Table 10- 4. In the third column change your focus and enter a more positive thought.

Situation	Thoughts at the Time	A Better Way to Think

2. Evaluate your habits which may alleviate performance anxiety:

   Do you have enough sleep each night? If not, how can you arrange your schedule to decrease fatigue?

   What improvements can you make to your nutrition and diet?

   What is your regular exercise schedule? If less than three times weekly, make a plan to incorporate more exercise.

   Are you working in a study group with others?

   Are you planning study time into your daily schedule?

   Do you have adequate social and emotional support?

CHAPTER 11

Taking Control:
Self-Management Strategies

> *Rae, a single parent, looked at her daily planner and discovered that she had two written exams and a practical exam in the next week. She had offered to work extra hours to cover for a coworker on vacation and she noted that her two children would be off for one day for a scheduled school holiday. She wondered, "How am I going to get all of this done?"*

Student Role Stress

Over the years, research indicates that student attitudes and behaviors are influenced by many sources of stress.[1-3] These include:

* Demanding schedule and limited time.
* High workload and excessive course requirements.
* High expectations of self and self-doubts.
* Differing expectations of students and instructors.
* Less than optimal learning environment.
* Challenging student-instructor relationships.
* Uncertainty in future career plans.
* Financial concerns.
* Unmet personal needs.

Although these are frequent concerns of traditional students, today's nontraditional students face additional stresses and pressures. A recent study reported that almost 70% of today's physical therapist assistant (PTA) students are over 25 years of age and almost half have worked in another career prior to beginning their educational program. Many also have families, dependent children, and pre-existing commitments and responsibilities.[4] Many of these students face the pressures of maintaining employment, family and child care responsibilities while attempting to complete the educational program.

Time Management

Careful planning and budgeted use of time will be critical to your experience in PTA education. Check your own routines against those listed in Table 11-1.

There are a few strategies that students have found helpful.[5-6]

Spend Time Like Money—CAREFULLY

* Realize that it is one of your most precious resources and that once it's gone, you can't have it back again. Make each moment count.
* Budget and schedule your time, including time for yourself (for whatever you need—exercise, haircut, shopping, meditation, etc). Schedule that time on your calendar, treating that time as you would any confirmed appointment.
* Use a "tickler file" to note important deadlines, dates, and events. Give yourself a reminder several weeks before important deadlines by writing them on the calendar. Also write in birthdays and other personal events on your calendar. If you must do something once a year or every 6 months, make an appointment with yourself just as the dentist does. Do not rely on your memory. There are many integrated on-line planners which will automatically notify you of upcoming events. These planners also allow you to synchronize this function with e-mail accounts, address books, calendars, and to-do lists. Planning software is packaged with Personal Data Assistants (PDAs) or popular office software systems.
* By spending the time to organize a system, you will save more time later.

Prioritize On a Daily and Long-Term Basis

* Not everything and everyone is equally important to your personal well-being.

Table 11-1

ROUTINES OF GREAT TIME MANAGERS[5]

* Prepare a "to-do" list the night before.
* Be realistic about time allocations, including time for school, work, study, play, family, and personal matters, as well as regular time for yourself. Balance your life.
* Use a personal organizer or PDA. You want to be able to access your schedule, telephone numbers, and key information easily. Write EVERYTHING down in this one location. Keep it with you always.
* Schedule classes, study times, meetings, deadlines, and tasks in your organizer. Write them down. Don't rely on your memory. Write addresses and phone numbers in one location. Use sticky notes for one time directions and information.
* Focus your energies on one thing at a time, for a specified period of time.
* Make yourself unavailable to others; avoid distractions.
* Change the way you do it. Organize yourself. Use a computer for tasks like banking, updating important records, and addresses.
* Do it right the first time, rather than having to do and redo a task. However, be careful that you are not falling into a perfectionism trap.
* Avoid becoming side-tracked by details or by lower priority requests which demand your time and talent.
* Finish what you start; there is satisfaction in knowing that you have completed what you set out to do.
* Periodically review whether what you are doing is a good use of your time. If not, drop the activity and move onto the next scheduled task or project. Review your accomplishments at the end of the day.

---

* Determine essential information/skills you will need to succeed in the ways you spend the most time and make sure that you have access to this information (eg, computer skills, automobile maps, library orientation). It takes less time to attend an orientation or training session than the countless hours you will spend later on trying to figure it out on your own.
* Plan and prioritize your schedule by the day, week, month, and year. Make prioritizing part of your daily routine.

Be Selective

* Spend less time on unimportant obligations and concentrate on people who really matter to you. Stop thinking that you need to know everything, be all things to all people or absorb all the information which comes your way.
* While reading, write summarizing notes in the margins of the page or take simultaneous notes of major points and definitions on another page. All of these activities (especially taking notes) help you to process and learn the material at the same time that you are reading it.

Learn to Say "No"

* This is a hard one for many people. The habits that you develop now will stay with you throughout your life. Say yes only if you have the time or it is imperative that you become personally involved in the activity.
* Resist the urge to be a volunteer with multiple projects.

Reduce Your Standards

* Let go of perfectionism. Compromise with yourself and relax your standards on how you do things.
* Don't make it mandatory that you "know it all."
* Prioritize what is most important to know.
* Use others as resources.
* Function effectively and efficiently. Focus on the results, rather than the method used to get there.

Delegate as Much as You Can

* It is often worth it to pay someone else to do a task, if it will save you time. Also, it may be worth paying an expert, rather than spending

your time learning how to do a task that can be completed in minutes by a trained person.

* Organize family members, roommates to divide household work.

Consolidate Similar Files, Things, Tasks, or Errands in One Location[7]

* Keep class notes and projects organized in the same folder or location. Dedicate book case space, file drawer space, and an area of your home that will not be disturbed. It will save time in having to locate materials to begin studying. Organize materials in loose-leaf notebooks while they are still active. Store materials from previous courses in files.

* Organize computer files on separate labeled floppy disks, with a retrieval system that makes locating files easy. Back-up hard-disk files on floppy disks, zip disks, or CD-ROMs. If you revise a document, be sure that you save the revised file with a new date or name. Throw away all drafts when the project has been completed. Be sure to save the finished project with a name like "FINAL" and other identifying information.

* Avoid making several trips, when you can do several errands in one trip, even if it means delaying action for several days. Consolidate phone calls to be returned for one sitting.

Confront Issues and Problems Early, Before They Compound

* Deal with problem people and events early on.

* Get help in courses, make appointments to talk with faculty, work out group project responsibilities at the first sign of trouble, rather than waiting until the situation is irreconcilable. It will take far less time to deal with a problem in its early stages than to wait and deal with a more serious situation.

Don't Waste Time Worrying

* Focus your energies on productive studying, constructive thoughts, discussion, and review before exams.

* Cut off negative thoughts when you recognize them. Replace them with more positive images (See Table 10-4).

When You Make a Mistake, Don't Dwell on It

* Don't waste time feeling guilty about mistakes you made, things you didn't do, or opportunities that you let pass by.

* Try to remember that a mistake is another way to do things, no more. AND, avoid making the same mistake TWICE.

Overcome Procrastination

* Make commitments for your time and stick to them.

* Don't offer excuses for why something is not done or accept that past habits are unchangeable.

* Be accountable for your time and efforts. Set deadlines and stick to them. Use the buddy system, where a friend or colleague checks in with you to ask about your progress.

* Do a little on big projects everyday. Spend time on the most difficult parts first. Reward yourself at the end of a specific time you have spent by doing something more pleasurable. Be strict with yourself.

Make Meetings Count

* Always have an agenda and a defined objective for the meeting. Set a quitting time in advance. Keep the meeting on track if the subject wanders. Start and end on time.

* Move meetings along toward the assignment of tasks.

* Summarize decisions made, tasks assigned, and direction developed in writing and distributed to all concerned after the meeting.

Remember That Working Hard is Not the Same as Working Smart

* Working smart involves delegation, project planning, finding new ways to do things, accepting help from others, and giving up perfectionism.

* Being "busy" is not an end in itself. Re-evaluate what you are actually accomplishing.

Table 11-2			
HOURLY WAGE CHART			
Hourly Wage	*Time Per Week (Hours)*	*Semester Wages (15 Weeks)*	*Sample Take Home Pay**
$6.00	5	$450.00	$352.13
$6.00	10	$900.00	$704.25
$6.00	15	$1350.00	$1056.38
$7.00	5	$525.00	$410.81
$7.00	10	$1050.00	$821.63
$7.00	15	$1575.00	$1232.44
$8.00	5	$600.00	$469.50
$8.00	10	$1200.00	$939.00
$8.00	15	$1800.00	$1408.50
$9.00	5	$675.00	$528.19
$9.00	10	$1350.00	$1056.38
$9.00	15	$2025.00	$1584.56
$10.00	5	$750.00	$586.88
$10.00	10	$1500.00	$1173.75
$10.00	15	$2250.00	$1760.63

*less FICA @6.75% and federal taxes @15%

Financial Management

Sasha had worked for 4 years as a clerk in a busy physical therapy outpatient clinic. She had recently been promoted to the position of Billing Coordinator. Her new job description included 30 hours per week of office work, some driving, and evening meetings several times per month. She felt that her job would perfectly complement her studies in the PTA program, and anyway, she was unwilling to give up her steady income now that she had worked her way up to a supervisory position. What would make this a manageable plan?

Just as you can plan for use of your time, you can plan for use of your financial resources. It is unlikely that you will have the time to work in a job which will provide for all of your school-related and living expenses. Review Chapter 4 regarding the investment that you are making and financial aid options. Explore alternatives that may be available in your institution, such as a tuition fee waiver, work-study, or special programs that may be available for a select group of students.

Whether to Work

Many students wonder if, when, and how much they can work while in school. It is important to look carefully at how much your time is worth and whether working in a minimum wage job is a good use of your time. In addition, you must look carefully at what contacts, skills, and/or knowledge you are gaining and whether that exposure will benefit you in the long run.

For example, a physical therapy aide position in a physical therapy clinic may be quite beneficial in the long run, given the career networks and exposure involved, even if the pay is low. An entry-level clerical position in a university office may not provide that same benefit for the same wage and time commitment.

Further, you need to consider how much time you will have available to study if you work; studying "at work" usually does not work. Constant distractions interfere with effective studying. In addition, your employer will expect your attention to the job!

Time vs Money

Your time may be more valuable to devote to succeeding in your studies. In Table 11-2, you can see that a student who works 15 hours per week and

Table 11-3

SAMPLE BUDGET
(FAMILY OF FOUR WITH TWO WAGE EARNERS)

Expenses	Monthly	Annual	% of Total Income
Rent and utilities	$1200	$14,400	38.5%
Insurance	$125	$1500	4.0%
Savings	$50	$600	1.6%
Other	$10	$120	0.3%
Tuition and fees	$120	$1440	3.9%
Books and supplies	$100	$1200	3.2%
Food and beverages	$400	$4800	12.8%
Household operations and maintenance	$50	$600	1.6%
Childcare	$600	$7200	19.3%
Furnishing and equipment	$50	$600	1.6%
Clothing	$150	$1800	4.8%
Personal allowance	$50	$600	1.6%
Transportation	$50	$600	1.6%
Medical care	$60	$720	1.9%
Recreation, entertainment	$50	$600	1.6%
Contributions, donations	$5	$60	0.2%
Credit card payments	$30	$360	1.0%
Total expenses	$3100	$37,200	99.5%
Income			
Salary (after taxes)	$2150	$25,800	69.0%
Scholarships	$167	$2,000	5.3%
Loans	$800	$9600	25.7%
Total income	$3117	$37,400	100.0%
INCOME LESS EXPENSES	$17	$200	

makes a wage of $10.00 per hour brings home less than $2000 each semester. It may be well worth taking out a loan for the same amount of money.

Budgeting

A budget is a planning tool that can both reveal problem spending areas and help fine-tune your cash flow. The mere process of gathering information to begin or maintain a budget can help you control your spending, quantify your needs for financial aid and make plans to save, invest, or pay off debt.[8] Table 11-3 illustrates budget categories that might be useful for a growing family.

Basic Budget Guidelines

1. A monthly budget is often the most useful; since some expenses and income items are paid less frequently, figure their annual or semi-annual amounts and then divide by 12. The goal is an estimated picture of your future cash flow.

2. List all of your income and expenses. Take a look at the budget categories below to assist you.

3. As one of your regular expense items you should include payments into a savings (or investment) account (otherwise known as paying yourself first). A good minimum savings goal is 10% of your gross income. The importance of this step

---

Table 11-4

RECOMMENDED BUDGET ALLOCATIONS[8]

Budget Category	Recommended Average Percentage of Gross Income
Housing and utilities	25 to 40%
Taxes	20%
Transportation and related costs	15%
Food	10%
Clothing	5%
Savings	10% and up
Entertainment and vacations	5%
Debt (credit cards, personal loans)	5%
Other expenses	5% and up

---

cannot be stressed enough; given enough time, it can literally bring you financial independence or save you in an emergency.

4. Subtract expenses from income. You should have a positive amount remaining; this is your bottom line and cushion for unforeseen expenses. A negative bottom line is a sign that you need to work at reducing your expenses or increasing your income.

Table 11-4 illustrates average budget allocations as a percentage of gross income for each general expense category. They are meant as guidelines and suggested maximums. Educational expenses are likely to account for 15 to 50% of a student's budget. Realistically, few students can absorb these expenses without making compromises in other areas. Easy on-line home budget systems are available in money management software packages.

Managing Guilt

Students who are single parents or have families with children often struggle with the demands of the academic program and juggling multiple responsibilities. These students often feel guilty that they are unable to be as accessible to their children or families, their employers and also succeed academically. At the same time, as members of their families make sacrifices to support their education, students report feeling selfish in spending the time needed to complete the academic program.

Although this is a temporary situation with a positive long-term outcome, many students need exten-sive support in the short-term to assist with unexpected emergencies, transportation needs, family illnesses, and financial crises.

There may be services on campus that can assist students to access available support. Neighbors and friends may also be available to help. Chapter 15 offers many ideas for students coping with the stresses of completing an educational program.

Support Systems

Students often encounter barriers that can become a source of frustration, confusion, and disappointment. A strong support system serves as a powerful mediator of the stress involved in an intensive educational program. Your family and friends can certainly provide emotional support and encouragement. They may also provide a welcome relief from the rigors or studying, writing papers, and practicing clinical techniques.

Peer Support

Peer support involves sharing experiences and reactions with those who have had or are having common experiences. Peer support can provide valuable mediation of stress experienced during the educational process and later during the transition from school to work.[9,10]

During your PTA education experience you will have opportunities to both receive support and to give support. It is important that you realize how powerful collegial support is in going through this process together.

Peer support involves:

* Discussing feelings about similar experiences and emotions
* Validating goals
* Sharing information, tips, and resources
* Participating in social and recreational activities
* Empowering your colleagues to take effective action
* Practicing skills
* Collaborating on projects

This doesn't mean complaining and griping with your friends. It involves listening and acknowledging the feelings and beliefs and relating your own experiences.

Providing support involves:

* *Empathy*: Understanding of the other person's feelings, experiences, and goals, and knowing how to correctly communicate this understanding to the other person(s). Being caring, sensitive, and responsive are basic to establishing a supportive relationship.
* *Respect*: Respect for the experience and feelings of the other person.
* *Sincerity*: Honesty and genuineness.
* *Trustworthiness*: Honesty and willingness to maintain confidentiality and be consistent.
* *Self-disclosure*: Relating to one's own experiences and feelings

Take Action

The Buddy System

Having a "buddy," "peer mentor," a "big sister," or "big brother" is the way that many educational programs arrange for a peer support relationship to develop. If a program exists in your university, use it. If not, you may want to suggest developing one.

Rest and Relaxation

Even though the demands of the academic program are great, you can relax occasionally and participate in social activities with your classmates and future colleagues. Identifying a class "social chair" is often a way to formalize regular social events outside of class. Again, scheduling social events is as important as scheduling your exercise commitments and personal priorities.

Celebrate!

Many landmark events occur during the educational process. Important exams, first clinical experiences, papers, projects, and presentations are just a few examples. It is important to celebrate your achievements during the process and acknowledge and recognize the positive accomplishments of your classmates.

Involving Significant Others

Significant others, the people who are closest to you, are critical to your support and well-being while going through the program, yet they are often left out due to the tremendous demands that the education program places on your time, effort and attention. Keep significant others involved as much as possible and help them to know how they can best support you.

Keep the Memories Forever

Photos, videos, and other records of the time your class has spent together will solidify the supportive experience and provide a long-lasting memory of the time you spent in your educational program. Appoint a class photographer or class historian to spearhead this effort.

Summary

Students face many sources of stress and uncertainty during the educational process. Time management, financial management, and peer support strategies are valuable and proven ways to gain a sense of control over the sometimes overwhelming demands of the educational program.

References

1. O'Meara S, Kostas T, Markland F, Previty J. Perceived academic stress in physical therapy students. *J Phys Ther Educ.* 1994;8:71-75
2. Hayward LM, Noonan AC, Shain D. Qualitative case study of physical therapist students' attitudes, motivations, and affective behaviors. *J Allied Health.* 1999; 28(3):155-64.
3. Graham C, Babola K. Needs assessment of non-traditional students in physical and occupational therapy. *J Allied Health.* 1998;27(4):196-201.
4. Stewart SR, Pool JB, Winn J. Factors in recruitment and employment of allied health students: preliminary findings. *J Allied Health.* 2002;31(2):111-6.

5. Curtis KA. *PH TH 120 Professional Orientation*. Fresno, Calif: California State University, Fresno; Fall, 1999.

6. Culp S. *Streamlining Your Life: A 5-point Plan for Uncomplicated Living*. Cincinnati, Ohio: Writer's Digest Books; 1991.

7. Pollar, O. *Organizing Your Workspace—A Guide to Personal Productivity*. Menlo Park, CA: Crisp Publications, 1992.

8. Financial Planning. The Importance of a Budget web page. Available from: http://www.smilebuilder.com/budget.htm. Accessed July 30, 2000.

9. Lees S, Ellis N. The design of a stress-management programme for nursing personnel. *J Adv Nurs*. 1990;15(8):946-61.

10. Curtis KA. Survival training for clinical practice. *Rehab Management*. 1991;4(2): 78-79.

PUTTING IT INTO PRACTICE

Consult your textbooks and the American Physical Therapy Association Web site to answer the following questions about the physical therapy profession:

1. Evaluate your personal habits in regard to time management. What changes can you make in each of the following areas that will save you time?

Time Management Strategy	Ideas for Improvement
Writing a daily to-do list?	
Keeping a current appointment book with addresses and phone number?	
Scheduling sufficient time for personal needs, studying, and exercise?	
Doing things once well, so that they don't have to be done over again?	
Lowering standards of perfectionism?	
Taking notes while you are reading assignments?	
Saying no?	
Delegating tasks to others?	
Organizing work space and study materials?	
Addressing high priority tasks first?	
Using an agenda for all meetings?	

2. Create a personal home budget following the guidelines presented. What changes do you need to make to manage your finances while in your educational program?

Expenses	Monthly Income	Annual Income	% of Total Income
Rent and utilities			
Insurance			
Savings			
Other			
Tuition and fees			
Books and supplies			
Food and beverages			
Household operations and maintenance			
Childcare			
Furnishing and equipment			
Clothing			
Personal allowance			
Transportation			
Medical care			
Recreation, entertainment			
Contributions, donations			
Credit card payments			
TOTAL expenses			
Income			
Salary (after taxes)			
Scholarships			
Loans			
Part-time employment			
TOTAL income			
INCOME LESS EXPENSES			

3. Evaluate your support network. How can you improve your support to others? How can you improve the support available to you?

To whom do you give support?

From whom do you receive support?

From whom do you request support?

CHAPTER 12

Legal and Ethical Considerations

Tara sat in her Systems/Problems in Health Care course and listened to the professor. She was surprised to hear that it was both illegal and unethical for physicians to tell patients that they are receiving "physical therapy" when it is provided by aides in their office. The outpatient work injury center in which she had worked for several years prior to her admission to the physical therapist assistant program had a physical therapist on the premises only two days a week. The on-the-job trained aides provided the physical therapy treatment activities. She wondered why they didn't know that this was illegal.

Laws, Regulations, and Ethics

There are many types of legal and regulatory influences that control health care practice. *Laws* are created to protect citizens from unsafe practices. *Regulations* have to do with the fair distribution of goods and services which often relates to service delivery and reimbursement in health care. The laws and regulations by which health care providers must abide are becoming increasingly complex and numerous. This coupled with the legalistic society in which we live, intensifies the need for health care providers to be astutely aware of the various laws, regulations and standards of practice that apply to their profession and practice setting.

In contrast, *ethical standards* deal with conduct and moral choices, which arise from professions, society, religion and culture. Ethical behavior is about doing the "best" or "right" thing in a given situation. This binds health care providers to the highest level of care possible. Therapists may find themselves struggling to balance proper patient care (doing the "right" thing) with cost containment realities of the health care environment (various laws/regulations). An *ethical dilemma* is defined as making performance decisions between unfavorable options.[1] Ethical dilemmas are typically resolved on an individual level because one's morals (values, principles, beliefs) are intensely related to identifying the dilemma, as well as plausible resolution options.

Laws

There are four sources of law in the United States.[2]

CONSTITUTIONAL LAW

The US Constitution guarantees personal rights and liberties in the Bill of Rights. In general, these laws take precedence over all other laws and regulations.

STATUTORY LAW

Statutes are laws that are established through legislation at either the state or federal level. For example, physical therapy practice acts are state laws; every state's practice act is different.

COMMON LAW

Common laws are derived from judicial decisions that create legal precedent in areas which are not covered by previously enacted statutes. Previous cases provide the basis for common laws.

ADMINISTRATIVE LAW

Administrative agencies are authorized by executive and legislative branches of government to establish and enforce *administrative law*, the rules and regulations which govern many of the daily activities of health care professionals. For example, the Center for Medicare and Medicaid Services (CMS) is charged with establishing the regulations by which the Medicare system is administered. These laws must be followed by health care providers for services rendered to be paid. Additionally, Medicare holds each *provider* responsible for any claim that is billed to be in accordance with all established regulations. Medicare deems the provider to be committing fraud if billing is not done in accordance with its regulations.

Private Regulatory Authorities

In additional to the four sources of laws, private agencies such as the Joint Commission on Accreditation of Health Care Organizations (JCAHO) establishes standards to which member organizations subscribe. The American Physical Therapy Association defines *Standards for Practice for Physical Therapy* (see Appendix 4) which defines acceptable standards for delivering physical therapy services. *Institutional policies and procedures* typically reflect the standards set by the regulatory agencies which monitor their service delivery. Achieving and maintaining accreditation is considered the benchmark of quality and tied to reimbursement for most health care entities.

Third Party Payers

The organizations that provide reimbursement for health insurance plans establish standards that require health care providers to practice in specified ways. A third party payer creates and enforces *policy* that governs the operation of the organization. For example, third party payers publish forms requiring specific types of information. Although this is not a statute, it is required if the provider is to be paid for his or her services from the third party payer.

Record Notice

Most government, administrative and third party agencies impose responsibility on the individual physical therapists and physical therapist assistants (PTAs) to comply with new laws as they take effect. This assumes one has ample "notice" once the change appears in an official document. For example, when Medicare regulations change, they are published in the Federal Register. It is up to the practicing therapists to insure the facility in which they work stays abreast of such changes and are communicating these changes accurately to all those impacted.

Code of Ethics

Professions establish their own codes of conduct, called a *code of ethics*. Codes of ethics are specific to the particular discipline governed by the code, represent the value set of that group, and are enforced by the profession.

A code of ethics serves several purposes.[3,4]

* *Standards for behavior*: A code of ethics provides standards for professional behavior. For example, Principle 4 of the Standards of Ethical Conduct for the Physical Therapist Assistant adopted by the American Physical Therapy Association states: "A physical therapist assistant shall comply with the laws and regulations governing physical therapy."
* *Protection of the public*: A code of ethics provides mechanisms for the protection of patients, clients, their families, and the public. See if you can find a principle in the APTA Standards of Ethical Conduct for the Physical Therapist Assistant (Appendix 2) which protects the rights of recipients of physical therapy services.

Each of the principles in a code of ethics represents one or more of the following ethical principles (Table 12-1).

APTA Code of Ethics

The American Physical Therapy Association has jurisdiction over 65,000 member physical therapists and PTAs. The APTA Code of Ethics and accompanying Guide for Professional Conduct of the physical therapist and Standards of Ethical Conduct for the Physical Therapist Assistant and accompanying *Guide for Conduct of the Physical Therapist Assistant* (Appendix 3) protects the rights of patients and client, establishes standards for autonomy and supervision, defines standards for peer review and reimbursement for services and outlines expectation and responsibilities for members of this organization.

In addition, there are disciplinary processes to submit complaints of suspected ethical violations by association members. While technically, only members of the American Physical Therapy Association can be found "unethical" in the eyes of the professional Association, many state practice acts include language that holds each licensed therapist and therapist assistant bound to the ethical standards espoused by the profession. Indeed, if one's conduct is deemed unethical, a violation of law may have occurred as well.

State Physical Therapy Practice Act

Each state has jurisdiction over the definition and legal requirements for the practice of physical therapy in the state. Although all state practice acts differ, the Model Definition of Physical Therapy for State Practice Acts (Appendix 1) provides a standard for the definition of physical therapy.

Table 12-1
ETHICAL PRINCIPLES AND TERMINOLOGY[5,6]

Term	Definition
Nonmaleficence	To "do no harm" (even if we cannot do good)
Beneficence	To promote good
Justice	To distribute benefits and burdens fairly
Autonomy	To make one's own choices
Veracity	To speak and act truthfully
Fidelity	To keep promises and commitments
Informed consent	To present benefits and risks of planned interventions to patients
Duty	Obligations that an individual has to society
Confidentiality	Keeping sensitive patient information in confidence
Paternalism	Failure to respect the autonomy of another person

---

Physical Therapy[7]

Physical therapy is the care and services provided by or under the direction of a physical therapist.

Licensure

Each state practice act differs. A physical therapist must apply for licensure in each state in which he or she will practice. Some states do not license or register PTAs. The American Physical Therapy Association is diligently working toward resolving this inconsistency. Some states do not allow practice by qualified physical therapist or assistant license applicants (new graduates) until they have taken and passed the state licensure examination and received a license to practice. Some states offer temporary licenses and other states define the role of a *physical therapist (or assistant) license applicant*. An on-line directory to state practice acts is available at: http://www.apta.org/Govt_Affairs/state/state_practice

Each of the 50 states, the District of Columbia, Puerto Rico, and the Virgin Islands has specific requirements for licensure of physical therapists and most for PTAs. The following web-site provides links to each of these 53 licensing boards: http://www.fsbpt.org/directory.cfm.

Direct Access

Direct Access (Definition)[8]

The right of the public to directly access physical therapists for evaluation, examination, and intervention. The public is best served when access is unrestricted.

Direct access to physical therapy (without requiring a referral from another health care provider) is another professional practice issue that is governed by state law.

Direct access to physical therapy services, physical therapist evaluation, examination, and intervention varies from state to state. In 38 states, the public may directly access physical therapists' services.

The state statutes governing direct access to physical therapy services can be classified into two categories: omission and provisions. *Omission* means that no referral language exists in state statute. *Provision* means that the public may access a physical therapist in a defined manner, which may include stipulations regarding a time frame, therapist years of experience, and the nature of the patient's problems.[8]

Of these 38 states, 12 states have direct access by omission, 26 states have direct access under provisions.[8] Download the following file http://www.apta.org/pdfs/gov_affairs/directalaws.pdf for a listing of states and check in which category your state falls.

Roles of Physical Therapy Personnel

In addition to governing the access to physical therapy, state practice acts govern the supervisory requirements of physical therapy personnel. State practice acts often define the roles of physical therapists in the supervision of PTAs, physical therapy aides, physical therapy students, physical therapy license applicants and other support personnel (massage therapists, athletic trainers). Some state practice acts are entirely silent on the use of support personnel other than the PTA. While this may be due to an oversight when the act was originally written or due to the philosophy that no other extender of care is to

---

Table 12-2

SAMPLE EXCERPT FROM STATE PRACTICE ACT[9]

CALIFORNIA CODES
BUSINESS AND PROFESSIONS CODE
SECTION 2630-2640

2630. It is unlawful for any person or persons to practice, or offer to practice, physical therapy in this state for compensation received or expected, or to hold himself or herself out as a physical therapist, unless at the time of so doing the person holds a valid, unexpired, and unrevoked license issued under this chapter. Nothing in this section shall restrict the activities authorized by their licenses on the part of any persons licensed under this code or any initiative act, or the activities authorized to be performed pursuant to Article 4.5 (commencing with Section 2655) or Chapter 7.7 (commencing with Section 3500). A physical therapist licensed pursuant to this chapter may utilize the services of one aide engaged in patient-related tasks to assist the physical therapist in his or her practice of physical therapy. "Patient-related task" means a physical therapy service rendered directly to the patient by an aide, excluding non-patient-related tasks. "Non-patient-related task" means a task related to observation of the patient, transport of the patient, physical support only during gait or transfer training, housekeeping duties, clerical duties, and similar functions. The aide shall at all times be under the orders, direction, and immediate supervision of the physical therapist. Nothing in this section shall authorize an aide to independently perform physical therapy or any physical therapy procedure. The board shall adopt regulations that set forth the standards and requirements for the orders, direction, and immediate supervision of an aide by a physical therapist. The physical therapist shall provide continuous and immediate supervision of the aide.

The physical therapist shall be in the same facility as, and in proximity to, the location where the aide is performing patient-related tasks, and shall be readily available at all times to provide advice or instruction to the aide. When patient-related tasks are provided to a patient by an aide, the supervising physical therapist shall, at some point during the treatment day, provide direct service to the patient as treatment for the patient's condition, or to further evaluate and monitor the patient's progress, and shall correspondingly document the patient's record.

---

be providing skilled therapy services, omission of any direction about the appropriate utilization of non-licensed physical therapy support personnel can leave much to interpretation and may not be in the best interest of the physical therapist-PTA preferred relationship.

Take a look below at the how the state law illustrated in Table 12-2 defines the number of aides allowed and nature of supervision required for a physical therapy aide.

Ursula, a licensed physical therapist (PT) in California, was delayed arriving at the office following a corporate breakfast meeting. Wayne and Vic, physical therapy aides in her private office, greeted the first patients of the day and started the patient's treatments by having them begin their therapeutic exercise programs by warming up on the treadmill in the gymnasium. Are they in violation of state law? (Check Table 12-2 to read the excerpt of the California State Practice Act which applies and make an interpretation).

If you answered yes, you are absolutely correct. They are in violation of state law. There are several issues involved in this case.

First, by state law, only one aide may be engaged in patient-related tasks and under Ursula's supervision. This may already be a violation in that two aides are employed and work simultaneously. Only one may provide patient-related services under Ursula's immediate supervision.

Second, the law states that "The aide shall at all times be under the orders, direction, and immediate supervision of the physical therapist. Nothing in this section shall authorize an aide to independently perform physical therapy or any physical therapy procedure."

And finally, the law states that "the aide must be supervised by a physical therapist in the same facility as, and in proximity to, the location where the aide is performing patient-related tasks, and shall be readily available at all times to provide advice or instruction to the aide." Ursula is not in the facility.

They may prepare the patients for treatment by taking them to a treatment room, or prepare the treatment area for treatment before Ursula returns to the clinic, but they may not initiate treatment.

The explicit language related to the supervision of the PTA significantly differs between state practice acts. It is imperative that each physical therapist and PTA have a clear understanding of the wording and interpretation by the regulatory board in that state as to the specific boundaries set forth in the law. Examine Table 12-3 to see how the excerpts from two state practice acts differ and completely alter job responsibilities and practice patterns.

> Yvette, a licensed PTA, learned that Alexandra, her supervising physical therapist, was suddenly called out of town for the day due to a family emergency. While Yvette had wanted to confer with Alexandra about a couple of patients' progress, there were no new evals or patients close to discharge today. Would Yvette be able to treat the existing case load today?

As you can see from comparing these two state's laws, Yvette would be able to treat the patients if she lived in Oklahoma, but would not be able to do so until another physical therapist arrived if practicing in Arizona. Direct supervision is required of PTAs in Arizona whether newly graduated or having practiced for 15 years. *Direct supervision* is required of student physical therapists and student PTAs, as well as those who have successfully graduated but are working under a temporary license. Ignorance of the laws governing practice where you work is unacceptable. Imagine the consequences if you were a PTA whose job required crossing state lines on a daily basis. Adherence to the specific practice act in each state may differ yet remains obligatory.

APTA Standards of Practice

The *Standards of Practice for Physical Therapy* is a document published by the APTA which defines the conditions and performance that is essential for high-quality physical therapy. The Standards cover conduct in compliance with legal and ethical guidelines, expectations of physical therapist and PTA roles, scope of responsibilities, and administration of physical therapy service delivery. The level of expectation found in this core document may surpass the explicit language of a state's physical therapy practice act. The practice act identifies minimally acceptable behavior; the Standards are frequently cited by

licensure boards and courts of law as to what are acceptable standards of care for the profession. Take a few moments to review the *Standards of Practice for Physical Therapy* in Appendix 4.

Legal and Ethical Issues for Student Physical Therapists and Physical Therapist Assistants

Student Responsibilities

The actions of student physical therapists and student PTAs are regulated by state law, the *Code of Ethics*, the *Guide for Professional Conduct*, and the *Guide for the Conduct of the Affiliate Member*.

Student Rights

The rights of students are protected under many Federal and State laws. Educational institutions must establish policies to address the provisions of federal and state legislation that influences many aspects of its programs and operations. Colleges must also provide information regarding channels to pursue for inquiries and complaints.

There may also be specific educational regulations that reflect laws requiring health immunizations and screening tests, such as rubella and measles immunizations. Here are some of these laws:

STUDENT PRIVACY IN EDUCATION RECORDS

The federal *Family Educational Rights and Privacy Act of 1974* established requirements designed to protect the privacy of students concerning their education records maintained by universities. This statute governs access to student records maintained by an educational institution and the terms for release of such records. The law requires that the institution must provide students access to records directly related to the student and an opportunity for a hearing to challenge such records on the grounds that they are inaccurate, misleading, or otherwise inappropriate. The law also requires the conditions under which written consent of the student be received before releasing personally identifiable data about the student. The law provides that the university is authorized to provide access to student records to campus officials, employees and related agencies and organizations that have legitimate educational interests in such access. The policies of individual institutions should reflect compliance with this legislation.

Table 12-3

COMPARISON OF SUPERVISION LANGUAGE FROM TWO STATE PRACTICE ACTS

Arizona

Arizona Codes 10
Revised Statutes Chapter 19
Section 32-2043.

Supervision

A. A physical therapist is responsible for patient care given by assistive personnel under the physical therapist's supervision. A physical therapist may delegate to assistive personnel and supervise selected acts, tasks, or procedures that fall within the scope of physical therapy practice but that do not exceed the education or training of the assistive personnel.

B. A physical therapist assistant shall function under the on-site supervision of a licensed physical therapist and as prescribed by board rules.

C. A physical therapy aide and other assistive personnel shall perform patient care activities only under the on-site supervision of a licensed physical therapist.

D. A physical therapist is responsible for patient care given by assistive personnel under the physical therapist's supervision. A physical therapist may delegate to assistive personnel and supervise selected act, tasks or procedures that fall within the scope of physical therapy practice but that do not exceed the education or training of the assistive personnel.

E. A physical therapist assistant shall function under the on-site supervision of a licensed physical therapist and as prescribed by board rules.

F. A physical therapy aide and other assistive personnel shall perform patient care activities only under the on-site supervision of a licensed physical therapist.

Oklahoma

State of Oklahoma Physical Therapy Practice Act
Title 59 O.S. Section 887.1 – 887.18
Section 435:20-7-1.

Supervision of Physical Therapist Assistants

A. Direct clinical on-site supervision. Direct clinical on-site supervision is personal management and control of the clinical practice of the physical therapist assistant. The physical therapist delineates the specific tasks and duties to be performed. Direct clinical on-site supervision is in effect during the licensure process when a physical therapist signs the Form #5, Verification of Supervision. The physical therapist is on the premises, readily available to respond and direct clinical supervision. Such supervision shall be sufficient to assure that the assistant is practicing under the direction of a physical therapist.

B. General Supervision. General supervision is the responsible supervision and control of the practice of a licensed physical therapist assistant by the physical therapist. The supervising physical therapist is regularly and routinely on-site. When not on-site, the supervising therapist is on call and readily available physically or through direct telecommunication for consultation. In general supervision where the physical therapist is not routinely on-site, the supervision of the physical therapist assistant shall include the following:

1. A physical therapist must be responsible for and participate in each patient's care. The physical therapist must perform an initial evaluation, identify problem areas, develop a written plan of care, and write or review and approver a written discharge summary.

2. A current written treatment plan will be formulated for each patient under the care of the physical therapist. Appropriate for the practice setting, but no less frequently than every 30 calendar days, the physical therapist will document that the treatment plan has been reviewed and/or revised, stating revisions.

3. The physical therapist assistant will respond to acute changes in the patient's physiological state and report these finding promptly to the physical therapist.

NONDISCRIMINATION

Gender

Title IX of the Education Amendments of 1972 and related amendments administrative regulations prohibit discrimination on the basis of gender in education programs and activities of a university. This legislation provides equal opportunities to male and female students in all campus programs, including intercollegiate athletics.

Sexual Harassment

In addition, Title VII of the Civil Rights also prohibits discrimination on the basis of sex. Sexual harassment violates Section 703 of Title VII. *Sexual harassment* is defined as:

"the unwanted imposition of sexual attention usually in the context of a relationship of unequal power, rank, or status, as well as the use of one's position of authority in the university to bestow benefits or impose deprivations on another. Harassment can include verbal, nonverbal, and/or physical conduct that has the intent or effect of unreasonable interference with individuals' or groups' education or work performance. This may also include actions that create an intimidating, hostile, or offensive working or learning environment. Both men and women can be the victims of sexual harassment."[11]

Disability

Section 504 of the Rehabilitation Act of 1973 and related amendments and regulations and the Americans with Disabilities Act (1990) prohibit discrimination on the basis of disability in admission or access to, or treatment or employment in, a university's programs and activities. See Chapter 13 for a more detailed discussion of student rights related to disabilities.

Equal Opportunity

Most institutions publish policies regarding their commitment to equal opportunity for all, regardless of race, color, national origin, gender, age, marital status, religion, disability, or sexual preference. The provisions of Title VI of the Civil Rights Act of 1964 and the Americans with Disabilities Act address equal opportunity in employment, admissions, recruitment, financial aid, placement counseling, curricula, and housing for students.

Student Misconduct and Disciplinary Action

> Brad was not a "morning person." It was difficult for him to arrive on time for his 7:30 AM class. In the previous class, the instructor reminded the students to review the syllabus regarding late arrivals and said that he would be closing and locking the classroom door at 7:30 AM. promptly so that the students in class would not be interrupted by latecomers. Brad arrived at 7:40 AM, and saw the classroom door was closed. He knocked on the door softly. There was no response. He began to pound on the door, shouting, "Open this door! I've paid money for this class!" The instructor, inside the classroom, called the campus police and reported that Brad was disturbing the class in session. Brad had no idea that this was student misconduct. The faculty of the PTA program had serious concerns about Brad's judgment and recommended that he be placed on probation.

Colleges publish policies regarding student conduct. Student misconduct, on or off-campus, involving any of the following activities might result in expulsion, suspension, or probation, in addition to consequences of violating state and local laws.

* Cheating and plagiarism
* Forgery or alteration of documents
* Misrepresentation or providing misinformation
* Obstructive or disruptive behavior
* Physical abuse or the threat of physical abuse
* Theft or nonaccidental destruction of property
* Unauthorized entry or use of campus property
* Sale or possession of drugs except under specific medical or research purposes
* Possession of explosives dangerous chemicals or deadly weapons
* Lewd, indecent, or obscene behavior on campus
* Abusive behavior toward another or hazing

The college catalog is a good place to look for a list of policies. Students in health occupation programs, such as, the PTA, are subject to the regulations and disciplinary actions that apply to all students. Most programs issue a *Physical Therapist Assistant Program Handbook* that outlines specific behavioral and performance standards expected of you as you enter the physical therapy profession. It is not uncommon to sign a myriad of consent and acknowledgment forms during the program orientation or the first days of classes.

Cheating, Plagiarism, and Copyright Infringement

> Carley and David had become good friends during their first semester. They often studied together. When they were faced with writing up their first patient case study, they worried about what to write. A student from the previous year's class emailed them a sample of model paper that the professor had given to students the year before. They copied the history and tests they would assist the therapist with and wrote an intervention, sampling liberally from the excellent examples on the model paper. Each student submitted the same paper, with only a different cover sheet. The professor returned the papers a week later. They each received a zero on their paper and a note to meet with her after class. They were shocked when the professor explained that they had cheated and this would be noted in their student record.

Reports of academic dishonesty are on the rise in this country. Students entering the health professions must be specifically aware of issues involving academic dishonesty, in actions such as cheating, plagiarism, and copyright infringement.

CHEATING

Cheating occurs when students use fraudulent or deceptive means to improve a grade, obtain course credit, or gain an unearned academic advantage.[12] When in doubt, ask faculty members. Receiving old exams from members of last year's class without the professor's knowledge is cheating. Misrepresenting clinical experience on an evaluation form is cheating.

Do NOT tolerate cheating of any kind in academic or clinical education. Remember, that ultimately, students who cheat are cheating the public, patients, and clients (ie, the consumers who will rely on their care and the profession that they are entering).

If you are ever tempted to cheat, ask yourself which part of therapy you would like someone treating your mother or your grandmother to have cheated on and not be fully competent.

PLAGIARISM

Plagiarism is a serious form of academic fraud when one misrepresents work of another, whether published or unpublished as one's own work.[13] This may involve such obvious acts as downloading term papers from the internet to more subtle forms of plagiarism such as using phrases of other authors without proper citation. Students sometimes do not understand that they can also plagiarize themselves, in turning in work done for one class as original

work for a subsequent class. To avoid plagiarism, always cite your sources.

COPYRIGHT INFRINGEMENT

> Esther was concerned about the high cost of books. One book that was required for their modalities class cost $25.00 and was only 300 pages long. She thought, "I could photocopy this book for only $15.00 at the office supply store that advertises photocopies for 5 cents." She thought further, "I could even make a little money if I charged my classmates $20.00 per book. That would still beat the bookstore's prices."

Copyright infringement is a form of theft. Copyrights are protected by the US Constitution and by the federal copyright statute and protects not only authors of literary works, but also artistic works, sound recordings and computer software.[14] Copying a book, an illustration, videotape or a portion of a videotape, a published graph, cartoon or photograph, computer program, or sound recording without permission are all examples of copyright infringement. Be careful... even copying a photograph from an Internet site into a computer slide presentation is a copyright infringement. Charging admission to view a rented videotape or taped sports presentation without paying royalties is also a violation.

It is important to understand that copyrights are property rights of the author which may be sold or transferred to another entity, such as a publisher. Authors or those to whom they have transferred their copyrights hold the rights to copy, create new works, distribute and display their works. To avoid copyright infringement, make sure that you have permission to use the work of the author.[14] Write to the author or publisher and request permission. And be aware that although many authors are happy to share their work for educational purposes, some authors and their publishers ask for a fee. You have the choice to pay the fee or not use the material. See samples of letters requesting permission to use copyrighted materials in Tables 12-4 and 12-5.

FAIR USE

Libraries and copy centers can advise you regarding policies for "fair use" of copyrighted materials for educational and research purposes. An excellent resource on "fair use" exists on-line at http://fairuse.stanford.edu.

Remember, when in doubt, ask!

Table 12-4

SAMPLE COPYRIGHT PERMISSION REQUEST TO USE PREVIOUSLY PUBLISHED MATERIAL

Student Name
Address
City, State, Zip Code

May 14, 2004

SLACK Incorporated
Attn: Permissions
6900 Grove Road
Thorofare, NJ 08086

To Whom It May Concern:

I am writing to request your permission to include the material described below in a manuscript entitled "Developing Culturally-Sensitive Education Materials in Physical Therapy," as part of the requirements for a course in my physical therapist assistant education program.

I would like to reproduce three tables relating to cultural competence in physical therapy from one of your publications, Curtis & Newman's *PTA Handbook: Keys to Success in School and Career for the Physical Therapist Assistant*. The material I would like to have permission to reproduce is:

p. 186—Table 18-2.

p. 187—Table 18-3.

p. 188—Table 18-4.

Please advise as to whether reproduction of this material will be permitted. I will give full credit to the author and original source. If there is an additional source that I must contact for permission to use the above material, I would appreciate any information you can forward to me. If I can answer any questions, you can reach me at [phone] or by e-mail at the following address: [email address].

I will look forward to hearing from you.

Sincerely,

Student name,

Student Physical Therapist Assistant

Name of Physical Therapist Assistant Education Program

Educational Institution

Attachments: pp 186, 187, 188, Curtis & Newman's *PTA Handbook*.

(attach copies of the requested material)

Avoid Academic Dishonesty!

To avoid plagiarism, always cite your sources!

To avoid copyright infringement, make sure that you have permission to use the work of the author.

Research on Human Subjects

The rights of subjects in research studies conducted by faculty, staff and students at academic or clinical institutions are well-protected. Each institution must establish standards for the conduct of research

---
Table 12-5
SAMPLE COPYRIGHT PERMISSION REQUEST TO USE MATERIAL FROM AN INTERNET WEB SITE

Date: Fri, 23 Jul 2004 11:52:46 -0700

To: Publisher/Author or Web master [look for this link at bottom of a site's home page]
       webmaster@domain.com

From: [your email address]

Subject: Permission to reproduce materials from your site

cc: [include your faculty advisor here]

I am a physical therapist assistant student at [college] studying physical therapy. I am doing a presentation on shoulder pathologies for my class, Orthopedic Management and found the diagrams on your Web-site to be perfect. I would like your permission to electronically reproduce this graphic and use it in a electronic slide presentation. The material I would like to have permission to use is Histology Atlas, Shoulder Joint at the following URL: http://www.sru.edu/depts/pt/histo/shoulder1.htm.

Please advise as to whether reproduction of this material will be permitted. If there is an additional source that I must contact for permission to use the above material, I would appreciate any information you can forward to me. If I can answer any questions, you can reach me at [phone] or by e-mail at the following address: [email address].

I will look forward to hearing from you.

Sincerely,

Student name,

Student Physical Therapist Assistant

Name of Physical Therapist Assistant Education Program

Educational Institution

(Attach the material to the email)

---

that employs or influences humans and/or animals. All research must comply with these provisions. Students should familiarize themselves with the provisions for the protection of human subjects before they undertake any research efforts.

Informed Consent

Students must be clear to identify themselves as students or interns when working with patients or clients in academic, clinical, or research situations. They must also be aware that the patient or research subject has the right to refuse participation and that they must respect that right. Inform appropriate clinical or academic faculty and research principal investigators if a patient client or subject does not want to participate or does not want to work with a student. Do not take it personally.

Supervision During Clinical Education Experiences

Students enroll in courses that may encompass clinical training, cooperative education, and service learning. PTA students may practice the techniques and problem solving activities they are learning as part of their education while enrolled in such courses, in compliance with state laws governing the practice of physical therapy and supervision of student PTAs.

Regardless of practice setting or proximity to graduation, physical therapy and PTA students require the *continuous on-site supervision* of the supervising physical therapist or PTA as allowed by state law. This means that the student cannot provide care in a single therapist clinic if the supervising therapist or licensed PTA (if permitted by state law) is out for lunch or at a conference off-site. Similarly, the student may not visit a patient in their home to provide physical therapy services, unless supervised on-site by the physical therapist, or licensed PTA where permissible by state law.

In summary, to provide patient-related physical therapy services, physical therapy or PTA students completing program coursework require the continuous on-site supervision of a supervising academic or clinical faculty member. The supervising clinical instructor cannot transfer this responsibility to a physician, athletic trainer, aide, or other health care provider even for a few hours.

Student Employment Situations

Many students work in clinics on a part-time basis during school or during the summer months. Students must remember that their status as a PTA student only extends to those situations in which they are enrolled in program coursework and the clinical staff provides instruction and appropriate supervision.

For all other situations, unless students already hold a state license in another licensed health profession, they are *unlicensed personnel*, usually functioning in the capacity of a physical therapy aide, personal care attendant, or personal trainer. Be careful that you are not practicing physical therapy without a license. Know your state laws!

In addition, there are always potential violations of the APTA Code of Ethics and Standards of Practice inherent in these types of employment situations.

If you are instructed to see patients and/or write notes signed as a student PTA, it is vital that you explain why you cannot do so. Speak to the supervisor of the facility and your program director or academic coordinator of clinical education at your earliest convenience to insure no further confusion exists.

Working as a Physical Therapy Aide

Physical therapy aides are any support personnel who perform designated tasks related to the operation of the physical therapy service.[15] They do not independently deliver physical therapy services in any setting. Physical therapy aides do not perform evaluations, determine what they should do with a patient or client, and/or perform techniques that require clinical decision making or clinical problem solving. They do not make judgments or clinical decisions. Aides may function only with the *continuous on-site supervision* by the physical therapist or, in some states, by the PTA.

Athletic trainers, massage therapists, personal trainers, and kinesiotherapists are considered aides when performing designated physical therapy tasks

within the clinical setting. They, too, are to follow the physical therapy aide job description.

Chiropractors and physicians may not provide supervision for *"physical therapy"* aides who provide patient-related services if it is being represented as physical therapy or physiotherapy. State practice acts, as well as, core documents published by the professional association have specific language that protects the title *"physical therapy." Physical therapy* is to be represented by and billable only when provided by a physical therapist or by a PTA appropriately supervised by a physical therapist.[8]

This means that physical therapy aides, *who also happen to be physical therapy or PTA students*, may not perform the skills they are learning as part of their education, at any point in their education, unless it is as a part of their enrollment in a course or program-supervised activity. Students should be wary of inadvertently practicing physical therapy without a license which is illegal and does a disservice to the patient and the profession.

Providing Attendant Care or Home Exercise Programs

Some students also work as personal care attendants for persons with disabilities. Personal care attendants (PCAs) are unlicensed personnel as well, usually hired directly by a person who needs such services. The same issues may arise in providing personal attendant care, as students can easily overstep their legal boundaries.

When a family or person with a disability hires a physical therapy or PTA student to carry out a home exercise program or personal care routine, the student must be very careful that the program was established by a licensed health care provider or professional staff caring for the patient. The PCA should be carrying out a program of care that could be performed by anyone. It is not the role of the PCA to make clinical judgments, modify or progress the program. The student should be careful to refer the patient or client back to licensed health care providers for any problems or alterations to the care program.

Providing Personal Training in Health Clubs or Fitness Facilities

Students who provide consultation or advice regarding weight training or fitness must also exercise caution. Performing strength and flexibility assessments, setting training goals and providing exercise interventions to address client needs is not physical therapy.

Further, personal trainers are not physical therapists and may not use the initials "PT." Students who work as personal trainers must be very clear to disclose their limitations and their role in working with clients. Practicing physical therapy without a license is a violation of state law. Be sure that you are not in violation of state law, ethical, and other published professional guidelines.

You be the judge of the following situation.

> Federico responded to an advertisement in his local newspaper stating: *Busy physical therapy practice seeks physical therapy aide for afternoon and evening hours.*
>
> He interviewed and the employer was delighted to find out that he was a PTA student only months away from graduation. The employer gave him a list of patients to treat and his own laptop to document patient care. Federico was elated at first, but then wondered, "am I practicing without a license?" What do you think?

The answer:

When enrolled in a course, students are able to function with direct and immediate supervision of clinical faculty and perform tasks which are indicated by their level of education and the objectives of the clinical experience.

In employment situations in the physical therapy field while in school, the student is restricted to a role as a physical therapy aide, regardless of knowledge or skills acquired in academic or clinical courses... unless the student holds a current state license to practice.

Therefore, Federico in the case above, should not agree to perform functions which clearly go well beyond the scope of duties of a physical therapy aide.

AFTER GRADUATION

In some states a new graduate PTA may work in a special status as a PTA license applicant (PTALA) or may work under a temporary license only after the requirements of licensure have been met and an application has been filed. In most cases the PTALA or temporary licensure status is valid only until the first opportunity to take the state licensing examination. Other states do not permit practice until the license has actually been received. Most states have strict supervision requirements for personnel in this status. It is important to know the regulations of your state.

Summary

Students must be aware of ethical and legal issues involved in academic, clinical education, and part-time employment situations. Federal and state laws,

professional codes of ethics and other practice guidelines must become part of the working knowledge of the PTA student. Integrating accurate, up-to-date laws, regulations and practice standards into daily practice not only serves to safeguard you from malpractice liability, it demonstrates your commitment to delivering quality patient care!

References

1. Barnitt R, Partridge C. Ethical reasoning in physical therapy and occupational therapy. *Physiotherapy Research International.* 1997;2(3):178-192.
2. Scott RW. *Promoting Legal Awareness in Physical and Occupational Therapy.* St. Louis, Mo: Mosby, 1997.
3. Scott R. *Professional Ethics: A Guide for Rehabilitation Professionals.* St. Louis, Mo: Mosby, 1998.
4. Swisher LL, Krueger-Brophy C. *Legal and Ethical Issues in Physical Therapy.* Boston, Mass: Butterworth Heinemann, 1998.
5. Kornblau, BL, Starling SP. *Ethics in Rehabilitation. A Clinical Perspective.* Thorofare, NJ: SLACK Incorporated; 2000.
6. Purtilo R. *Ethical Dimensions in the Health Professions.* 3rd ed. Philadelphia, Pa: WB Saunders; 1999.
7. APTA. *Guide to Physical Therapist Practice.* Rev 2nd ed. Alexandria, Va: American Physical Therapy Association; 2003.
8. APTA. Direct access. Available at: http://www.apta.org/Govt_Affairs/state. Accessed August 30, 2004.
9. State of California Department of Consumer Affairs. Business and professions code section 2630-2640. Available at: http://www.leginfo.ca.gov/cgi-bin/waisgate?WAISdocID=96625829484+3+0+0&WAISaction=retrieve. Accessed September 22, 2004.
10. Arizona Board of Physical Therapy. Arizona revised statutes. Chapter 19 Board of Physical Therapy article 32-2043. Available at: http://www.ptboard.state.az.us. Accessed August 31, 2004.
11. Oklahoma Board of Medical Licensure & Supervision. Physical Therapy Practice Act. Oklahoma Administrative Code, Title 59 O.S., Section 887.1–887.18. Available at: http://www.okmedicalboard.org/miscFunction.php?filename=PTRules.pdf. Accessed August 31, 2004.
12. California State University Fresno. *General Catalog 2003-2004.* Policies and regulations. Available at http://www-catalog.admin.csufresno.edu/current/policies.html. Accessed August 31, 2004.
13. University of Indiana Writing Resources. Plagiarism: what it is and how to avoid it. Available at: http://www.indiana.edu/~wts/wts/plagiarism.html. Accessed August 31, 2004.
14. Stanford University Libraries. Copyright and fair use. Available at http://fairuse.stanford.edu. Accessed August 31, 2004.

15. APTA. Provision of physical therapy interventions and related tasks HOD 06-00-17-28 (Program 32). Available at: http://www.apta.org/pdfs/governance/hod/hodPolicies.pdf. Accessed September 17, 2004.

PUTTING IT INTO PRACTICE

1. Using the ethical principles in Table 12-1, identify which of these principles are represented in each of the Standards of Ethical Conduct for the PTA and Guide for Conduct of the PTA (Appendix 2).

Term	Definition
Nonmaleficence	To "do no harm" (even if we cannot do good)
Beneficence	To promote good
Justice	To distribute benefits and burdens fairly
Autonomy	To make one's own choices
Veracity	To speak and act truthfully
Fidelity	To keep promises and commitments
Informed consent	To present benefits and risks of planned interventions to patients
Duty	Obligations that an individual has to society
Confidentiality	Keeping sensitive patient information in confidence
Paternalism	Failure to respect the autonomy of another person

Cite particular ethical principles above that apply in each of the Standards of Ethical Conduct of the PTA.

Ethical Principle(s)	APTA *Standards of Ethical Conduct of the PTA*
Nonmaleficence	A PTA shall respect the rights and dignity of all individuals and shall provide compassionate care.
veRAcity	A PTA shall act in a trustworthy manner towards patients/clients.
INFoRmeD CONSeNt	A PTA shall provide selected physical therapy interventions only under the supervision and direction of a physical therapist.
DUTy	A PTA shall comply with laws and regulations governing physical therapy.
BeNeficence	A PTA shall achieve and maintain competence in the provision of selected physical therapy interventions.
-AUtoNoMy-	A PTA shall make judgments that are commensurate with their educational and legal qualifications as a PTA.
CONfideNtiality-	A PTA shall protect the public and the profession from unethical, incompetent, and illegal acts.

2. Of the 38 states that have direct access to physical therapy, 12 states have direct access by omission, 26 states have direct access under provisions.[7] Download the following file http://www.apta.org/pdfs/gov_affairs/directalaws.pdf for a listing of states and check in which category your state falls.

3. Find your state practice act by accessing the Web site: http://www.apta.org/Govt_Affairs/state/state_practice.

   Download provisions relating to the roles of and supervision requirements for physical therapy and therapist assistant students, temporary licensees or license applicants, PTAs and physical therapy aides. Summarize those provisions below:

Role	Role Definition	Supervisory Requirements
Student physical therapist or therapist assistant _Follow_	responsible for patient care given by assistive personnel under PT supervision clinical instructions instructed to follow	A student PT and PTA would work under the supervision of a PT/PTS
Physical therapist and physical therapist assistant license applicant or temporary licensee) (if this status exists)	evaluation - examination intervention- may delegate to assist tasks/procedures that fall in the realm - but do not exceed the training -education articipate in patient care	supervision for PTA would be under the PT
	providing skilled therapy services - can leave much to interpretation	A PTA would work under the supervision of a PT
	therapy aides patient care activities - un support personnel who rform tasks related to operation of PT service function only with continuous on site supervision by PT/PTA may not perform skills they are learning -	an aide may be in engaged in patient related tasks under under a PTs supervision- - must be under the orders + directions & immediate supervision of the PT an aide must be supervised by a PT in the same facility as, and in proximity to, the location where the aide is performing patient related tasks - & shall be readily available at all times to provide advice or instruction to the aide.

APTA can respond to acute changes in patient's physiological state & report these finding promptly to the physical therapist

PART FOUR

Support for Special Student Needs

CHAPTER 13

Students With Disabilities

Greg had become interested in physical therapy during his own rehabilitation after an automobile accident at age 15. Following a very serious left lower leg fracture, his surgeons performed a below-knee amputation. He wears a prosthesis and maintains an active lifestyle. In fact, he competed in football and hockey in high school and currently plays intramural basketball. He hoped that he would be able to help others with amputations in the future.

Higher Education and Students With Disabilities

Federal and state laws and most institutional policies require a higher education institution to provide reasonable accommodation in its academically-related programs to students with disabilities. This applies to students in health professions education.[1-12]

University academic accommodations and support services are intended to provide students equal access by reducing the negative impact of their disabilities. The key federal legislative acts that support the rights of students with disabilities are Section 504, the Rehabilitation Act of 1973 and the Americans with Disabilities Act (1990).

Section 504, Rehabilitation Act of 1973

The Rehabilitation Act of 1973 states that "No otherwise qualified individual with a disability in the United States, as defined in section 706 (8) of this title, shall, solely by reason of his or her disability, be excluded from the participation in, be denied the benefits of, or be subjected to discrimination under any program or activity receiving Federal financial assistance or under any program or activity conducted by any Executive agency or by the United States Postal Service." Institutions of higher education are included in the definition of institutions receiving federal financial assistance.[13]

Americans With Disabilities Act

The Americans With Disabilities Act (ADA) was signed July 26, 1990. It prohibits discrimination based on disabilities in the areas of employment, public services, transportation, public accommodations, and telecommunications. It requires all affected entities (businesses) to provide "reasonable accommodation" to persons with disabilities.[14,15]

The Americans with Disabilities Act defines *disability* as "(a) a physical or mental impairment that substantially limits one or more of the major life activities of such individual; (b) a record of such impairment; or (c) being regarded as having such an impairment."[13]

What is a Disability?

This legislation applies to persons with disabilities such as amputation, arthritis, autism, blindness, burn injury, cancer, cerebral palsy, cystic fibrosis, deafness, head injury, heart disease, hemiplegia, hemophilia, respiratory or pulmonary dysfunction, mental retardation, mental illness, multiple sclerosis, muscular dystrophy, musculoskeletal disorders, neurological disorders (including stroke and epilepsy), paraplegia, quadriplegia and other spinal cord conditions, sickle cell anemia, specific learning disability, and end-stage renal disease. The disability must substantially limit a major life activity.[13,14] (This is not an all-inclusive list.)

What is an Accommodation?

Accommodation refers to the provision of services that ensure equal access to a student with a disability (eg, providing extended examination time for a student who processes information more slowly than other students because of a learning disability).[14,15]

Table 13-1

EXAMPLES OF SERVICES FOR STUDENTS WITH DISABILITIES[16]

Adaptive equipment	Housing assistance	Real-time captioning
Assistive listening devices	Interpreters	Registration assistance
Campus orientation	Mobility assistance	Special materials
Campus van service	Notetakers	Support groups
Computer lab	Peer mentoring or counseling	Test proctoring
Computer technology	Priority enrollment	Tutoring
Disability counseling	Readers	Workshops
Disability parking		

Academic accommodations and support services are determined on an individual basis. Each accommodation is based on documented functional limitations and designed to meet a student's needs without fundamentally altering the nature of the student's instructional program(s) or altering any directly related licensing requirement.

Appropriate academic accommodations may include readers, note-takers, access to adaptive technology, part-time enrollment or relaxed time frame for completion of degree requirements, substitution of coursework required for graduation, and testing accommodations.

What are Academic Support Services?

Appropriate disability-based support services may involve services such as disability-related counseling, priority enrollment, referral to faculty, staff, campus resources and community agencies, mobility assistance, and assistance in compensatory strategies for reading, writing math, and basic study skills.

Campus Resources for Students With Disabilities

Most campuses provide an office that coordinates services to students with disabilities. These services focus on encouraging independence, assisting students in realizing their academic potential and eliminating barriers to their participation in the academic environment. Services are provided in accordance with the specific documented needs of the student. Tables 13-1 and 13-2 show examples of the types of services available on college campuses for students with disabilities.

Requesting Accommodation

Student Responsibilities

Students are responsible for disclosing and defining their disabilities and requesting accommodation(s). In other words identifying that you have a disability and asking for accommodation are personal decisions.

If a student requests accommodations, he or she is likely to be responsible for registering with the appropriate on-campus office and making his or her specific needs for accommodation known.

Most on-campus offices for students with disabilities require that students take responsibility for providing documentation of the disability and making specific requests for reasonable accommodations and academic support services. A sample of student responsibilities for requesting accommodations is shown in Table 13-3.

Documentation of Disabilities

Students requesting accommodations and/or support services under the Americans with Disabilities Act (ADA) and/or Section 504 of the Rehabilitation Act of 1973 must provide documentation of the disability that substantially limits a major life activity. In order to accurately determine the appropriate accommodations, the documentation must be current and reflective of the adult's current functioning.[14,15]

Physical Disabilities

Documentation of physical disabilities must be based on appropriate diagnostic evaluations administered by trained and qualified (ie, certified and/or

---

Table 13-2
EXAMPLES OF DISABILITY-SPECIFIC SERVICES[17]

Learning disability services	Disability-related counseling with a learning-disability specialist, taped textbooks, extended time for tests, alternative test formats, notetakers, taped lectures, adaptive technology, tutoring, support groups, learning skills workshops, and peer counseling.
Deaf and hard-of-hearing student services	Sign language interpreters, notetakers, real-time captioning, assistive listening devices, disability-related counseling, and tutoring.
Mobility assistance program	Transportation services, orientation and mobility assistance for students with visual impairments, disability parking.
Note-taker services	Note-taker services are for students with disabilities which limits their abilities to take notes.
Reader services	Tape recorded assigned classroom readings
Testing accommodations	Test-taking conditions (longer time periods, distraction-free rooms). Test proctoring to insure test security and that indicated conditions are in place.
Priority enrollment	Priority enrollment for access to certain classes.
Special materials and equipment	Written materials and textbooks in alternative formats such as: enlarged print, Braille, raised-line drawings, and tape recordings.
Technology and resources	Adaptive equipment and assistive computer technology including: scanners, voice-synthesizers, reading machines, voice recognition programs, large screen displays, Braille screen displays, and printers.

Table 13-3
SAMPLE OF STUDENT RESPONSIBILITIES IN REQUESTING ACCOMMODATION[17]

1. Supply supporting clinical documentation to the Office of Disabled Student Services (DSS) in advance of the semester to determine appropriate services and accommodations. For students registering with a learning disability, documentation needs to be current within the last 3 years.

2. Request accommodations from DSS in person with at least 2 weeks notice of the accommodation need. If less than 2 weeks notice is given, every effort will be made to provide reasonable accommodations, but accommodations are not guaranteed.

3. Confirm the adequacy of accommodations as soon as possible and notify DSS whenever they encounter unsatisfactory conditions.

4. Approach faculty and staff in a confidential setting to discuss accommodations requested and deliver, in person, letters for request of accommodation from DSS to faculty or staff.

5. Obtain syllabi and lists of course materials for reproduction in alternate formats.

6. Adhere to deadlines established by the DSS, Residential Life, faculty, Registrar, etc for submission of medical documentation and requests for accommodations.

7. Pursue financial aid or state vocational rehabilitation support for accommodations and personal equipment needs.

8. Notify DSS of pre-registered classes for the following semester so accessible space can be arranged if necessary.

licensed) professionals (eg, medical doctors, ophthalmologists, psychologists, neuropsychologists, audiologists). Disability diagnosis categories include:

1. Orthopedic disability
2. Blind or visual impairment
3. Deaf or hard-of-hearing
4. Traumatic brain injury and
5. Other health-related/systemic disabilities

The diagnostic report must include a clear diagnosis and history, including secondary conditions, results of diagnostic tests, associated symptoms, medications, and functional manifestations. This must include substantial limitations to one or more major life activities and indicate the degree of severity. The report should also include recommendations and the rationale for accommodation. If the accommodation recommendations are specific to limitations in learning, an appropriate evaluation of a learning disability must also be performed. Students should always check well in advance regarding deadlines for required documentation, as late submissions may result in delays in service delivery.

Learning Disabilities

The National Joint Committee on Learning Disabilities defines the term "learning disabilities" using the following definition.[18]

Learning disabilities refers to a heterogeneous group of disorders manifested by significant difficulties in the acquisition and use of listening, speaking, reading, writing, reasoning, or mathematical abilities. These disorders are intrinsic to the individual, presumed to be due to central nervous system dysfunction, and may occur across the life span. Problems in self-regulatory behaviors, social perception, and social interaction may exist with learning disabilities but do not by themselves constitute a learning disability. Although learning disabilities may occur concomitantly with other [disabling] conditions (for example, sensory impairment... serious emotional disturbance) or with extrinsic influences (such as cultural differences, insufficient or inappropriate instruction), they are not the result of these conditions or influences.

Many students with learning disabilities typically have average to superior ability, yet experience marked difficulty in one or more academic areas as a result of a significant information processing disorder. To be considered a disability that warrants accommodation, the disorder must substantially interfere with the student's participation in the educational process.

The student who requests disability-related services must provide a current and comprehensive written evaluation of his/her learning disabilities. Extensive print and video resources are available at the Association for Higher Education and Disability website at: http://www.ahead.org.

There must be clear and specific evidence and identification of the student's disability(ies). Individual learning or processing differences do not, by themselves, constitute a learning disability.

The determination of a learning is disability is based on:

a. An educational history
b. Behavioral observations
c. Clearly specified and significant intracognitive and cognitive-achievement discrepancies
d. Current functional limitations imposed by the learning disability in the academic setting
e. Evidence that the disorder substantially interferes with the student's educational progress[18]

Standards of Performance in Physical Therapist Assistant Education

Individual academic programs are responsible to define standards of performance and request that students inform them if they require reasonable accommodation to meet those standards.

Essential functions are key duties (Table 13-4) that student physical therapist assistants (PTAs) must be able to complete, with or without accommodation.[19]

Employment Issues for Physical Therapist Assistants With Disabilities

The Americans with Disabilities Act (ADA) requires employers to *make reasonable accommodations* for a qualified individual with a known physical or mental disability. Examples of reasonable accommodations include job restructuring, reassignment to a vacant position, part-time or modified work schedules, assistive technology, or aides or qualified interpreters. The ADA does not require employers to make accommodations that pose an "undue hardship"(defined as significantly difficult or expensive). Tax credits are available to businesses who remove architectural barriers, target jobs for individuals with disabilities, or provide assistive technology or interpreters to workers with disabilities.[20]

Table 13-4
ESSENTIAL FUNCTIONS FOR THE PHYSICAL THERAPIST ASSISTANT STUDENT[19]

1. Read, write, and spell at the collegiate level.
2. Demonstrate common sense, problem solving abilities, and sound judgment.
3. Achieve "Health Provider" level CPR.
4. Stand for 8 hours.
5. Sit for 8 hours.
6. Perform skills requiring manual dexterity, fingering, and feeling.
7. Maintain good standing balance on all surfaces.
8. Administer manual exercises.
9. Perform skills requiring walking.
10. Make simple mechanical adjustments and repairs of therapy equipment.
11. Safely transfer patients from all surfaces.
12. Measure vital signs.
13. Lift up to 25 lbs frequently.
14. Lift up to 100 lbs infrequently.
15. Squat, stoop, kneel, and/or crawl.
16. Transport patients with wheelchairs and carts by pushing and pulling.

Reprinted with permission from Oklahoma Community College. Informed consent program participation. *Oklahoma Community College Physical Therapist Assistant Program Handbook*. Oklahoma City, Okla: Oklahoma Community College; 2003.

Table 13-5
ESSENTIAL FUNCTIONS[20]

Essential functions are the basic job duties that an employee must be able to perform, with or without reasonable accommodation.

Factors to consider in determining if a function is essential include:

* Whether the reason the position exists is to perform that function
* The number of other employees available to perform the function or among whom the performance of the function can be distributed
* The degree of expertise or skill required to perform the function

Reprinted from US Equal Employment Opportunity Commission. The ADA: your responsibilities as an employer. Available at: http://www.eeoc.gov/facts/ada17.html.

Employers are required to make reasonable accommodation for qualified individuals with a disability, who are defined by the ADA as individuals with a disability, who satisfy the job-related requirements of a position held or desired, and who can perform the *essential functions* of such position, with or without reasonable accommodation (Table 13-5).

The employer identifies the job's essential functions. Job descriptions are prepared before an individual is interviewed or selected for a position giving evidence of a job's essential functions. If the individual cannot perform an essential function, even with accommodation, the individual is not considered a *qualified individual with a disability* under the law.

The employer and employee determine the type of accommodation that will enable the employee to perform the essential functions of the position. Accommodations of a personal nature (such as a guide dog for a visually impaired employee, or a wheelchair) would not be the employer's responsibility.

Employers must provide a list of essential functions of a job. The essential functions listed in Table 13-6 are an example of essential functions for the PTA in an employment situation.

Table 13-6

EXAMPLE OF ESSENTIAL FUNCTIONS
FOR THE PHYSICAL THERAPIST ASSISTANT[21]

TITLE: *Physical Therapist Assistant*

General Summary

Under general supervision of a Physical Therapist performs physical therapy treatments directed toward relieving pain and/or restoring physical functions.

Essential Functions

1. Performs directed physical therapy procedures as selected by the physical therapist (ie, therapeutic exercises) to maintain and restore strength, range of motion, endurance, coordination, and function by:

    * Discussing the treatment plan as outlined by the physical therapist with patients and their families to allay anxieties and elicit cooperation.

    * Administering treatments using therapeutic equipment, machines, or assistive or supportive devices as outlined by the physical therapist.

    * Preparing progress notes, recording daily treatment statistics, writing charge slips for billing purposes and completing other forms, letters, and instructions.

    * Training and directing patients in the use and care of wheelchairs, braces, canes, crutches, and other special equipment.

    * Observing reactions and responses of patients and reporting observations to the physical therapist, physician, or allied health care personnel.

    * Assisting the physical therapist to perform tests and evaluations to determine the patient's functional level in performing activities.

    * Informing the appropriate physical therapist of changes in the patient's condition, which may lead to modification of the treatment plan.

2. Contributes to the overall efficiency of the department by:

    * Instructing members of other health care disciplines in standard methods of performing tasks such as: transfers, ambulation, positioning of patients, and body mechanics.

    * Completing other job-related duties as assigned.

Knowledge, Skills, and Abilities

1. Requires a basic knowledge of physical therapy techniques and theory and experience in applying these techniques.

2. Demonstrates analytical skills necessary for evaluation of the patient's condition in order to make accurate observations and report changes in patient behavior and performance.

3. Demonstrates interpersonal skills necessary to interact effectively with patients, families and staff members in a professional, courteous, friendly, sincere, and understanding manner which projects a positive image consistent with hospital guest relations standards.

4. Requires the physical ability and stamina to remain on feet and/or walk for long periods of time, push wheelchairs and carts, lift or pull patients or supplies, provide CPR, perform specified treatment modalities, train for activities of daily living, etc.

5. Requires fine motor skills for manipulation of highly technical equipment used to meet patient care needs and the visual acuity and manual dexterity to perform the essential functions of the position.

6. Requires the physical ability to perform the essential functions of the position.

continued

Table 13-6 (continued)

Example of Essential Functions for the Physical Therapist Assistant[21]

The above level of knowledge, skills, and abilities are normally acquired through the successful completion of a 2-year college level program for Physical Therapy Assistant and certification, or certification eligibility, to practice in the State of [state name].

Working Conditions

Works in a patient care environment requiring physical exertion, frequent changes in job demands, certain undesirable patient care activities, possible exposure to bio-hazards and normal hazards encountered in a community environment.

Adapted from Memorial Hospital and Health Care System. Physical therapist assistant job description. Available at: http://www.job-smichiana.com/memorialhospital/view_job.php?jobid=2997. Accessed July 13, 2003.

Clinical Education Issues

Hilary was diagnosed with multiple sclerosis during the first semester of the PTA program. A year later, she was in remission, however she often felt fatigued with physical exertion. Although she tried to conserve energy, she found herself wiped out at the end of an 8-hour clinical day. She requested an 18-week clinical assignment, instead of the usual 9 weeks and requested that she attend the clinic from 8:00 AM. to noon daily.

Clinical education courses are usually held in off-campus clinical sites. Those clinical sites, through their agreements with the PTA program agree to make accommodations for student learning. Changes in the type of assignment, daily hours or duration of the assignment would all be reasonable accommodations.

The student, however, is always responsible for requesting accommodations that will assist him or her to meet the essential job functions. The clinical and academic faculty are responsible to insure that all educational conditions meet national and state laws and are in compliance with ethical guidelines for the practice of physical therapy.

Summary

Federal and state legislation mandate accommodation for students with disabilities. An understanding of the types of services available for students with disabilities and the educational program's requirement to provide those services will assist students with disabilities to successfully complete PTA education.

References

1. Colon EJ. Identification, accommodation, and success of students with learning disabilities in nursing education programs. *J Nurs Educ.* 1997;36(8):372-7.

2. Watson PG. Nursing students with disabilities: a survey of baccalaureate nursing programs. *Prof Nurs.* 1995;11(3):147-53.

3. Helms LB, Weiler K. Disability discrimination in nursing education: an evaluation of legislation and litigation. *J Prof Nurs.* 1993;9(6):358-66.

4. Shuler SN. Nursing students with learning disabilities: guidelines for fostering success. *Nurs Forum.* 1990;25(2):15-8.

5. Shomaker TS. The Americans with Disabilities Act and family practice residency programs. *Fam Med.* 1999;31(9):622-3.

6. Losh DP, Church L. Provisions of the Americans with Disabilities Act and the development of essential job functions for family practice residents. *Fam Med.* 1999;31(9):617-21.

7. Smith JJ, Gay SB. Disabled residency candidates and federal law: implications of the Americans with Disabilities Act. *Acad Radiol.* 1998;5(3):207-10.

8. Reichgott MJ. "Without handicap": issues of medical schools and physically disabled students. *Acad Med.* 1996;71(7):724-9.

9. Helms LB, Helms CM. Medical education and disability discrimination: the law and future implications. *Acad Med.* 1994;69(7):535-43.

10. Ward RS, Ingram DA, Mirone JA. Accommodations for students with disabilities in physical therapist and physical therapist assistant education programs: a pilot study. *J Phys Ther Educ.* 1998;12(2):16-21.

11. Hendrickson-S; Lyden S, Tarter C, Banaitis D, Cicirello N. Implementation of the Americans With Disabilities Act into physical therapy programs. *J Phys Ther Educ*. 1998;12(2):9-15.

12. Rangel A, Wittry A, Boucher B, Sanders B. A survey of essential functions and reasonable accommodations in physical therapist education programs. *J Phys Ther Educ*. 2001;15(1):11-19.

13. US Department of Labor. Section 504 Rehabilitation Act of 1973 Web page. Available from: http://www.dol.gov/oasam/regs/statutes/sec504.htm. Accessed September 22, 2004.

14. US Equal Opportunity Commission. Facts about the Americans with Disabilities Act web page. Available at: http://www.eeoc.gov/facts/fs-ada.html. Accessed September 22, 2004.

15. Job Accommodation Network. *Americans with Disabilities Act Document Center. The Americans with Disabilities Act: A Brief Overview*. Available from: http://www.jan.wvu.edu/links/ adasummary.htm. Accessed September 22, 2004.

16. University of California, Los Angeles. *Office for Students with Disabilities at UCLA* Web page. Available from: http://www.saonet.ucla.edu/osd. Accessed September 22, 2004.

17. Brown University Disability Support Services. *Student's Responsibility* Web page. Available at: http://www.brown.edu/Student_Services/Office_ of_Student_Life/dss/registering_students.html. Accessed September 22, 2004.

18. Brinckerhoff LC, Shaw SF, McGuire JM. *Promoting Postsecondary Education for Students with Learning Disabilities: A Handbook for Practitioners*. Austin, Tex: Pro-Ed; 1993:67-87.

19. Oklahoma Community College. Informed consent program participation. *Oklahoma Community College Physical Therapist Assistant Program Handbook*. Oklahoma City, Okla: Oklahoma Community College; 2003.

20. US Equal Employment Opportunity Commission. The ADA: your responsibilities as an employer. Available at: http://www.eeoc.gov/facts/ada17. html. Accessed September 22, 2004.

21. Memorial Hospital and Health Care System. Physical therapist assistant job description. Available at: http://www.jobsmichiana.com/memorialhospital/view_job.php?jobid=2997. Accessed July 13, 2003.

PUTTING IT INTO PRACTICE

1. Write down the contact information for your campus office for students with disabilities. If there is a Web site, also write down the URL address.

   Name of Director:

   Campus Location:

   Telephone:

   Web site:

2. If you have a disability, write down any accommodations that you will request to enable you to complete your professional education in physical therapy.

   If you do not have a disability, consider the accommodations that the following students requested. From your understanding of the provisions of the ADA, discuss whether these are reasonable. Why or why not? What services might be of value to these students?

   Case A:

   Selena had been hard-of-hearing since early childhood. She had never experienced difficulty before in her academic work. When she received an "F" on her first kinesiology test, she requested that the instructor prepare a written transcript of each lecture prior to the lecture so that she could read it as the instructor spoke in class.

   Case B:

   Karen's asthma was worse than usual this semester. The chemicals in the anatomy lab seemed to trigger her chemical sensitivities and cause increased shortness of breath. She requested a rebreathing mask, similar to that used by firefighters to eliminate this as a problem.

   Case C:

   John fractured his left tibia in a rollerblading accident during summer break. His cast was removed two weeks prior to beginning his final clinical internships. He began his first internship and found his foot swelling at the end of the day. He found it impossible to continue at the pace required in the clinic. He requested an 8-week leave of absence from the program and went to recuperate at his parent's home.

CHAPTER 14

When Speaking and Writing English is a Challenge

> *Isabella bought her books during the first week of class and was frightened by the size of the books and how small the writing was. Although she had studied English as a second language in an intensive course last semester, she was afraid that she wouldn't be able to keep up with her reading assignments.*

Common Issues for Second Language Speakers

Non-native English speakers face a double challenge. Students must not only master the physical therapy content but they must do so in English, comprehending and learning what they read and using this new vocabulary in written and spoken communications.

There are many strategies for learning which may help the non-native English speaker cope with the challenges of physical therapist assistant education.

Medical Terminology and Lay Language

First, it is important to understand that physical therapist assistant students are learning a new language, using medical terminology, abbreviations, and terms that have meaning only to those in the health professions. Everyone who is learning the language of a profession struggles initially to communicate using both lay language with patients and clients and medical terminology with colleagues.

Be aware that there are terms that are appropriate for use in health care communication and terms that would not be appropriate. For example, compare these statements which both describe the same event: *Medical terminology*—the patient consulted the orthopedic surgeon for treatment of his left ulna fracture and *lay language*—the patient went to the doctor to get a cast on his broken arm.

Reading

There are strategies that students can use to improve both their vocabulary and comprehension of reading assignments.[1] It may help to also review the active learning strategies suggested in Chapter 9.

Survey and Skim First

Determine a structure of the material. Before you read, look for the main ideas and points. Examine how a chapter or article is organized. Look at headings and points of emphasis, often in italics or bold print. Look for summaries. Try to identify a few main ideas. Before you read thoroughly, write a sentence that expresses the main idea of what you will read.

Look for words like first, second, finally to indicate a progression and sequence of topics and transitions between different ideas.

Identify Your Purpose

Why do you need to read this? Is it for the general idea or for details? You will adjust your reading strategy accordingly.

Assess Difficulty and Choose What to Read

How difficult is this material? Do you know the vocabulary? Choose a few sentences to read thoroughly. If it will be too time-consuming to read word by word, look for the sentences that start and conclude a section of text. There are some additional strategies for reading difficult material in Table 14-1.

Table 14-1

HOW TO READ A DIFFICULT BOOK[2]

1. *Study the table of contents* to get a general sense of the book's structure. Note the subtitles and other indications of the content of the chapter.

2. *Look at the title page of each chapter.* Often the first few paragraphs create a structure for the chapter.

3. *Read the conclusion of the chapter.* There is often a summary that will denote key terms and concepts in the chapter.

4. *Check the glossary and index of the book as you encounter new terms.* This will give you an idea of the relationships of concepts and it may help to see its application later in the book. Use your English and Medical dictionaries to assist you.

Table 14-2

TIPS FOR IMPROVING YOUR ENGLISH READING SPEED[3]

1. *Do not pronounce words as you read.* If you speak or whisper as you read, you will be able to read only as fast as you can speak. Your speed will be two to three times faster if you read silently. Focus on speaking only key terms as you try to improve your reading speed.

2. *Avoid rereading the same material.* If you have skimmed the material first, then you have looked for the key phrases in a paragraph or section. If you do not understand a passage, then find some material later that you do understand. Most writers make a statement and then give examples and then restate the information in a conclusion. Try to pick up the main idea in what you read, not every detail.

3. *Read in phrases, not word by word.* Meaning is conveyed by a phrase in a context, not by the definitions of individual words.

Choose What to Read in a Systematic Way

Identify statements, definitions and formulas that you must understand completely and remember precisely. Look for definitions, highlighted areas, and text, which accompanies figures, graphs and tables. These usually summarize the major ideas and facts of a chapter. Check the strategies for improving your reading speed in Table 14-2.

Build Your Vocabulary of Medical Terminology at the Same Time

Use a medical dictionary. Write down unfamiliar terms and phrases and their definitions on a separate sheet as you do your assigned reading. Review these terms later. Look for these words in your reading. Write down questions that arise as you are learning new terms. Make it a point to use these words in a new sentence or question.

Test Your Comprehension

Make up questions about the material. Write the question. Answer the question in writing. Talk about the material with others. These steps in thinking about the material after reading it are the key to remembering it.

Listening

There are many strategies that will improve your listening comprehension.[1]

Become Familiar with the Material First

Skim the assigned reading. Look for key words and ideas. These phrases will be very important to your recognizing the topic being discussed and keeping up in class.

Choose a Good Seat in the Classroom

Sit in the front of the classroom. There will be fewer distractions and it will be easier to hear and see. Arrive early so that you have your choice of seats.

Attend All Classes and Take Notes

Never miss a class. Take notes in the classroom and review your notes later. Organize your notes by date and keep them in one place. Do not try to write down everything the instructor says. Leave spaces in your notes so that you can add to them later.

It may also be helpful to tape record lectures and use the recording to help review and edit your notes. Be sure to ask the instructor or any guest speakers if you have their permission to tape their lectures to help you study the material later.

Use Outlines and Course Syllabi

Use outlines, handouts, and other materials that the instructor provides to orient you during a lecture. If you are not understanding all of it do not worry about what you have missed. Listen and write what you can. You can fill in the details after the lecture.

Identify the Most Important Points

Listen for cues as to important points, transitions from one point to the next, repetition of points for emphasis, changes in voice inflections, or lists of a series of points. Most instructors present a few major points and several minor points in a lecture. Much of the remaining material explains those points.

Write Down What is on the Board

Write down everything that the instructor writes on the board. This is a good way to prioritize the key concepts and vocabulary related to the subject.

Use All of Your Senses

Use all of your senses (seeing, hearing, feeling) to learn. Focus on visual materials and demonstrations in addition to what is in writing. Practice skills by moving and saying instructions out loud.

Eliminate Distractions

Focus 100% of your attention and concentration during lectures and while studying. Take a break when needed to revitalize and refresh your mind.

Writing

It is often very helpful to see samples of work that previous students have done. Ask the faculty member for good examples of the kind of work he or she expects.

Ask for feedback prior to submitting your final paper. Many faculty members are willing to review your written work in a draft form and give you feed-

back. In fact, this type of feedback is frequently the most helpful in revising your writing.

Use on-campus writing resource centers to assist you in presenting your ideas. Your writing style will be concise, directed toward a specific purpose and often follows a predefined format. Review Chapter 8 for examples of the requirements of different types of writing assignments.

Express Yourself

You should use a writing style that will improve the reader's understanding of your thoughts and ideas. English writing styles change with the type of writing and purpose of the assignment.

Professional writing tends to be goal-directed, concise, and clear. Writing assignments in the physical therapist assistant program may differ considerably from a student's past experience. Some guidelines are presented in Table 14-3. You may find it helpful to review Chapter 8 as well.

The Voice of Your Writing

The active voice is simpler and more effective in conveying your ideas. Many cultures and languages commonly use the passive voice. Consider the differences between the passive and active voices presented in Table 14-4. How does the active voice improve your understanding of what has been written?

Essentials of English Grammar

An inexpensive, classic reference is *The Elements of Style*.[5] This is a key resource for your library. This simple book contains rules of grammar and provides the key requirements of English writing style. It concentrates on the fundamental rules of usage and principles of composition most commonly violated.

Proofreading

Jiro received his paper back and it was covered with red ink. How could it be possible that he had made so many errors? He felt embarrassed and went to the see the instructor during office hours to discuss his grade on the paper.

Proofreading is essential for all writers. All writers make errors. Using the following strategies may help to find those errors.[6]

Table 14-3
GUIDELINES FOR PROFESSIONAL WRITING IN ENGLISH[3,4]

Strategy	Explanation
Outline and organize your ideas before you begin writing.	Review the assignment and establish a writing outline that follows the directions of the assignment.
Provide connections between your ideas or indicate a progression of points.	Use words that indicate similarities and differences, such as "Similarly,…" or "In contrast,…" or "Next,…"
Give examples and evidence of the statements you make.	Follow an introductory sentence with one or two sentences that illustrate the initial idea of the paragraph. Use statistics, facts, and outside references to support the points you make.
State your purpose.	Identify the purpose of the paper in the first few paragraphs. "The purpose of this paper is to examine the evidence that supports the use of ultrasound as a therapeutic modality."
Use headings and sub-headings to orient the reader.	Help the reader to follow your ideas by making brief titles to describe the sections of your paper (examples: APTA Position, Interview Findings).
Use the active voice.	Avoid passive verbs. Identify an actor for the actions you present in your sentences (See Table 14-4 for more examples).
Use appropriate language; avoid slang.	Use phrases like "many" instead of "a lot of" or "I must go to work" instead of "I've got to go to work."
Take a stand. Be clear about why you have made a decision, have an opinion or position.	State your decision or position and the reasons and rationale that support your position. Indicate your thought processes. "It is important to monitor blood pressure because nonweight bearing ambulation puts a much higher demand on the cardiovascular system."
Follow referencing styles.	If there is not a referencing style indicated in the instructions, inquire as to what style the faculty prefers that you use.
Make sure that your work is free of spelling and grammatical errors.	Use a spell-checker to check your work. Check the tables below for examples of common grammatical errors.

Table 14-4
SAMPLES OF PASSIVE AND ACTIVE VOICE

Passive Voice	Active Voice
The patient was interviewed before beginning the treatment.	The instructor interviewed the patient before beginning the treatment.
We were given the assignment on Thursday.	The instructor gave us the assignment last Thursday.
The students were asked to complete a three-page questionnaire.	The students completed a three-page questionnaire.
I was told that you called yesterday.	Janet, our receptionist, told me that you called yesterday.

Table 14-5

COMMON ENGLISH ERRORS FOR NON-NATIVE ENGLISH SPEAKERS[7,8]

Type of Error	Incorrect Form	Correct Form
Absent determiners (the, a, an).	She is good physical therapist assistant. What is answer?	She is a good physical therapist. What is the answer?
Incorrect choice of preposition. (in, on, with, over, above, below, beside)	My lab coat is stained in coffee.	My lab coat is stained with coffee.
Incorrect verb sequences, especially involving tense agreement.	The patient should have recover by now.	The patient should have recovered by now.
Incorrect choice of verb to use with the infinitive.	I wouldn't mind to take a vacation.	I would like to take a vacation.
Disagreement between determiners and nouns.	He ate many tomato on Wednesday. She identified some abnormal neurological finding yesterday.	He ate many tomatoes on Wednesday. She identified some abnormal neurological findings yesterday.
Sentence fragments	Sending the letter yesterday.	She sent the letter yesterday.
Irregular verbs, nouns, and adjectives, such as go/went/gone, drive/drove/driven, think/thought, send/sent, and child/children.	He sended the report of the evaluation to the physician. I thinked about that answer for a long time during the test.	He sent the report of the evaluation to the physician. I thought about that answer for a long time during the test.
Subject-verb agreement errors.	The results of the test was negative.	The results of the test were negative.
Commonly confused words, such as to/too/two, except/accept, effect/affect, which/that, then/than, piece/peace, and its/it's.	Their are to many patients. Everyone is turning there work in on time accept for John.	There are too many patients. Everyone is turning in their work on time except for John.

Read Very Slowly

Read out loud if possible, one word at a time. Read what is actually on the page. Proofread more than once and if possible have someone else check your work. Repeat after you have finished.

Identify Common Mistakes and Look for Them

Look for common spelling errors using a "spell-check" function in your computer word processing program. It will be more difficult, but not impossible, to find common errors in usage that are spelled correctly.

English is a complicated language with many irregularities. The grammatical errors that non-native English speakers make fall into several common categories. Be careful of these errors (Table 14-5).

An excellent on-line resource is available from the Purdue University Online Writing Lab at: http://owl.english.purdue.edu/handouts/esl/eslstudent.html.

Test-Taking

Non-native English speakers face some particular challenges during examinations. Often a single word may change the meaning of a question. Review Chapter 7 as test-taking strategies apply here as well. Be careful of some common problems (Table 14-6) that are particularly difficult for non-native English speakers.[9]

Table 14-6

COMMON TESTING ERRORS FOR NON-NATIVE ENGLISH SPEAKERS

Error	How is this error made?	Example
Missing a double negative in a sentence	Words like not, lack, or absence are easy to find and these indicate the negative condition. It is more difficult to find whole words that indicate the negative condition, such as illogical or uncertain. Remember that these words also indicate a negative condition. Two negative words together indicate a positive condition.	Which of the following situations are NOT illegal? A. Not having the patient sign the consent form B. Offering to change the dates on the insurance claim C. Lack of consideration of the patient's request for an appointment in the morning D. Leaving an unsupervised aide in the clinic while you go for lunch To correctly answer this question, the test-taker must look for the only situation which is not illegal, or in other words, legal.
Missing a qualifying word	Single words such as always, never, just, only, and except change the meaning of a phrase (and may also indicate an unlikely correct choices). Extreme words (always, never, totally) are frequently associated with incorrect answers.	A patient with a blood pressure of 90/60 will always complain of dizziness upon standing (FALSE). Although it is true that a patient with a blood pressure of 90/60 might feel dizzy, the word *always* is an important clue in this question.
Confusing look-alike options	Be careful to read all of the options, as a phrase may be repeated in a similar way, with the intent to mislead you. Be aware of details.	The most reliable sign of hypertension is: A. Resting systolic blood pressure over 90 B. Resting diastolic blood pressure over 90 C. Resting heart rate over 90 D. 90-point difference between systolic and diastolic blood pressure Don't be fooled! Look for the correct term (diastolic) and which matches with the repeated value (90).

Cultural Adjustments for International Students

On the first day of class, Katrina was surprised when her instructor told the class to call him by his first name, "Tom" She thought to herself, "I want to treat my instructors with respect. I just don't feel right about doing that."

International students may find that teaching and learning methods and social customs are very different than those practiced in their home country. International students are often surprised to see differences in relationships between students and instructors and expectations of students. In addition, differing social customs such as dress, informality in relationships, and what is acceptable behavior in many academic and work situations may differ considerably. This is a predictable and common reaction to immersion in a different culture where the behavior and values seem to be so different.

In addition, international students often observe behaviors such as competitiveness, materialism, or hurrying in American culture. Some of these behaviors may seem rude. It may be difficult to adjust to different standards of behavior.

Sociologists define this as *culture shock*. Students often feel lonely, alienated, and exhausted. They may feel frustrated and angry. They may withdraw and hold back from participating fully in the new culture.[10]

Coping With Culture Shock

Coping with such feelings is essential to progress with your education. Try some of the following strategies.[10]

* *Avoid stereotyping*: Try not to stereotype the characteristics of "Americans" based on your experiences with a few individuals. Try to look at each situation as new and each individual as unique.
* *Express your feelings*: Talk about your feelings and observations with others in the same situation. Ask others if they have experienced similar feelings at some times.
* *Open yourself to the experience*: Try to learn about the history and culture of community in which you live. Think of this experience as an adventure. Focus on "now," not yesterday or the future.
* *Use humor*: Maintain a sense of humor and a friendly outlook. Find amusement in your observations. You may feel better if you try to maintain a positive outlook.
* *Join the group*: Group activities which involve your classmates will be very helpful to develop the kind of friendships that will help you to overcome culture shock.
* *Relax and be patient*: This is a common reaction. Assume that these feelings will pass and don't dwell on them. You are not alone and you will find it easier if you remind yourself that this is not permanent.

What's the Hurry?

Time is highly valued in physical therapist assistant educational programs. Tardiness is often not tolerated and may be interpreted as a sign that a student does not value the time of others.

Always strive be early or on time or early for both classes and clinical experiences. Be careful to turn assignments in when they are due and to write down deadlines and appointments in a calendar or appointment book.

Web Resources for International Students

The US Department of State provides a comprehensive web site for international students that helps to explain many aspects of US culture, education and issues of everyday living at http://www.educationusa.state.gov/living.htm.[11]

Another useful site for tips on living in the US is Edupass, the Smart Student Guide to Studying in the United States at http://www.edupass.org.[12]

Summary

International students often face unique challenges in struggling through the educational program in a second language (English). Non-native English speakers will benefit by using strategies for reading and taking notes that maximize attention to key concepts in the written material. Proofreading is an essential step in the writing process as non-native English speakers are likely to make errors that must be corrected prior to handing in the assignment. Student-instructor relationships and expectations of students may be quite different in the US higher education system. Students should take active measures to cope with culture shock so that it does not cause problems in their academic pursuits.

References

1. Carter C. Bishop J. Kravits SL. *Keys to Effective Learning*. Upper Saddle River, NJ: Prentice-Hall; 1998.
2. Virginia Polytechnic Institute and State, Cook Counseling Center. How to read a difficult book. Available at: http://www.ucc.vt.edu/stdysk/stdyhlp.html. Accessed September, 2004.
3. Gocsik K. Cultural Difference and its impact on rhetoric: an overview. *Dartmouth Writing Program* Web page. Available from: http://www.dartmouth.edu/~writing/resources/tutor/problems/esl.html#overview. Accessed August 30, 2004.
4. Holt S. Responding to Non-Native Speakers of English. Available from: http://cisw.cla.umn.edu/faculty/responding/pdfs/nn_speakers.PDF. Accessed August 11, 2003.

5. Strunk W, White EB, Angell R. *The Elements of Style*. 4th ed. Needham Heights, Mass: Pearson Higher Education (Allyn and Bacon); 2000.

6. Purdue University Online Writing Lab. *Proofreading Strategies* Web page. Available at: http:// owl.english.purdue.edu/handouts/general/gl_ proof.html. Accessed September 22, 2004.

7. Edupass. The smart student guide to studying in the United States. *Common Usage Errors* Web page. Available at: http://www.edupass.org/english/ errors.phtml. Accessed September 22, 2004.

8. Gocsik K. Common ESL errors: the top ten list. *Dartmouth Writing Program* Web page. Available at: http://www.dartmouth.edu/~writing/resources/ tutor/problems/esl.html#overview. Accessed September 22, 200.

9. University of Victoria Learning Skills Program. Strategies for reading exam questions. Available at: http://www.coun.uvic.ca/learn/program/hndouts/Readexam.html. Accessed September 22, 2004.

10. Scheider K. Cultural differences: international students coping with culture shock. Available at: http://www.uwec.edu/Counsel/pubs/ shock.htm. Accessed August 11, 2003.

11. Bureau of Educational and Cultural Affairs, US Department of State. *Living in the United States* Web page. Available at: http://www.educationusa.state. gov/living.htm. Accessed August 11, 2003.

12. Kantrowitz M. *Edupass: The Smart Student Guide to Studying in the United States* Web page. Available from: http://www.edupass.org. Accessed September 22, 2004.

PUTTING IT INTO PRACTICE

Consult your textbooks and the American Physical Therapy Association Web site to answer the following questions about the physical therapy profession:

1. Identify a reading assignment in one of your classes. Give yourself only 5 minutes. Skim the assignment. Write down all the key words and phrases you can find in that time.

2. Correct the following sentences:
   I can to give her the assignment tonight.

   Many student talked to me after class today.

   I go to the clinic yesterday.

   He want more exercises to practice.

3. Many international students are surprised about various aspects of life in US higher education. Write down an observation that was surprising to you. How have you coped with this difference? Have you changed your expectations? Do you look at this differently now?

CHAPTER 15

Re-Entry and Career Transition Students

Tina Buettell, MPT

A *re-entry student* is loosely defined as any student age 25 or older.[1] The concept of re-entering the academic arena also implies that a student has not been continuously enrolled full-time at the college level.[1,2] The term *nontraditional student* is commonly used synonymously with re-entry student, but more specifically refers to students who do not fit the traditional profile of full-time attendance, ages 18 to 22, with on-campus residency.[1,2]

A nontraditional student is alternately defined as having multiple roles and at least 1 year in a nonacademic role between high school or last college experience and present enrollment in college.[3] Frequently, nontraditional or re-entry students are beginning a second career.[4]

Changing Demographics

Student demographics at community colleges have shifted to include more diverse, older, female, part-time students who work full-time and attend college in the evenings. For example, in 1970, women comprised 40% of students attending community college. Almost 30 years later, 1999 statistics show that 59% of community college students were women; the average age of these community college students was 29. Similarly, there are more part-time students (61%) and minority students (33%) now enrolled in community college than ever before. [5]

Career Transitions

With a social trend toward adult career changes, a career as a physical therapist assistant (PTA) offers a practical, meaningful vocation where life experience tends to enhance applicable decision-making and communication skills. PTA students tend to be older, female students, seeking a second-career. In fact, these students may succeed because of their maturity, experience, and motivation.[6]

25, 35, 45...

Younger re-entry students, ages 25 to 34, have much in common with traditional students. Many are still single and without dependents, although this is also the classic marriage-childbirth-divorce age group. Time since previous schooling is minimal, and interests and activities are broad, often involving group trips and athletic recreation.

Middle re-entry students, ages 35 to 44, are frequently in committed relationships, or have been, often have children to care for, have multiple outside interests or steady employment, and may own a home or have other major responsibilities or debts. These students often have been out of school for many years and often find it difficult to make time for classes and assignments in their already full lives.

Older re-entry students, ages 45 and over, are a distinct minority. They may have established careers, teenage or grown children, and elderly parents. They are beginning to deal with issues of aging and may have begun to consider financial planning for retirement. They are old enough to be their younger classmates' parents and have few socio-historical bonds with students a generation younger.

Predictable Strengths and Benefits

Success and retention, the big concerns for pre-admission screening, are not big issues for most re-entry students. Re-entry students tend to be highly motivated, grounded, goal-oriented students who are eager to learn and have a sense of purpose and dedication.[1-4] Findings that nontraditional students more eagerly attend classes and do homework may suggest their higher enthusiasm for learning after time spent away from classrooms.[3] This often is their second chance, so there is no backing out. This is particularly true of older students who may feel career time running out.

Older or nontraditional students tend to see themselves as more applied and process-oriented than their concrete, task-focused, traditional classmates who may be more interested in short-term goals.[7] Other unique attributes of re-entry students may include a more serious view of education and a high value placed on positive working relationships with faculty.[7]

One study comparing nontraditional female students with housewives found that the returning students experienced greater self-respect and respect from others, a more diversified life, and less boredom.[3] Service to community, enhancement of quality of life, personal career satisfaction, and acquisition of a practical skill are reasons given by re-entry students for taking the leap.[4]

Can I Learn As Quickly As My Younger Classmates?

Contrary to the popular notion that adult age and cognitive abilities are inversely related, recent longitudinal studies suggest that mean cognitive performance may not significantly decline until late adulthood (age 65 and older).[8] Vocabulary increases with age, and performance on language ability tests has been shown to be more strongly associated with the subject's educational level than with his or her age.[9] Additionally, students with vast life experience have more finely tuned their social and communication skills through years of practice in diverse settings.

Helen Hislop has written about the importance of "productive dissent" and the "ability to listen to opposing perceptions in a nonjudgmental manner, to deal with different ideas with an open mind..." versus rigidity and resistance to dissent.[10] Older or multi-role students often have encountered a greater variety of people and ideas than their more youthful classmates. They also have had more time to solidify rigid beliefs, but either way, they have experienced many decision-making challenges. These experiences may prepare them to accommodate for clinical ambiguity, "the uncertainty principle that intrudes into every human interaction between patient and therapist," and facilitate their development of clinical intuition.[10]

Predictable Challenges and Sacrifices

Technology and You

In spite of their many positive qualities, re-entry students can face challenges when it comes to current technology and recent schooling trends. Most did not grow up with computers as students do today. Papers were written on manual typewriters using carbon paper for copies. Library card catalogs used to consist of wooden drawers of 3" x 5" cards, and the index for journals was the voluminous, hardbound *Reader's Guide to Periodical Literature*.

Similarly, older students may remember using trig tables and slide rules for math and chemistry classes instead of today's ubiquitous calculators. There were no Web sites and no computerized testing. For students who completed prerequisites 10 or 15 years before re-entering, certain subjects may be distant memories. Test-taking can feel terrifying, and sitting for hours in a classroom may be unfamiliar as well as uncomfortable.

What school was like 20 years ago is not what it's like upon re-entry. Trivial, everyday procedures for most students can be traumatic at first for a returning student.

Years ago, Sally attended a technical college to train as a medical assistant. Returning to college at age 40 was exciting, yet perplexing. Sitting at her first kinesiology exam, the unfamiliar scantron upside down on the desk, wearing reading glasses for the first time, wedged between two other students, surrounded by what seemed like dozens of younger students, feeling insecure about putting her backpack up front, Sally felt like an alien and remembers saying to herself, "This is crazy; I can't believe I'm doing this."

Reevaluating the stressful situation, Sally requested a different seating arrangement and left her backpack in her locker for the next exam. By the end of the semester she was tutoring fellow students and received an A on the final exam, but it was a rough start.

Physical and Social Challenges

Older students may experience physical challenges such as worsening eyesight, slower thought-processing, and increased sensitivity to noise, time pressures, crowding, and bedlam. Middle-aged female students may be experiencing peri-menopausal symptoms. Multirole students may resent the tedium of class meetings, birthday announcements, and busywork assignments knowing they have a sick child at home or a long night ahead at a job. They may share little in common with younger students involved in dating and struggles with roommates.

Time and Stress Management

Time and stress management are challenges for all students; re-entry students are just more experienced at coping with them. Fortunately so, because they often have less time and potentially more stress than their traditional classmates. Various studies have replicated findings that nontraditional students' complex time and role demands are sources of anxiety and tension.[3] They have more responsibilities at home, less time spent with friends and peers, and less vacation time than traditional students.[3]

Financial Needs

Starving students also can be found at all echelons, but for re-entry students financial woes are usually more complex than just paying rent and borrowing a little more from parents. Re-entry often means job loss that means downward mobility for adults accustomed to a steady income with health insurance and other benefits. Dependents further complicate matters, especially if they also have college expenses. Home owners may have mortgage payments as well as maintenance and homeowner's insurance to continue to pay.

Unpredictable Struggles and Growth

Returning to full-time study can be an enormous transition. "You are settled, stable, and competent in what you do. Everyone's reaction is, You want to do what?[11] What may have begun as an off-chance of qualifying for a long-postponed dream suddenly looms as a dire threat to financial, marital, and mental stability. There may be an overwhelming sense of "Help! I can't really do this," or "Oh my gosh, what have I gotten myself into?"

Older Students, Younger Faculty

In spite of expecting skills to be a little rusty, the shock of suddenly sitting in a science fiction classroom where chalkboards are history and TV monitors beam down from opposite corners can be unsettling. Additionally, even faculty and staff are no longer similar to memories of previous school days. Whereas traditional students look up to faculty as older and wiser, students who are the same age or older than their faculty may have a hard time submitting to the conventional faculty-student hierarchy. In their own areas of prior expertise and training, re-entry students may have specific skills superior to those of some faculty. Some older students also may have more experiential wisdom than their younger faculty.

High Expectations

Expectations are another pitfall. Re-entry students have been through a lot to get where they are, and may be demanding, impatient, and judgmental of faculty shortcomings that are viewed as impediments to their own goals. They may feel more competitive than cooperative. In a recent study, nontraditional students reported greater frustration from poor teaching than did their traditional counterparts.[3] Re-entry students may cope with these perceptions with arguments, direct confrontation of authority, refusal to follow instructions, and endless unsolicited suggestions for improvement and change.

Relationships

What about friendships? Outside of school, faculty and older students may have mutual friends and common bonds, and would be inclined to socialize, but role boundaries may limit social contact between faculty and students. Older students may have more in common with faculty their own generation than with students two decades younger but are segregated by artificial barriers. Where are the limits? Faculty may be well aware of their own roles and boundaries, but newly returning students unaccustomed to academia may find it initially confusing to differentiate between acceptable friends (classmates) and friendly authorities (faculty, clinical instructors, staff).

Support Systems

At the same time re-entry students are trying to foster a support system on campus, they must redefine their support network at home and beyond. One re-entry student remarked, "The magnitude of support I've had to find boggles my mind. I don't think I'd have dared to try this if I'd known how much help I'd need."

> Melody, a 36-year-old married mother of three, works part time at a suburban health center near her home. Interested in furthering her education, she accepts her employer's incentive to pay tuition and fees for her to upgrade her skills. She applies and is accepted for the PTA program at the community college 25 miles away. At the new student picnic, she talks to a re-entry student in the second year class about her concerns. "Will I be able to keep up with classes if I have children at home? It sounds great, but how difficult are the courses? My computer skills are weak. I have a 40-minute commute; I don't know how I'll manage evening classes. Can I live at home during my clinicals?"
>
> The second year student confesses that the first year was a struggle, but she has survived. "Sure, give it a try. Do you have enough support?" The new student answers that she plans to arrange after-school child care 3 days per week, her husband is employed full-time, and she's saved a little money for books and supplies. "Not enough. You'll need more help at home, more flexibility, and campus resources. Better see a re-entry counselor."

Support is more than tacit approval and occasional child care. Assumption of homemaker duties by other family members, residential relocation, noninvolvement in children's school activities, extreme economizing, tutoring needs, scheduling nightmares, psychological counseling, aging issues, extended family participation, vacations spent barely catching up, zero recreational time, bouts of self-doubt, and major lifestyle disruption may be some of the challenges a re-entry must contend with in addition to academic demands.

Multilevel support is crucial to transcend the demoralizing realization that the best one can do is to get by a day at a time. Professional and personal support can be key to recapturing the vision that originally brought one to college and to making "insurmountable hurdles become just another day's adventure..."[11]

And a Midlife Crisis Too?

To add to the complexities of re-entry, middle-age is often developmentally a time of reevaluation, spiritual growth, searching, or midlife crisis for many adults. This may be what inspires a second-career decision in the first place. A 45-year-old student may have a very different perspective on the meaning of his or her chosen field of study than a 22-year-old traditional student who thought PTA education sounded like an interesting program and hopes it will pay well. The following re-entry student statement is typical:

> I needed to change my life. I knew I could do more, and I didn't want to get stuck where I was forever. I'd always wanted to go back to school but money, family, or other commitments got in the way. I finally just had to make the leap; small steps weren't getting me there, and time was running out. It was terrifying, but I'm glad I did it. I wasn't really sure it was possible, after so many years and with so many obstacles, but I had to find out. I would always have wondered and regretted the missed opportunity. Some days I wake up very surprised that I'm here.

These subtle surprises create unsubtle confusion for re-entry students who are already feeling slightly lost and overwhelmed. Returning students may repeatedly think, "This is silly. This shouldn't be a problem. I'm mature and experienced. I can handle this." When re-entry students experience conflicts for speaking out or being different, or burnout from being pulled in too many disparate directions, they need help. It is important to identify students at risk for stress and burnout related to personal and environmental factors in order to initiate appropriate preventive measures.[12]

Strategies for Re-Entry Students

Professional Counseling

Competent professional counseling can make all the difference in the world. In a study of role strain of nontraditional women students, "Psychological support was found to be a significant factor in feelings of satisfaction for women who were re-entering the academic world."[3] This may be related to another finding that women re-entering after an average absence of 10 years had depression symptom scores twice as high as a normative population.[3]

Re-entry students who seek campus counseling services often report they are dissatisfied with the support they receive, commenting for example, "The counselor is younger than I am and doesn't understand my problems," or "When I explained what I was dealing with, the counselor seemed overwhelmed by its complexity." Campus services are geared primarily to traditional students and often rely on counseling student interns. Finding a good fit between counselor and counselee is sometimes difficult. If dissatisfied, talk directly to your program director or the head of the counseling center.

Financial Aid

Financial aid and scholarships can be lifelines. Talk to a financial aid counselor. Submit applications on time. Research scholarships for which you are uniquely qualified, Plan ahead; have essays and references ready well ahead of deadlines. Explore private loans from friends or relatives. Barter. Temporarily down-scale; this won't last forever. Work as a student assistant to integrate earning and learning.

Use Re-Entry Program Services

Re-entry programs exist at some colleges. Consider applying to schools that can offer re-entry services including counseling, scholarship guidance, peer support groups, quiet study areas, tutoring, speaker programs, family activities, and the support of other re-entry students. Find a few students with similar concerns; get together regularly for support and problem solving. Network with same-age, same-interest students at other schools.

Solicit the Support of the Faculty

Faculty are allies. Appreciate them, trust them, work with them. Help them think of ways to help you. Tell them what you need and what you'd like to try. Be patient. Get involved with student clubs and professional associations.

Collaborate With Your Classmates

Your classmates of all ages can be treasures. Find a few with whom to work closely and have fun. Seek out other returning students. Welcome opportunities to work with students unlike yourself to expand your awareness and understanding. Trade skills— help those you can, ask for help as needed. Be a good group member; do your share or more and use your maturity to help facilitate good group process and to resolve conflicts quickly and effectively. Model appropriate behavior—honesty, trustworthiness, reliability, and clear communication.

Involve Your Family and Significant Others

If you are parenting very young children, carefully evaluate whether this is the best time to return to school. You may miss a substantial part of your child's first few years.

Family members need to play a part in your educational experience. Elicit broad support. Clearly explain the potential benefits for everyone of your success. Give every family member a role to play. Primary school children can help label supplies, color charts, sort laundry, and unpack groceries. Older children can help locate library and Internet materials, organize tapes, create quizzes, critique practice presentations, and assist with meals and cleaning. Establish quiet study hours. Organize routine chores for maximum efficiency. Share lots of hugs.

Spouses or significant others can make it or break it for a re-entry student, especially if there are dependents who need care. Household help, multifaceted child or elder care and transport, school liaison, meals, laundry, car care, banking, bills, and shopping can eat up oceans of time. Reassurance and pep talks may be vital, and general organizational help is essential. Assistance with typing, proofing, printing, collating, photocopying as well as being on hand for deadline crunches can be sanity-preserving for the overloaded student.

Siblings, parents, or friends can help by providing loans or special gifts such as children's piano lessons, orthodontist care, soccer shoes, or summer camp. Child care, meals, shopping, and transportation assistance may also help. Everyone can give moral support. Invite family to special presentations and include them in your accomplishments and celebrations. Ask for what you need. Remember to express appreciation, and when you can, return the favor, or the money.

Acquire Computer Skills

Become computer literate. Beg, borrow, or buy a functional computer to use at home and be able to problem solve its idiosyncrasies. Know how to create documents and files, how to share disks and avoid viruses, and how to use the Internet. Invest in high-speed Internet access to allow unlimited e-mailing, and use of distance learning and library search engines. Practice new computer skills prior to panicky deadlines. Acquaint yourself with the campus computer lab, for inevitable hardware breakdowns at home. Join a Users' Group or find a reliable friend to help you learn and keep learning. Have faith; it's all possible.

Be an Active Learner

Assert your desire to learn. Ask questions. Question discrepancies. Follow your interests. Share your enthusiasm and thinking. Get involved in interesting projects. Initiate. Explore. Seek out like-minded individuals. Accept opportunities.

Use All Your Best Survival Strategies

Do what you need to do to succeed. Sit in front in classes, tape lectures, find a tutor, schedule time with faculty, borrow materials, buy a computer, hire child care, eat healthy snacks, wear the glasses, and get comfortable. Don't waste energy worrying about not fitting in. In the long-run, it won't matter and may even be an advantage.

Don't Take Yourself Too Seriously

Relax. Sure you're different, but don't dwell on it. You're probably more okay and acceptable than you imagine. Contribute your perspective; so much the better if it is unique and interesting. Be yourself. Focus on what you can do rather than what you can't do. Smile a lot, stay sane, and do the best you can.

Be Your Best Ally

YOU are your own best friend and advisor. Listen to your inner self. Believe in yourself. Trust your intuition. Take care of your health—physical, mental, emotional, and spiritual. Make choices that support your success. And let yourself enjoy this fantastic opportunity.

Summary

Re-entry students face both academic, social, and family challenges as they enter physical therapy education. A positive attitude, combined with careful planning can help to reduce some of the predictable stresses involved in juggling academic and family demands. Students may benefit from using available on campus services such as counseling, child care, and financial aid to assist in meeting their needs.

References

1. Re-entry Center, California State University, Fresno. Fresno, CA; 2003.
2. *Return to College, A Resource and Planning Guide for California State University, Hayward Adult Students.* Hayward, CA: Adult Re-entry Services, California State University, Hayward; 1989.
3. Dill PL, Henley TB. Stressors of college: a comparison of traditional and nontraditional students. *J Psychol.* 1998;132(1):25-32.
4. Lawrence LP. The path to PT. *Phys Ther.* 1999;7(1):46-55.
5. USDOE. *Digest of Education Statistics.* Washington DC: United States Department of Education, National Center for Education Statistics; [2003].
6. Hayes SH, Fiebert IM, Carrol SR, Magill RN. Predictors of academic success in a physical therapy program: is there a difference between traditional and nontraditional students? *J Phys Ther Educ.* 1997;11(1):10-16.
7. Bradshaw MJ, Nugent K. Clinical learning experiences of nontraditional age nursing students. *Nurs Educ.* 1997;22(6):40,47.
8. Finkel D, Pedersen NL, Plomin R, McClearn GE. Longitudinal and cross-sectional twin data on cognitive abilities in adulthood: the Swedish adoption/twin study of aging. *Dev Psych.* 1998;34(6):1400-1413.
9. Ardila A, Rosselli M. Spontaneous language production and aging: sex and educational effects. *Int J Neurosci.* 1996;87(1-2):71-78.
10. Hislop HJ. Clinical decision making: educational, data, and risk factors. In: Wolf SL. *Clinical Decision Making in Physical Therapy.* Philadelphia, Pa: FA Davis Co; 1985.
11. Cole BH, Brunk Q. Six rules for computers and other stumbling blocks to obtaining an advanced degree. *J Contin Educ Nurs.* 1999;30(2):66-70.
12. Balogun JA, Hoeverlein-Miller ES, Katz JS. Academic performance is not a viable determinant of physical therapy students' burnout. *Percept Motor Skills.* 1996;83(1):21-22.

Additional Resources

National Association of Student Personnel Administrators (NASPA). *Adult Learner Network* Web page. Available at: http://www.naspa.org/network/ADULT.HTM. (This site provides national and regional network contact names and addresses for re-entry programs.)

Adult Learners/Commuter Students and Distance Learning Listserv. (To subscribe send email to listmanager@listserv.naspa.org with "join adult-learn" in body of message [no quotes].)

Joint Task Force on Student Learning Draft Position Paper, Web page. Available at: http://www.naspa.org/special/jointtask/draftpap.htm.

PUTTING IT INTO PRACTICE

1. Write down the contact information for your campus counseling center. If there is a web page, also write down the URL address.

   Name of Director:

   Campus Location:

   Telephone:

   Web site:

2. Interview another student in your class.
   What did he or she do prior to entering the PTA education program?

   What changes has your colleague made in his or her life since entering the program?

   Who else was influenced by your colleague's decision to enter the PTA education program?

   What emotional, academic, relationship, and/or financial stresses has this decision created?

   What similarities do you recognize in your own life?

   What differences have you experienced?

PART FIVE

Planting the Seeds
for a Bright Future

CHAPTER 16

Evidence-Based Practice in Physical Therapy

> *Nadine decided to do her paper on the effectiveness of magnet therapy, an alternative technique for pain management gaining considerable exposure in the medical literature. She collected articles and thought, "Even in the face of all this evidence, many people still don't believe that it works."*

Critical Thinking and Clinical Problem-Solving

Physical therapists (PTs) engage in critical thinking processes. *Critical thinking* involves the discipline, ability, and willingness to assess evidence and claims, to seek contradicting as well as confirming information, and to make objective judgments on the basis of well-supported reasons as a guide to belief and action.[1]

Physical therapist assistants (PTAs) work closely with physical therapists in *clinical problem-solving* in the work environment, within the context of delegated activities and within the established plan of care. Problem-solving activities involve recognition and identification of the problem, description of the problem, identification of possible solutions, and the consequences of those solutions. The PTA seeks assistance and consultation as needed prior to implementation of a solution.[2]

Both critical thinking and problem-solving require an active awareness of the thinking process. *Metacognition* is the process of monitoring and considering one's thoughts while in the thinking process. Awareness of choices and active involvement in determining the best way to make choices are key parts of the metacognitive process.[1]

Critical thinking requires the thinker to use a process characterized by clarity, accuracy, precision, consistency, relevance, sound evidence, good reasons, depth, breadth, and fairness. In contrast, clinical problem-solving exists within a carefully defined context and within limits of role and environmental constraints.

Remember that PTAs implement delegated patient interventions and modify those interventions within the *PT's established plan of care*. The problem-solving functions of the PTA involves the following components:[2]

* Within the process of patient management established by the PT, the PTA adjusts or withholds intervention based on patient status as determined through observation, data collection, and interpretive processes.
* The PTA possesses the requisite knowledge to identify the situation, weigh alternatives, and select appropriate responses within the plan of care established by the PT.
* The PTA demonstrates problem-solving skills.
* The PTA participates in patient status judgments by reporting changes to the supervising PT and requesting patient re-examination or revisions to interventions.

Evidence-Based Practice

> *Dr. Jenkins praised Nadine for her thoughtful and thorough analysis of the evidence supporting magnet therapy. He noted that consumers may have driven this movement. She approached Dr. Jenkins after class and asked, "I wanted to talk with you about your comment on my paper; how can I help consumers to get this information?" Dr. Jenkins suggested that she write an article for the campus newspaper summarizing the major findings reported in the literature.*

Evidence is information that tends to support something or show that something is true, such as clinical research or objective changes in function. Evidence-based practice involves the use of current best evidence in making decisions about the care of individual patients.[3]

Evidence-based practice de-emphasizes intuition, unsystematic observations of clinical experience, and the opinions of "authorities."[4] Evidence-based practice requires the critical analysis of evidence.

PTs who use evidence-based practice blend their individual clinical expertise and judgment with the best available external evidence. Thus, evidence might involve information about:

* The accuracy and precision of diagnostic tests and screening examinations (including clinical observations).
* The prediction of outcomes from various clinical findings.
* The efficacy and safety of therapeutic and preventive interventions.[2]

The demand for "evidence" comes from growing consumer-driven cost-consciousness, combined with increased accountability across the health care professions. Consumers and third-party payers have largely driven this movement, as information has become more widely available, across the Internet, through television and print media.

Types of Evidence

In describing evidence-based practice approaches, some authors have suggested several types of evidence:[1]

Empirical Evidence

Empirical evidence is obtained by objective observation, rather than reasoning or feeling. This is the type of evidence provided by research studies that meet currently accepted standards of design, execution, and analysis. Strong empirical evidence is derived from outcomes of experiments using rigorous controls and having clear, unequivocal outcomes.

Analogical Evidence

Analogical evidence involves comparing known similarities between two systems and hypothesizing that a relationship shown to exist in one system but unknown in the other also exists in the other. For example, this type of evidence might apply the findings of animal studies to justify interventions with humans. This type of evidence is considered weaker than empirical evidence because effects are hypothesized but not tested.

Anecdotal Evidence

An anecdote describes an experience in an individual or situation. A case report is an example of anecdotal evidence. Anecdotal evidence is considered the weakest of the three because it is difficult to repeat and difficult to draw any conclusion regarding the cause of an outcome. Even multiple case studies do not substantially add to the strength of anecdotal evidence.

Reviewing Scientific Merit

Research articles can be evaluated for their scientific merit.[5] Not everything that is written should be accepted as evidence. Researchers and clinicians can evaluate an article by examining the supporting theories and the design of studies that test a particular intervention approach.

Researchers are constantly challenged to meet stringent criteria. Not many studies of complex human phenomena such as education or rehabilitation are able to meet these criteria. When researchers design studies to test "real-life" conditions, they often must live with the constraints and ambiguities that everyday life presents. This is quite different than working with animals in a laboratory setting.

Further, the base of knowledge of what underlies the practice of physical therapy is vast and has been drawn from multiple disciplines over time. Theories are often contradictory and confusing. In addition, there is the problem of how to measure and what is measurable and what is not.

Qualitative researchers argue that there are other types of research that have scientific merit besides the randomized controlled clinical study.[6] Others contend that the complexity of the human condition is impossible to document with the requisite scientific rigor. Even if we believe it exists, we lack the tools at this point in time to measure energy flow, emotional discharge, or subtle changes in subjective well-being.[6,7]

The answer may lie in the approach that we take to thinking, decision making, and problem solving. Training in critical thinking and making good decisions are as important as understanding the mechanisms of physiology or pathology which underlie the approaches that we choose to take.

Evidence in Physical Therapy

Pamela Duncan was one of the first to write about evidence-based practice in physical therapy:

Advances in physical therapy will be possible only if we critically evaluate our assumptions and shift our paradigm. Although scientifically based models for interventions do exist in physical therapy, the current paradigm for practice is based for the most part on expert opinion and clinical experience. It is driven by many assumptions that guide education, clinical practice, and research.[8]

This paradigm shift involves the following.

Recasting the Role of Authority

Evidence-based practice places a much lower value on "authority." Opinions offered by experts can be evaluated using available evidence. Some argue that the knowledge and skill one gains from experience can never be measured in randomized controlled studies. The key here is that the importance of what authorities offer must be appraised and evaluated in the context of underlying evidence.

Peer-reviewed medical journals in many disciplines and specialty areas publish studies that provide such evidence. Physical therapists must look to the literature and to other disciplines in many cases for evidence supporting their practice.

Practicing by the Guide

In the absence of strong empirical evidence, we can refer to clinical practice guidelines. Clinical practice guidelines, such as those published in the *Guide to Physical Therapist Practice*, are written to assist practitioner and patient decisions about appropriate care for specific clinical circumstances. These guidelines were developed by consensus, by teams of clinicians and educators without an interest in a specific physical therapy intervention approach.[9] Practice guidelines assist in defining the boundaries of practice and provide an external reference when there is disagreement regarding the benefits of various interventions.

Looking at the Context in Which Evidence Exists

Just as a physical effect may be dependent on ambient conditions of temperature, light, and humidity, the mechanisms of response to a physical therapy intervention may be dependent on complex *biopsychosocial* phenomena that are more difficult to measure than objective physical phenomena.

The *biopsychosocial model* integrates theory from biology, psychology, anthropology, and sociology as an explanatory theme for health and health care. This model includes issues of health and wellness; spirituality; psychoneuroimmunology; methods of coping with disability, illness, or injury; ways to reduce stress; and smoking cessation.[10]

For example, many PTs would predict a better outcome for a patient with strong social support (such as a family) system to provide care. Most PTs would also rate a patient's prognosis more favorably if they were functioning independently prior to an illness or injury. How are these factors measured, or even considered in choosing a physical therapy intervention duration or a discharge destination?

We cannot draw conclusions about the consequences of the PT's decisions or the effects of physical therapy intervention without also considering evidence and the factors that may influence those outcomes. Valid, reliable, standardized assessment tools provide the best hope of quantifying the many factors that may interact to influence an outcome.

Comparing the Costs to the Benefits of Intervention

How much change in a condition can be expected? How much time and effort will it take to achieve and/or sustain that change? How expensive is the physical therapy intervention compared to the potential benefit that the patient will gain? Medicine is often accused of applying technology because it exists and has some small chance of changing an outcome. It often feels better to do "something" than to do nothing.

Timing It Right

The cost-benefit issue applies on an even larger scale when it comes to prevention. It is often far less costly to provide an intervention that *prevents* a disability than to treat that disability once it has developed. It may be even less costly to provide widespread screening to identify those at greatest risk for developing a disability and then provide individual physical therapy intervention to selected high-risk individuals.

The costs of providing care are usually calculated on an individual basis... the *costs to society of preventing* people from needing those services in the first place are unknown.

The Future

The future is clear... PTs must seek evidence to justify the physical therapy intervention they recom-

---
Table 16-1

EXAMPLES OF CLINICAL MANAGEMENT TASKS IN PHYSICAL THERAPY[2,12,13,14]

Typical Tasks for the Physical Therapist

Establish a differential diagnoses for patients across the lifespan based on evaluation of results of examinations and medical and psychosocial information.

Communicate or discuss diagnoses or clinical impressions with other practitioners.

Determine patient or client prognoses based on evaluation of results of examinations and medical and psychosocial information.

Collaborate with patients, clients, family members, payers, other professionals, and individuals to determine a realistic and acceptable plan of care.

Establish goals and functional outcomes that specify expected time duration.

Define achievable patient or client outcomes within available resources.

Deliver and manage a plan of care that complies with administrative policies and procedures of the practice environment.

Monitor and adjust the plan of care in response to patient or client status.

Typical Tasks for the Physical Therapist Assistant

Assist with data collection; assist the PT in performing components of tests and measures.

Communicate observations and data collected with the PT and with patient, family, and other health care professionals as appropriate.

Progress patients through the plan of care as established or delegated by the PT.

Offer suggestions to the PT based on the PTA's observations of patient status and performance.

Discuss indicators in patient status/performance related to goals that may result in need for PT to change plan of care.

Consider the influence of reimbursement policies on outcomes.

Follow established policies and procedures of the clinical setting.

Request patient re-examination or revisions to interventions when the patient's status warrants.

Reprinted with permission from APTA. *A Normative Model of Physical Therapist Assistant Education Version 99*. Alexandria, Va: American Physical Therapy Association; 1999; Evaluative Criteria for Accreditation of Education Programs for the Preparation of Physical Therapists [press release]. Alexandria, Va: American Physical Therapy Association; 1996. Available at: http://www.apta.org/pdfs/accreditation/ AppendixB-PT-Criteria.pdf.; Evaluative Criteria for Accreditation of Education Programs for the Preparation of Physical Therapist Assistants; and APTA. *Normative Model of Physical Therapist Professional Education. Version 2004*. Alexandria, Va: APTA; 2004, with permission of American Physical Therapy Association. This material is copyrighted, and any further reproduction or distribution is prohibited.

---

mend. Costly and time-consuming interventions without demonstrable effects are likely to be denied by third-party payers and refused by consumers.

In their *Vision 2020* statement, the American Physical Therapy Association House of Delegates addressed evidence-based care[11] (see Chapter 1 for the full statement):

> Guided by integrity, life-long learning, and a commitment to comprehensive and accessible health programs for all people, physical therapists and

> physical therapist assistants will render evidence-based service throughout the continuum of care and improve quality of life for society.

Evidence and Physical Therapy Clinical Management

In what instances do PTs and PTAs apply evidence to solve clinical problems? What evidence underlies the decisions that they make? Table 16-1 lists typical clinical problem-solving tasks in physical therapy practice, with distinction as to the roles of the PT and PTA.

Chapter 9 discussed information processing and ways to improve your attention to and understanding of the wealth of information available in the clinical environment. To what you pay attention may make a tremendous difference in sifting through and processing information. Let's look at the following tasks.

Setting Goals

Adam listened as his instructor said, "The physical therapist sets goals that are functional, realistic, measurable and achievable within time and resource constraint..." He thought to himself, "How do the patient's goals affect treatment planning?"

Who Cares and So What?

A goal "belongs" to a person who has an active interest in achieving it. Often this is the patient or client; perhaps we could also include the larger circle of family and care givers in the group of people who care about achieving the goal. This provides the "who" of "who cares?" Goals are more easily achieved when the patient and family are involved in the goal-setting process.

The "so what" question is easy to ask. What do you want to be able to do differently? This may be sleeping through the night, being able to work an 8-hour day, being able to get on and off the toilet, or getting in and out of the shower independently.

Goal-setting is a complex process which on a very simple level answers the above two questions. Goal-setting determines where you are going. Just as it would be difficult to take a trip without having a destination, a goal defines a target for the therapeutic intervention. If we want to travel 20 miles, we may design a different route than if we want to travel 200 miles.

How does the PT set goals, especially in projecting realistic time frames for the achievement of these goals?

The PT considers the following factors:

PRIOR LEVEL OF FUNCTION

Function is defined as one's ability to perform daily activities such as self-care, walking, climbing stairs, shopping, cooking, and working outside the home.[9] There are various scales that measure function.

Most evidence indicates that a higher premorbid (preinjury or illness) level of function is predictive of achievement of a higher level of function post-intervention.[15] Thus, physical therapists are more likely to have higher expectations of function for a patient who functioned independently prior to the current injury or illness.

SOCIAL SUPPORT

Social support is a key factor in quality of life and speed of recovery from illness or injury. Care givers in the home are a critical factor that influences physical therapist decision making regarding discharge destination.[16]

COMORBIDITY

Many patients and clients have multiple medical disorders that coexist as chronic illnesses. They may change a patient's prognosis in that a disorder such as diabetes may slow wound healing time or heart or kidney disease may influence tolerance for activities. PTs always take comorbidity into account when determining the patient or client's prognosis.

DISCHARGE PLAN

Recommending a discharge plan is a key part of the physical therapist's decision-making process. The PTA plays a role in communicating closely with the PT while delivering the established plan of care.

Discharge destination may be a function of the efficacy of physical therapy services and may largely determine future access to physical therapy services.[16] Patient safety, judgment, and cognition are often just as important as the patient's physical function. Of course, social support plays a key role in discharge planning decisions.

Outcomes Assessment

Evaluating outcomes is a key activity to gather evidence of the efficacy of physical therapy intervention. PTAs often collect data to assist the PT in monitoring the outcomes of physical therapy intervention.

On the simplest level, outcomes are the measure of whether you've reached your destination (the goal). From a more complex perspective, we can look at how effectively we have used our time or resources. In other words, what did it cost in time or resources to reach the goal?

Efficiency

Suppose my goal is to reach a destination 20 miles away. I can travel on country roads or on the freeway to this destination.

How much time does it take to travel 20 miles on narrow winding country roads compared to driving the same distance on the freeway? I can travel 20 miles in 1 hour on the country road. In comparison I can drive 20 miles in less than 20 minutes on the freeway.

The distance divided by the time it takes is a measure of *efficiency*.

Low Efficiency	High Efficiency
20 miles at 20 miles per hour = 1 hour	20 miles at 60 miles per hour (or 1 mile per minute) = 20 minutes

How efficient is a physical therapy intervention? Use the example above. It takes less time to accomplish the same goal using a *highly efficient* treatment.

Value

How many gallons of gasoline will it take to travel 20 miles? If I have a motor home, it may take as many as 5 gallons of gas to travel 20 miles. A new compact car may use less than a gallon.

Low Value	High Value
20 miles at 4 miles per gallon = 5 gallons	20 miles at 30 miles per gallon = .66 gallons

How cost-effective is a physical therapy intervention? Using the example above, it takes *less gas* to accomplish the same goal using a *high value* intervention.

Value x Efficiency

Continuing with the same example, we could take the same motor home on country roads or on the freeway. There are four possible methods to reach the outcome:

1. Choosing to drive the motor home on country roads to our destination wastes time and resources.
2. Choosing to drive the motor home on the freeway may save time but still is at a high cost.

3. Choosing the compact car and driving on country roads will save gas but it still takes a long time.
4. The obvious best choice—choosing the compact car and driving on the freeway—will save both time and resources.

	Low Efficiency	High Efficiency
Low Value	Takes a long time, costs more money. WORST OPTION.	Time saved may be offset by high costs.
High Value	Money saved may be offset by time lost.	Takes short time, costs less money. BEST OPTION.

Clinical Applications

With the current emphasis on accountability and cost-effectiveness, why would we choose a method that takes a long time and costs more money? Good question.

PTAs add value in contributing their skills and observations and gathering and communicating information to support the physical therapist's clinical judgment.

Evaluating the value and efficiency of the interventions we provide are keys to understanding the best choices we can make. Just as we may regret missing the scenery of the country road or the comfort of the motor home by making these choices, we must make some hard decisions regarding the best use of limited time and resources to provide health care. PTs make daily decisions to maximize time and staff resources.

Although this is a very simple example, it is easy to understand the principles of using evidence to support our intervention decisions. Various clinical tools provide quantifiable measures of function, balance, strength, or quality of life. We can easily measure the duration or frequency of a physical therapy intervention and its associated costs and do simple division to determine the efficiency and the value of physical therapy intervention provided.

With this information, PTs can make informed decisions and we can choose to compromise when we need to take a detour or stop on our path to reaching the destination.

APTA Hooked on Evidence

A Web-based resource is now available at: http://www.apta.org/hookedonevidence/index.cfm.

American Physical Therapy Association members may search a database of article extractions relevant to the field of physical therapy to build support for evidence-based practice. Clinical practice guidelines based on systematic reviews of the literature are also included at the site.

Summary

PTAs are involved in a variety of clinical problem-solving activities including collecting data, identifying any changes in the patient's status, and notifying the PT in a timely manner. Evidence-based practice requires a PT's analysis of intervention goals and related outcomes. The types of evidence offered may influence clinical decision making. Comparison of the time and resources spent to achieve a physical therapy outcome allow us to choose the most efficient and cost-effective interventions.

References

1. Gay, JM. General terms for epidemiology and evidence-based medicine, clinical epidemiology, and evidence-based medicine glossary. Available at: http://www.vetmed.wsu.edu/courses-jmgay/GlossClinEpiEBM.htm#. Accessed August 14, 2004.

2. APTA. *A Normative Model of Physical Therapist Assistant Education Version 99.* Alexandria, Va: American Physical Therapy Association; 1999.

3. Sacket DL, Rosenberg WMC, Gray JAM, Haynes RB, Richardson WS. Evidence based medicine: what it is and what it isn't. *BMJ.* 1996;312:71-72.

4. Lindberg DA, Hart YM, Sackett DL, et al. Evidence-based medicine: a new approach to teaching the practice of medicine. *JAMA.* 1992;268:2420-2425.

5. Harris SR. How should treatments be critiqued for scientific merit? *Phys Ther.* 1996;76:175-181

6. Berger D, Davis CM. What constitutes evidence?. *Phys Ther.* 1997;76(9):1011-1012,1014-1015.

7. Dorko B, Spielholz NI. Outside of Science: Where are the Data? *PT.* 1997;5(3):60-64.

8. Duncan PW. Evidence-based practice: A new model for physical therapy. *PT.* 1996;4(12):44-48.

9. APTA. *Guide to Physical Therapist Practice.* Alexandria VA: American Physical Therapy Association; 2001.

10. Bernard LC, Krupat E. *Health Psychology: Biopsychosocial Factors in Health and Illness.* London: Harcourt Brace; 1994.

11. American Physical Therapy Association Press Release. APTA House of Delegates endorses a vision for the future. Indianapolis, In, June 16, 2000. Available from: http://www.apta.org/news/vision-statementrelease. Accessed September 3, 2000.

12. Evaluative Criteria for Accreditation of Education Programs for the Preparation of Physical Therapists [press release]. Alexandria, Va: American Physical Therapy Association; 1996. Available at: http://www.apta.org/pdfs/accreditation/AppendixB-PT-Criteria.pdf. Accessed August 13, 2003.

13. Evaluative Criteria for Accreditation of Education Programs for the Preparation of Physical Therapist Assistants [pressr release]. Alexandria, Va: American Physical Therapy Association; 2000. Available at: http://www.apta.org/pdfs/accreditation/AppendixA-PTA-Criteria.pdf. Accessed August 13, 2003.

14. APTA. *Normative Model of Physical Therapist Professional Education. Version 2004.* Alexandria, Va: APTA; 2004.

15. Curtis KA, Crawford M, Johnson H, Knowles S, Metelnikow L: The influence of perceived prior level of function and social support on physical therapist projections of patient functional outcomes (abstract). In: *Proceedings of the 12th International Congress of the World Confederation for Physical Therapy.* Alexandria, Va: American Physical Therapy Association; 1995:125.

16. Roach KE, Ally D, Finnerty B, Watkins D, Litwin BA, Janz-Hoover B, Watson T, Curtis KA. The relationship between duration of physical therapy services in the acute care setting and change in functional status in patients with lower-extremity orthopedic problems. *Phys Ther.* 78:19-24, 1998

PUTTING IT INTO PRACTICE

1. Review a few pages of one of your current textbooks. What statements provide evidence to support a proposed intervention or recommended technique? Refer to the author, title, and page of the book you use.

2. Actively consider the problem-solving approaches you take to every day decisions. Give an example of a way in which you use evidence or data to make an every day decision.

CHAPTER 17

Information Competence

> Oxana prepared to begin her research for her clinical in-service presentation. She turned on her computer and opened the PubMed Web site. She thought to herself, "I am so much better at this than I was when I started a year ago. I don't know what I would have done without the help of these great librarians."

What is Information Competence?

Information competence is the process of finding, evaluating, using, and communicating information.[1] Our world has mushroomed with respect to available information. We are bombarded daily with television advertisements, telemarketing opportunities, e-mail, and new Web sites, in addition to traditional print resources such as newspapers, magazines, and books.

Information competence is a critical process to master as our abilities to find, process, and use information are critically linked to being able to undertake and integrate the key processes listed below:

* Recognize the need for information.
* Determine information requirements in various disciplines for the research questions, problems, or issues.
* Use information technology tools to locate and retrieve relevant information.
* Organize information.
* Utilize current and relevant information.
* Communicate using a variety of information resources and technologies.
* Understand the ethical and legal issues surrounding information and information technology.
* Apply the skills gained in information competence to enable lifelong learning.[1,2]

Researching the Topic (MEDLINE, CINAHL, Internet, Interviews)

The first step in finding information is knowing what you need to know and where to look. Both of these processes may depend on your ability to conceptualize your needs in language that is consistent with the ways in which this information is stored.

Key words become critical in searching for information. Key words follow established conventions for searching that are universally accepted by librarians and others who establish and maintain databases.

Medical Subject Headings

Medical Subject Headings (MeSH) are the controlled vocabulary used by the National Library of Medicine for indexing articles, for cataloging books and other holdings, and for searching MeSH-indexed databases, including MEDLINE. MeSH terminology provides a consistent way to retrieve information that may use different terminology for the same concepts.[3]

The National Library of Medicine offers an on-line browser that provides a guide to terminology. This tool is designed to help quickly locate descriptors of possible interest and to show the hierarchy in which these descriptors appear. The browser shows MeSH records and also provides qualifiers that will narrow a search. The URL for the browser is www.nlm.nih.gov/mesh/MBrowser.html.

Databases

Databases are indexed lists of resources, journal articles, conference proceedings, and other materials that are often discipline-specific. Some of the most useful databases for the health-related fields are MEDLINE, CINAHL, and PSYCINFO.

Table 17-1
HEALTH-RELATED ON-LINE RESOURCES

APTA Hooked on Evidence
www.apta.org/hookedonevidence/index.cfm

A database of article extractions relevant to the field of physical therapy to build support for evidence-based practice. Site also includes clinical practice guidelines based on systematic reviews of the literature.

HSTAT
http://hstat.nlm.nih.gov

Health Services/Technology Assessment Text is a searchable collection of large, full-text clinical practice guidelines, technology assessments, and health information.

MEDLINE Plus
http://medlineplus.gov

MEDLINE Plus has extensive information from the National Institutes of Health and other trusted sources on over 600 diseases and conditions. There are also lists of hospitals and physicians, a medical encyclopedia and a medical dictionary, health information in Spanish, extensive information on prescription and nonprescription drugs, health information from the media, and links to thousands of clinical trials. Updated daily, there is no advertising on this site, nor does MEDLINEplus endorse any company or product.

Pubmed MEDLINE
www.ncbi.nlm.nih.gov/PubMed

The National Library of Medicine's MEDLINE and Pre-MEDLINE Database (WWW Access). This is the gold standard for MEDLINE searches.

MEDLINE: 1966 TO PRESENT

Provided by the National Library of Medicine, this database indexes thousands of medical journals published throughout the world. Primarily for health professionals, this is the most comprehensive database of medical literature available. Not all journals are indexed in MEDLINE. For example, although the journals *Physical Therapy* (*Phys Ther*) and *Journal of Orthopaedic and Sports Physical Therapy* (*JOSPT*) are indexed in this data base, *PT—The Magazine of Physical Therapy* is not.

CINAHL (CUMULATIVE INDEX OF NURSING AND ALLIED HEALTH LITERATURE): 1982 TO PRESENT

CINAHL contains over 250 000 references to journal articles, meeting abstracts, audiovisuals, and dissertations in nursing and allied health sciences. This index covers over 1000 nursing, allied health, biomedical, and consumer health journals. CINAHL also provides access to healthcare books, nursing dissertations, selected conference proceedings, stan-

dards of professional practice, and educational software in nursing. Additional physical therapy related resources are indexed in CINAHL.

PSYCINFO: 1967 TO PRESENT

The American Psychological Association's index to 1300 journals covering all aspects of psychology,. PSYCINFO also indexes books, chapters in books, technical reports, and dissertations. This is the first place to look for published research in psychology.

Most databases today exist on-line or on CD-ROM and are accessible in libraries. Take a look at the data bases listed in Table 17-1. Your access to a database, however, may be limited. There may be a fee or you may have to register as a student to gain access to a library's databases.

There are also many on-line databases that provide access to health-related literature. In addition, your library probably provides access to many additional resources. Consult with the reference librarian in your library to guide you to these resources.

Let's see how it works.

Table 17-2

SAMPLE MeSH BROWSER OUTPUT

MeSH Heading: Osteosarcoma

Tree Number: C04.557.450.565.575.650

Tree Number: C04.557.450.795.620

Annotation / blood supply / chem / second / secret / ultrastruct permitted; coord IM with BONE NEOPLASMS (IM) or specific precoord bone/neopl term (IM) or specific bone (IM) + BONE NEOPLASMS (IM)

Scope Note: A sarcoma originating in bone-forming cells, affecting the ends of long bones. It is the most common and most malignant of sarcomas of the bones, and occurs chiefly among 10- to 25-year-old youths. (From Stedman, 25th ed)

Entry Term: Sarcoma, Osteogenic

Allowable Qualifiers: BL BS CF CH CI CL CN CO DH DI DT EC EH EM EN EP ET GE HI IM ME MI MO NU PA PC PP PS PX RA RH RI RT SC SE SU TH UL UR US VE VI

Online Note: use OSTEOSARCOMA to search SARCOMA, OSTEOGENIC 1966-88

History Note: 89; was SARCOMA, OSTEOGENIC 1963-88

Unique ID D012516

Payton was preparing a case study on a 12-year-old-girl with whom she worked during her last clinical experience. The patient had a diagnosis of osteogenic sarcoma, a malignant bone tumor. She wanted to research the functional outcomes of limb-sparing surgical procedures in MEDLINE. On entering the term "osteogenic sarcoma," she initially found 14,198 articles!

Narrowing the Search

When there are too many references, we can have a database do the work for us. By using the MeSH browser, we can find the terms under which the best articles should be indexed.

For example, on entering the search term *osteogenic sarcoma*, the MeSH browser tells us that the correct terminology for searching MEDLINE is *osteosarcoma*. When this term is entered, the output in Table 17-2 results. It also gives us a possible qualifier "RH," which stands for rehabilitation. We can use this qualifier to narrow the search by placing "/RH" after our search term *osteosarcoma*.

Payton runs a MEDLINE search using the term "osteosarcoma/RH" and finds 32 articles. She selects three that seem most applicable. She searches through the key words (MH) in the output for other possible search terms.

The MEDLINE output of one of these articles is listed in Table 17-3. We can widen or further our search by using terms listed under MH. This is often

helpful, as there may be terms that we haven't used in initiating this type of search.

Internet Directories and Search Engines

To search the Internet, it may be helpful to use either a search engine and/or a directory. Not everybody understands the difference and when it's best to use one or the other.

Directories

Directories provide lists of Web sites, categorized by topic area with brief descriptions. The categories and descriptions are based on submissions by Web site masters, reviewed and edited by professional or volunteer editors. The following are examples of directories:

* Yahoo: http://dir.yahoo.com
* Librarian's Index to the Internet: http://lii.org

Search Engines

In contrast to a directory, which categorizes Web sites and contains very little information about them (just the description), a search engine indexes all the information on all the Web pages it finds.

A Web site might have a few, hundreds, or thousands of pages. The search engine sends out robot programs (called "crawlers") that bring back the full text of the pages they find.

Table 17-3
SAMPLE MEDLINE OUTPUT

One result of the search using osteosarcoma/RH

```
UI  -  93129098
AU  -  Frieden RA
AU  -  Ryniker D
AU  -  Kenan S
AU  -  Lewis MM
TI  -  Assessment of patient function after limb-sparing surgery
LA  -  Eng
MH  -  Adolescence
MH  -  Bone neoplasms/rehabilitation/surgery
MH  -  Child
MH  -  Early Ambulation
MH  -  Female
MH  -  Femoral neoplasms/rehabilitation/*surgery
MH  -  Gait
MH  -  Human
MH  -  Joint prosthesis/*rehabilitation
MH  -  Male
MH  -  Osteosarcoma/*rehabilitation/*surgery
MH  -  Outcome assessment (health care)
MH  -  Physical therapy/methods
MH  -  Range of motion, articular
MH  -  Sarcoma, Ewing's/rehabilitation/surgery
PT  -  JOURNAL ARTICLE
DA  -  19930211
DP  -  1993 Jan
IS  -  0003-9993
TA  -  Arch Phys Med Rehabil
PG  -  38-43
SB  -  A
SB  -  M
CY  -  UNITED STATES
IP  -  1
VI  -  74
JC  -  8BK
AA  -  Author
EM  -  199304
```

AB - Cancer rehabilitation is becoming more of a focus for the field of physiatry due to increased longevity and the side effects of treatment. In order to investigate the rehabilitation needs of patients undergoing limb-sparing procedures, chart analysis was conducted on 17 children treated for primary bone tumors by resection and an expandable endoprosthetic replacement. Each patient underwent a course of postoperative inpatient and outpatient physical therapy and was followed over an average of 2.5 years. Gait training was relatively straightforward and in seven patients required neither orthosis nor ambulatory aid. The other 10 patients walked with a knee orthosis, axillary crutches, or both. Until the time came for reoperation to lengthen the implant, a shoe lift of 1 in maximum was added to compensate for the limb length discrepancy. These findings compare favorably with the more complex requirements of high proximal amputees with external prostheses, including more difficult gait training and the need for frequent adjustments, as well as prosthetic replacement as the children grow. It is clear that children undergoing limb-sparing surgery have special needs that should be addressed, including early mobilization, gait training, adjustment to repeated brief hospitalizations for lengthening, and continued follow-up to monitor their activity restriction.

AD - Department of Rehabilitation Medicine, Mount Sinai Medical Center, Mount Sinai School of Medicine, New York, NY 10029.
PMID - 0008420518
EDAT - 1993/01/01 00:00
MHDA - 1993/01/01 00:00
SO - Arch Phys Med Rehabil. 1993 Jan;74(1):38-43.

Table 17-4
CRITERIA FOR EVALUATING ARTICLES[4]

1. How recent is this source? Is it written in the last 2 to 5 years? Are there more recent sources?
2. Is it a primary or secondary source? Is it a review article, a position paper, or a research report?
3. Is there a single author or multiple contributors? With what institution(s), universities, or medical centers are the authors affiliated?
4. Who is the intended audience? Is it a scientific or scholarly journal or a popular magazine or newspaper article?
5. What theoretical approaches or methodologies are used?
6. What findings, facts, or statistics are useful to you? What new information does this source provide?

The search engine indexes every word of every page found by its numerous crawlers. It organizes this information not just by the words, but by the order of the words, so you can search for phrases or entire sentences. The following are examples of search engines:

* Google: www.google.com
* AltaVista: www.altavista.com
* HotBot: www.hotbot.com
* Lycos: www.lycos.com

There are even search engines that search in multiple search engines simultaneously.

* DogPile: www.dogpile.com/info.dogpl. Searches 13 Web search engines, six Usenet sources, as well as two FTP archives.
* Ask Jeeves!: www.ask.com. User can enter his or her own language to search the Ask Jeeves database as well as other search engines.
* Hotsheet: www.hotsheet.com. Provides access to both search and multi-search engines, as well as links to wire services, investing services, and much more.
* MetaCrawler: www.metacrawler.com. Searches six search engines and produces a ranked, annotated list of sites.

Evaluating the Quality of the Information You Find (Refereed Journals, Books, Internet)

The various searches may turn up journal articles, Internet-based bibliographies, testimonials and commercial sources selling medical products. The next step is to evaluate the credibility of the source. Tables 17-4 and 17-5 below give some useful tips for evaluating articles and Internet resources.

Organizing Information

Once the search is done, the next step is to organize the information. It may be helpful to use outlines, two-dimensional grids, or more flexible mapping techniques.[5] Examples are given below:

Outline

An outline is useful to list and categorize information. This is always a good start to classify and list information.

Osteosarcoma

I. Prevalence and incidence
II. Pathology
III. Non-surgical treatment
    A. Radiation
    B Adjuvant chemotherapy
IV. Surgical treatment
    A.. Amputation
    B.. Limb-saving approaches
V. Rehabilitation issues
    A. Timing
    B. Gait training
    C. Complications
VI. Case study

Two-Dimensional Grid

This method is often useful to compare and contrast approaches, techniques or sources of information by pre-determined categories.

It might be useful in this case to contrast the outcomes of amputation and limb-saving procedures by some predetermined categories. Under each category, one could list articles that address the relevant categories (Figure 17-1).

Table 17-5

CRITERIA FOR EVALUATING INTERNET RESOURCES[4]

1. Who is the intended audience of the page, based on its content, tone, and style? Does this meet your needs?

2. What is the source of this information? Web search engines often amass vast results, from memos to scholarly documents. Many of the resulting items will be peripheral or useless for your research.

3. Is there an identifiable author/producer? Does this author have expertise on the subject or published credentials? You may need to trace back in the URL (Internet address) to view a page in a higher directory with background information.

4. What is the location of the site? Is it the site of a larger institution? Sponsor/location of the site is appropriate to the material as shown in the URL.

    Examples:

    .edu for educational or research material

    .gov for government resources

    .org for non-profit organization

    .info for individuals or businesses to publish information

    .com or .biz for commercial products or commercially-sponsored sites

    A name(~NAME) in the URL may mean a personal home page with no official sanction.

5. Is there a "Mail-to link" that is offered for submission of questions or comments?

6. Is the information referenced? Just because it is written, it is not necessarily true. Web sites are rarely refereed or reviewed, in contrast to scholarly journals and books. The source of the information should be clearly stated, whether original or summarized from elsewhere.

7. Is the information comprehensive, or does it cover a specific time period or aspect of the topic?

8. Is the information current? Has the site been updated recently?

9. Are links relevant and appropriate? Do they work? Is there a SEARCH function on the site?

Figure 17-1. Sample two-dimensional grid.

Surgical Treatment	Author, Year	Long-Term Survival	Sensory and Motor Function	Gait
Amputation				
Amputation				
Amputation				
Limb-saving procedure				
Limb-saving procedure				

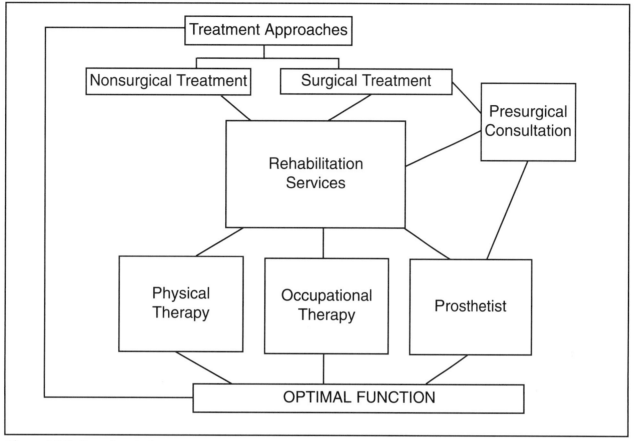

Figure 17-2. Sample mind map.

The Concept Map

The "mind-map" provides a flexible means to portray and relate information. The "mapper" sketches concepts and draws relationships between them. See the mind map above (Figure 17-2). The value of this approach to organizing information is the ability to include relationships, contingencies and feedback systems.

Summary

Acquiring, evaluating, and using information may be technically complex and overwhelming. Information competence involves using effective strategies for searching, organizing and presenting information. Attention to the technical aspects of searching literature and databases will accelerate the acquisition of relevant information. Developing skills in information competence will assist the student to effectively search the literature and use the information found appropriately.

References

1. Gavilan Community College Library. *Information Competence Plan for the California Community Colleges* Web page. Available at: http://gavilan.cc.ca.us/library/infocomp/intro.html#what Accessed September 28, 2004.

2. California State University, Northridge Library. Information Competence. *A Set of Core Competencies* Web page. Available at: http://library.csun.edu/susan.curzon/corecomp.html. Accessed September 28, 2004.

3. USDHHS. *Searching PubMed in Gratefully Yours.* Bethesda, Md: US Department of Health and Human Services, Public Health Service, National Institutes of Health, National Library of Medicine. 1998:7

4. Curtis KA. *Library assignment, UNIV 001, University Orientation.* Fresno, Calif: California State University, Fresno; 1998.

5. Carter C, Bishop J, Kravits SL. *Keys to Effective Learning.* Upper Saddle River, NJ: Prentice-Hall; 1998.

PUTTING IT INTO PRACTICE

1. Go the PubMed Web site: www.ncbi.nlm.nih.gov/PubMed:

2. Enter a topic (word or phrase) for a search:

3. Enter the number of articles you found:

4. Narrow the search using the MeSH browser, located at: http://www.ncbi.nlm.nih.gov:80/entrez/mesh-browser.cgi:

5. What MeSH terms are applicable for your topic?

6. Enter the number of articles you found using this term:

7. Narrow the search using a qualifier by following the MeSH term with /[qualifier].
   List of possible qualifiers:
   BL BS CF CH CI CL CN CO DH DI DT EC EH EM EN EP ET GE HI IM ME MI MO NU PA:PC PP PS PX RA RH RI RT SC SE SU TH UL UR US VE VI

8. Now how many articles did you find?

9. Select and print one or two of the abstracts that look most applicable to your interests.

CHAPTER 18

Diversity and Cultural Competence in Physical Therapy

> *Russell opened his mailbox and saw the letter from the physical therapist assistant program where he had applied. He opened the letter quickly and scanned the text. "You have been admitted, pending successful completion of all prerequisites courses prior to beginning the program." He ran into his apartment to tell his roommates. Only Sam was home. He congratulated Russell and asked if he would be the only African-American male in the program.*

Diversity in the Physical Therapy Profession

Who works in the physical therapy profession? Take a look at the demographics of the physical therapist assistant (PTA) and physical therapist (PT) membership of the American Physical Therapy Association (APTA) in Figures 18-1, 18-2, and 18-3. As you can see, the profession of physical therapy includes members of all age and ethnic groups. By these comparisons, we can see that the majority of PTAs and PTs are under age 45, female, and white.[1]

Almost 65% of PTs and 70% of PTAs fall between the ages of 25 and 44. In contrast, PTs are most likely to provide care to the elderly, 35 million strong and growing in numbers daily.[2]

Estimates indicate that there are approximately 120,000 licensed PTs and over 38,000 licensed PTAs in practice in the United States.[3] Even though that seems like a large number, this amounts to less than one PT or PTA for every 1700 people who live in the United States today. In sum, this amounts to a national average of 54.7 PTs and PTAs for every 100,000 people in our population.[2,3] Even though women outnumber men in physical therapy 2 to 1, recent surveys indicate that there are widespread inequities in salary and positions by gender.[4]

Comparing the Demographics of Those Who Provide Physical Therapy Services to the US Population

The US population estimates have quite different demographics when compared to the members of the physical therapy profession.[1,2,5] There are large differences between the distribution of PTs, PTAs, and the general population by age, gender, and ethnicity. It is likely that physical therapy staff will be providing *services to persons unlike themselves in age group, gender, or ethnic origins*. It is critical that PTs and PTAs have the skills to deliver physical therapy services across this diverse population.

The population of the United States is becoming even more culturally diverse. Over 30% of the US population is currently comprised of people from African-American/Black, Hispanic/Latino, Asian-American, Native Hawaiian or other Pacific Islander, and American Indian/Alaska Native backgrounds.[1] By 2050, projections are that people from the above groups will comprise 47% of the US population.[6] In contrast to the US population, there are *just over 10%* of APTA members (either PTs or PTAs) from these same backgrounds.[5]

Figure 18-1. Comparison of APTA members and US population estimates by age group (adapted from APTA. *Surveys and Stats* Web page. Available at: http://www.apta.org/Research/survey_stat. Accessed September 27, 2004 and US Census. Profile of General Demographic Characteristics, 2000. Available from: http://www.census.gov/Press-Release/www/2001/tables/dp_us_2000.PDF. Accessed September 24, 2004).

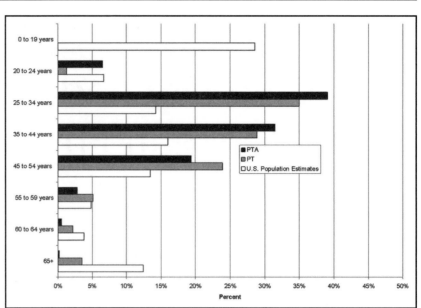

Figure 18-2. Comparison of APTA members and US population by gender (adapted from APTA. *Surveys and Stats* Web page. Available at: http://www.apta.org/Research/survey_stat. Accessed September 27, 2004 and US Census. Profile of General Demographic Characteristics, 2000. Available from: http://www.census.gov/Press-Release/www/2001/tables/dp_us_2000.PDF. Accessed September 24, 2004).

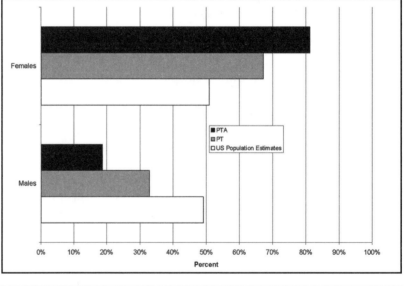

Figure 18-3. Comparison of APTA members and US population by ethnic group/race (adapted from APTA. *Surveys and Stats* Web page. Available at: http://www.apta. org/Research/survey_stat. Accessed September 27, 2004 and US Census. Profile of General Demographic Characteristics, 2000. Available from: http://www.census.gov/Press-Release/www/2001/tables/dp_us_2000.PDF. Accessed September 24, 2004).

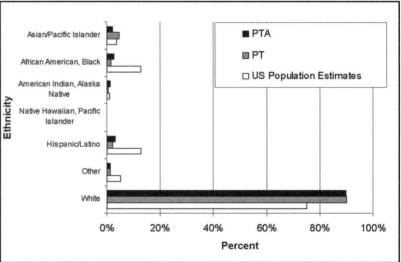

Table 18-1
ETHNICITY OF RECENT PHYSICAL THERAPIST ASSISTANT GRADUATES

| | Year of Graduation | | | | |
	1997	1998	1999	2000	2001
Number of Graduates	5090	5727	5455	3390	4433
African-American	3.1%	3.4%	3.9%	6.7%	5.5%
American Indian/Alaskan Native	0.5%	0.6%	0.5%	0.6%	0.4%
Asian/Pacific Islander	2.1%	3.0%	3.0%	3.4%	3.4%
Hispanic/Latino	4.2%	4.6%	5.4%	8.2%	7.3%
White	88.5%	86.3%	85.6%	81.3%	82.7%
Other	0.8%	0.8%	1.0%	0.7%	0.9%
Unknown	0.6%	0.8%	0.4%	0.4%	0.9%

Adapted from APTA. 2002 fact sheet physical therapist assistant education programs, December 2002. Available at: https://www.apta.org/pdfs/accreditation/PTAFactSheet2002.pdf. Accessed September 24, 2004.

Although it would be optimal to have comparable representation of all ethnic groups within the staff of the physical therapy setting, it is more important that physical therapy staff, regardless of their own ethnic background, become culturally competent.

Increased Minority Representation Among Students

The APTA is committed to enhancing cultural diversity and awareness of differences in the profession of physical therapy. The APTA's activities are directed toward promoting minority representation among the APTA membership and leadership; recruiting minority students, educators, and researchers; toward inclusion of issues of cultural diversity in physical therapy educational programs; and toward promoting physical therapy service delivery to minority group members. There are scholarships, educational materials, workshops, fund-raising events, and public relations efforts that are committed to realizing this agenda.

The news is improving as we look at who is graduating from PTA educational programs. Recent data indicates that 15% to 20% of PTA program graduates are members of minority groups[7] (Table 18-1). However, this encouraging data is only the beginning. Profession-wide initiatives will continue to foster increased minority participation in PT and PTA education and practice.[6]

Culture

> Tracy was assigned for a 3-week practicum to a clinic that provides health care services to migrant farm workers. Although many of the clinic staff members were bilingual, Tracy struggled to communicate in Spanish. Her patients seemed to appreciate her efforts and she was surprised on her last day when a patient and his wife brought her a large plate of tamales.

Culture provides a lens through which people see their world and largely determines the characteristics of their community and family life.[8-13] A *cultural group* shares values, norms, symbols, language, and living practices that are repeated and transmitted from one generation to another. Culture goes far beyond race and ethnicity. Where you live, your lifestyle, and age often form values that cross ethnic and racial lines.

We traditionally associate the term *culture* with the food, music, dance, and clothing that are unique to groups of people. Although cultures differ from one another, there are also subgroups within cultures. We don't always associate the concept of culture or subculture with the values of a professional group or roles within organizations. Yet we experience the effects of these cultures daily.

Table 18-2

CULTURAL VOCABULARY[8-11]

Beliefs	Acceptance of something as true.
Culture	The learned and shared knowledge, beliefs, and rules that people use to interpret experience and to generate social behavior. The guiding force behind the behaviors and material products associated with a group of people.
Cultural competence	A set of practice skills, knowledge, and attitudes that encompasses: 1) Awareness and acceptance of difference; 2) awareness of one's own cultural values; 3) understanding of the dynamics of difference; 4) development of cultural knowledge; 5) ability to adapt practice skills to fit the cultural context of the client or patient.
Cultural group	A group of people who consciously or unconsciously share identifiable values, norms, symbols, and some ways of living that are repeated and transmitted from one generation to another.
Culture shock	A form of anxiety that results from an inability to predict the behavior of others, or act appropriately in a cross-cultural situation.
Ethnicity	A group identity based on culture, language, religion, or a common attachment to a place or kin ties.
Ethnocentrism	The interpretation of the beliefs and behavior of others in terms of one's own cultural values and traditions with the assumption that one's own culture is superior.
Intracultural differences	Variations within a cultural group, possibly related to acculturation, socioeconomic status or individual, family, or regional differences.
Language	The form or pattern of speech (spoken or written) used by residents or descendants of a particular nation or geographic area or by any large body of people. Language can be formal or informal and includes dialect, idiomatic speech, and slang.
Norms	A standard, model, or pattern for a group.
Social customs	A usual practice carried on by tradition by a group.
Values	Acts, customs, and institutions regarded as especially favorable by a group.

Cross-cultural experiences involve our moving into a different culture. Although we often associate this term with experiencing the customs of a different ethnic group, we can use this term in many contexts. For example, students within universities live within a very specific subculture of the university; they often find it difficult to make the transition to the subculture of work upon graduation.

Cultural competence is a term that describes a set of skills that grow from the foundation that culture is the key force in shaping behaviors, values, and institutions, including some concepts like family and community.[8-10] Providers, clients, and patients have unique, culture-specific needs that influence service delivery. This perspective encompasses the view that people from different racial and ethnic groups can be best served by persons who are part of or sensitive to their culture.

A Culture of One

There is no "one way" to provide services for a person from a particular racial and ethnic group. We need instead to develop interventions that are individualized and offered to patients and families with their own unique needs in mind.

Despite a person's ethnicity, geographical area of origin, occupation, disability, sexual preference, gender, or age, he or she may be quite different from others who share these identifying characteristics. Appreciating the *culture of one* requires an appreciation of the unique characteristics of every person. There is wide variation within every culture (*intracultural differences*) and therefore a care provider must be sensitive, not only to the cultural context in which a person lives, but also sensitive to the individual's needs.

Table 18-3

CULTURAL AWARENESS EXERCISE

Answer the following questions to test your cultural awareness:

1. Someone in your workplace has practices different from your own. This might involve a religious practice, a style of dress or lifestyle. How do you react? Are you judgmental or critical of this person either openly or silently?

2. What diverse groups of individuals live in your neighborhood, or attend school or work with you? How are different cultural practices honored? How do you feel about a colleague requesting a delay of an examination or asking for a day off from work for celebration of ethnic or religious holidays?

3. How were you raised as a child? What are your cultural origins? What beliefs, stories, and values did your family share with you? How did your upbringing differ from those of your friends and neighbors? What did you learn about alternate lifestyles or belief systems? If you have children, what beliefs, stories, and values do you share with them? How would you feel about your children, nephews, or nieces learning about alternate lifestyles or belief systems? What might you teach them?

4. What health behaviors do you practice that are related to culture? How much are the foods you eat, your attitudes about sickness and health, and the care you seek when you are ill influenced by your cultural beliefs? How tolerant would you be of a patient or client who failed to change the behavior (such as a dietary habit) that resulted in a serious and preventable health problem?

5. What are your expectations in receiving health care? How do you feel about receiving expert care that is insensitive to your experience, beliefs, or family situation? What assumptions does your health care provider make about you or a family member? What recommendations of a health care provider have you or a family member ignored because they did not fit with your lifestyle, your traditional diet, or social customs?

See how aware you are of the language of culture. Which of the terms in Table 18-2 are familiar to you? Let's look more closely at your culture and how it may affect the expectations you have of others.

Assess your cultural awareness. The questions in Table 18-3 may stimulate you to critically assess your beliefs and practices with persons from cultures different from yours.

If some of the situations in Table 18-3 made you feel uncomfortable or question your tolerance, be assured that you are normal. Cultural competence involves gaining an awareness of your values and the common experiences around differences, so that you can develop the skills to provide culturally appropriate services.

The Continuum of Cultural Proficiency

Victor had grown up outside of Paris, as the son of a US diplomat. He considered himself an international and cultural expert. "All people are the same; I treat everyone equally, regardless of their race, ethnicity, religion or sexual preference." I am intolerant of anyone else who does not do the same.

Can you rate Victor's awareness of cultural issues on the scale shown in Table 18-4?

Although helping professionals are motivated to provide high quality care, they may approach this area with blinders. Although Victor acknowledges the value of culturally sensitive care, his assertion that all people are the same may prevent him from further developing his cultural proficiency. His "equal treatment for all" approach may limit his effectiveness as a clinician.

In contrast, the culturally proficient clinician accepts and respects difference and seeks innovative approaches to enhance cultural competence in service delivery.

Implications of Culture on Physical Therapy Practice

The following are just a few areas in which culture may have a profound influence in what PTs, PTAs, their patients, and clients experience.[9,10,13-16]

Table 18-4
The Continuum of Cultural Competence

Stage	Name	Definition
1	Cultural destructiveness	People are treated in dehumanizing manner and are denied services on purpose.
2	Cultural incapacity	Unable to work with patients from other cultures effectively; bias, paternalism, and stereotypes exist.
3	Cultural blindness	Presumption is that all people are the same and that no bias exists; policies and practice do not recognize the need for culturally specific approaches to problem solving; services are ethnocentric and encourage assimilation; patients are blamed for their problems.
4	Cultural precompetence	Committed to using appropriate response to cultural differences; weaknesses are acknowledged and alternatives are sought.
5	Cultural competence	Cultural differences are accepted and respected; continuous expansion of cultural knowledge and resources and continuous adaptation of services occur; continue self-assessment about culture and vigilance toward the dynamics of cultural differences exist.
6	Cultural proficiency	Cultural differences are highly regarded; the need for research on cultural differences and the development of new approaches to enhance culturally competent practice is recognized.

Adapted from Leavitt RL. Developing cultural competence in a multicultural world, part I. *PTmagazine of Physical Therapy*. 2002; 10 (12):36-48.

Health Beliefs

> Whitney felt the lump in her breast for months before she mentioned it to anyone. By the time she visited the clinic, the lump had doubled in size. A biopsy showed an invasive intraductal carcinoma, almost 2.0 cm in diameter. The oncology nurse encouraged the PTA students to explore the patient's beliefs to understand why she waited to seek attention.

Health beliefs are related to our perceptions of our vulnerability and the seriousness of an illness or injury. We also hold beliefs about our likelihood of recovery and the seriousness of the problem. Health beliefs and related fears may keep a person from taking action or may cause a patient to seek assistance for an alternative healer.

Cultural Beliefs

> Yasmine waited nervously in the chairs outside the clinic doors. Armando, the student PTA, called her name. She asked, "Excuse me, I'd prefer to be seen by a female therapist. Is that possible?" Armando asked Beatrice, his supervisor, to work with Yasmine. Beatrice, afterwards, complimented Armando on his cultural sensitivity and told him that the patient's religious beliefs did not permit her to disrobe in front of a man.

Cultural beliefs may dictate assignment of a physical therapy staff member of the same gender. It may not be acceptable for male staff to provide care to female patients or for female staff to care for male patients. Beliefs may also preclude some forms of physical therapy intervention.

Concepts of Time

Time is a culturally defined phenomenon. "Early" and "late" are cultural concepts. Physical therapy staff may be quite surprised or frustrated by the unexpected or delayed arrival of a patient.

Food and Lifestyle Habits

Diet, exercise, "Type A" behavior, stress, and expectations of ourselves are all influenced by culture. It may be very difficult to change behavior, even when unhealthy due to the strong influence of the family, the environment, social customs, and habits. Consider how difficult it would be to change foods when a certain dish symbolizes prosperity, love or hope.

Meaning of Illness, Aging, and Death in Patient Culture

The meaning of an illness or death within a culture largely determines actions around these events. You can imagine that advice regarding prevention or healing might be taken quite differently by people who see illness as the effect of an external force out of one's control and people who believe that illness has internal causes that can be controlled.

> Mrs. Chen fractured her hip in a fall in her bedroom. This was the third hospital admission in the past 6 months. Although the orthopedic team recommended placement in a subacute facility, her son and daughter-in-law insisted on home-based rehabilitation services. She was discharged 2 days later.

Are the elderly valued and revered or discounted as a burden? Cultural beliefs may determine the structure of the health care system as well. In some cultures, placing a loved one in a long-term care facility is an unthinkable option.

Health Disparities, Access, and Outcomes

The Institute of Medicine (IOM) in its 2002 publication, *Unequal Treatment: Confronting Racial and Ethnic Disparities in Health Care* reported that regardless of a patient's insurance status or income, individuals from racial and ethnic minority groups tend to receive a lower quality of health care than do members of nonminority group. The study documented that stereotyping, biases, and uncertainty on the part of health care providers all contribute to unequal treatment.[17]

A failure to recognize the influence of language or culture can easily lead to undesirable health outcomes. The IOM report documented numerous examples of poor outcomes related to language barriers and cultural misunderstandings.

For example, findings indicate that patients with limited English proficiency (LEP) are less likely to visit physicians and receive preventive services, regardless of economic status, source of care, literacy, health status, or insurance status.[17]

Patients with LEP also report lower rates of satisfaction with their care. Researchers have found that patients who did not speak the same language as their provider were more likely to miss appointments or drop out of treatment. Findings indicate that using interpreters seems to eliminate the likelihood of missed appointments.[17]

Developing Cultural Competence

Students will have many opportunities to develop cultural competence. Take this responsibility seriously. Culturally-sensitive care is your responsibility as a health care provider.

Developing cultural competency involves identification of personal cultural biases, understanding general cultural differences, accepting and respecting cultural differences, and the application of cultural understanding.[13] Study, practice, and reflection are essential processes to develop cultural competence. The following considerations are all important aspects of culturally proficient care.[8-16]

Show Respect

Demonstrate respect for the diverse cultures, heritages and experiences of the patients you encounter. Gain experience in working with racially, ethnically, and culturally diverse populations. Seek experiences which challenge you to work with individuals who are unlike yourself.

Develop Self-Awareness

> Dorian, a student PTA, was assigned to the spinal cord injury unit. Her patient had sustained a spinal cord injury just 2 weeks earlier. She was not hopeful that he would regain muscle function, as his injury was complete and he had no signs of neurological function below the level of the spinal cord lesion. She approached his room on Tuesday afternoon and was told a healing session was in progress and that he would not be finished for at least another hour. Dorian felt inconvenienced and wondered later why the hospital would allow such practices.

Examine the influence of the similarities and differences of your own culture, ethnicity, language, and/or race on your interactions with others. Identify how your own biases might influence service delivery. Examine how your values may conflict with the needs of the individual. Recognize the need to address these differences and possibly refer the patient to another provider to achieve the most desirable outcomes.

Learn As Much As You Can

Read about the differences in cultures related to history, traditions, values, belief systems, reasons for immigration, dialect, and language fluency. Examine particular stressors and traumas that a group of people may have experienced, related to war, trauma or violence, political unrest, racism, or discrimination. Identify unique aspects of cultural survival and maintenance, socioeconomic status, and culturally-based belief systems.

Communicate in Many Ways

Develop sensitivity to verbal and nonverbal language, speech patterns, and communication styles. Incorporate sensitivity to the potential influence of psychological, social, biological, physiological, cultural, political, spiritual, and environmental aspects of the patient or client's experience.

Services for the non-English speaking patient should include informing him or her that he or she has the right to receive no-cost interpreter services. Signs and commonly used written patient education materials should be translated for the predominant language groups in a service area.

Try to use the patient/client's preferred language whenever possible. Use interpreters as needed when bilingual clinicians are not available. Interpreters and bilingual staff should have bilingual proficiency and be trained in interpreting. They should have knowledge in both languages of the terms and concepts needed in the clinical encounter. Family members are not considered suitable substitutes for trained interpreters, as they usually lack these skills and knowledge. Avoid using a patient's children or grandchildren as interpreters.

Be Flexible Regarding Physical Therapy Intervention

Dorian reflected further on her patient's needs. She thought about her own beliefs and how she might react to a catastrophic injury. Would she cling to hope from anyone who offered it?

Acknowledge differences in the acceptability and effectiveness of various physical therapy interventions for individuals from different groups. Consider social, political, and economic conditions that may influence the nature of the intervention that you can provide. Seek ways to incorporate indigenous healing practices and the role of belief systems (religion and spirituality) in the intervention wherever possible.

See Through Cultural Lenses

PTAs and PTs must work closely to develop an intervention that fits the patient/client and family's concept of illness or injury. Create collaborative plans for service delivery that incorporate the culture, the family and community. Use resources that are culturally-appropriate, such as the family, clan, church, community members, and other groups.

Take Cultural Competence as Seriously as Other Clinical Skills

Develop and practice these skills as diligently as you would your clinical treatment techniques. It will make a big difference to all whose lives you touch.

Federal Standards for Culturally and Linguistically Appropriate Services

The US Department of Health and Human Services' (HHS) Office of Minority Health (OMH) addressed standards for culturally and linguistically appropriate services (CLAS) by publishing national standards in March, 2001[18] (Table 18-5). These standards were written for health care organizations and address Culturally Competent Care (Standards 1 to 3), Language Access Services (Standards 4 to 7), and Organizational Supports for Cultural Competence (Standards 8 to 14). Currently, all recipients of Federal funds are mandated to meet CLAS Standards 4, 5, 6, and 7. The full text of these important standards are available on the Office of Minority Health Web site.[18]

Summary

With increasing diversity in our population, it is likely that PTs and PTAs will frequently work with patients and clients of a different ethnicity, age, or gender group. Cultural competence involves the acquisition of skills that enable the physical therapy staff members to provide culturally and linguistically-sensitive services to the all persons.

Table 18-5

NATIONAL STANDARDS FOR CULTURALLY AND LINGUISTICALLY APPROPRIATE SERVICES IN HEALTH CARE (CLAS)[18]

CLAS Standards

Standard 1. Health care organizations should ensure that patients/consumers receive from all staff members effective, understandable, and respectful care that is provided in a manner compatible with their cultural health beliefs and practices and preferred language.

Standard 2. Health care organizations should implement strategies to recruit, retain, and promote at all levels of the organization a diverse staff and leadership that are representative of the demographic characteristics of the service area.

Standard 3. Health care organizations should ensure that staff at all levels and across all disciplines receive ongoing education and training in culturally and linguistically appropriate service delivery.

Standard 4. Health care organizations must offer and provide language assistance services, including bilingual staff and interpreter services, at no cost to each patient/consumer with limited English proficiency at all points of contact, in a timely manner during all hours of operation.

Standard 5. Health care organizations must provide to patients/consumers in their preferred language both verbal offers and written notices informing them of their right to receive language assistance services.

Standard 6. Health care organizations must assure the competence of language assistance provided to limited English proficient patients/consumers by interpreters and bilingual staff. Family and friends should not be used to provide interpretation services (except on request by the patient/consumer).

Standard 7. Health care organizations must make available easily understood patient-related materials and post signage in the languages of the commonly encountered groups and/or groups represented in the service area.

Standard 8. Health care organizations should develop, implement, and promote a written strategic plan that outlines clear goals, policies, operational plans, and management accountability/oversight mechanisms to provide culturally and linguistically appropriate services.

Standard 9. Health care organizations should conduct initial and ongoing organizational self-assessments of CLAS-related activities and are encouraged to integrate cultural and linguistic competence-related measures into their internal audits, performance improvement programs, patient satisfaction assessments, and outcomes-based evaluations.

Standard 10. Health care organizations should ensure that data on the individual patient's/consumer's race, ethnicity, and spoken and written language are collected in health records, integrated into the organization's management information systems, and periodically updated.

Standard 11. Health care organizations should maintain a current demographic, cultural, and epidemiological profile of the community as well as a needs assessment to accurately plan for and implement services that respond to the cultural and linguistic characteristics of the service area.

Standard 13. Health care organizations should ensure that conflict and grievance resolution processes are culturally and linguistically sensitive and capable of identifying, preventing, and resolving cross-cultural conflicts or complaints by patients/consumers.

Standard 14. Health care organizations are encouraged to regularly make available to the public information about their progress and successful innovations in implementing the CLAS standards and to provide public notice in their communities about the availability of this information.

Adapted from USDHHS. *National Standards for Culturally and Linguistically Appropriate Services in Health Care.* Washington DC: US Department of Health and Human Services, Office of Minority Health; 2001. Available at: http://www.omhrc.gov/omh/programs/2pgprograms/finalreport.pdf. Accessed Sep-tember 24, 2004.

References

1. APTA. *Surveys and Stats* Web page. Available at: http://www.apta.org/Research/survey_stat. Accessed September 27, 2004.

2. US Census. Profile of general demographic characteristics, 2000. Available at: http://www.census.gov/Press-Release/www/2001/tables/dp_us_2000.PDF. Accessed September 24, 2004.

3. Busse N, ed. *Jurisdictional Licensure Reference Guide, Federation of State Boards of Physical Therapy.* Alexandria, Va: Creative Publishing; 2002.

4. Rozier CK, Raymond MJ, Goldstein MS, Hamilton BL. Gender and physical therapy career success factors. *Phys Ther.* 1998;78(7):690-704.

5. APTA. Minority membership statistics. Available at: http://www.apta.org/Advocacy/minorityaffairs/minoritymembershipstats. Accessed September 24, 2004.

6. US Bureau of the Census. *Current Population Reports: Population Projections of the United States by Age, Sex, Race, and Hispanic Origin 1995 to 2050.* Washington, DC: Bureau of Census; 1996. Publication No. P25-1130. Available at: http://www.census.gov/prod/1/pop/p25-1130/p251130.pdf. Accessed September 24, 2004.

7. APTA. 2002 fact sheet physical therapist assistant education programs, December 2002. Available at: https://www.apta.org/pdfs/accreditation/PTAFactSheet2002.pdf. Accessed September 24, 2004.

8. Shaw-Taylor Y, Benesch B. Workforce diversity and cultural competence in healthcare. *J Cult Divers.* 1998;5(4):138-46; quiz 147-8.

9. Leavitt RL. Developing cultural competence in a multicultural world, part I. *PTmagazine of Physical Therapy.* 2002;10(12):36-48.

10. Leavitt RL. Developing cultural competence in a multicultural world, part II. *PTmagazine of Physical Therapy.* 2003;11(1):56-70.

11. Bureau of Primary Health Care. Office of Minority and Women's Health. What is Cultural Competence? Web page. Available at: http://158.72.105.163/cc/7domains.htm. Accessed July 16, 2000.

12. Leavitt RL, ed. *Cross-Cultural Rehabilitation: An International Perspective.* London: WB Saunders; 1999.

13. Black JD, Purnell LD. Cultural competence for the physical therapy professional. *J Phys Ther Educ.* 2002; 16(1):3-10.

14. Monahan B . The quest for diversity in the classroom. *PT.* 1997;5(1):72-77.

15. Noorderhaven NG. Intercultural differences: Consequences for the physical therapy profession. *Physiotherapy.* 1999;85(9):504-510.

16. Padilla R, Brown K. Culture and patient education: challenges and opportunities. *J Phys Ther Educ.* 1999; 13(3):23-30.

17. Institute of Medicine of the National Academies, (Smedley BD, Stith AY, Nelson AR, eds). *Unequal Treatment: Confronting Racial and Ethnic Disparities in Health Care.* Washington DC: National Academies Press; 2002.

18. USDHHS. *National Standards for Culturally and Linguistically Appropriate Services in Health Care.* Washington DC: US Department of Health and Human Services, Office of Minority Health; 2001. Available at: http://www.omhrc.gov/omh/programs/2pgprograms/finalreport.pdf. Accessed September 24, 2004.

19. APTA. FSBPT Advisory statement: physical therapist assistant regulation, October 1998. Available at: http://www.fsbpt.org/pdf/Advisory_PTA.pdf. Accessed September 21, 2003.

PUTTING IT INTO PRACTICE

1. How would you define your culture? Consider shared values, norms, symbols, language, and living practices that are repeated and transmitted from one generation to the next.

2. In what ways do the similarities and differences of your own culture, ethnicity, language, and/or race influence your interactions with others?

3. Take the Cultural Diversity and Competence Exam at www.quia.com/jq/17648.html.

4. Plan a visit to a local physical therapy clinic. What evidence would you look for as indicators of culturally-sensitive care? After the visit, summarize your observations below.

CHAPTER 19

Collaboration: You're on the Team

Ebony, a physical therapist assistant, was carefully reviewing Mr. Grey's chart when Faye, a registered nurse, asked, "Are you heading in to see Mr. Grey any time soon? I could really use some help in getting him up so I can change his bed." Ebony answered, "Yes, that's who I hoped to see next." Overhearing this conversation, Hailey, an occupational therapist, commented to Ebony, "Perhaps we can work with him together as I'd like to see him transfer before working on shaving at the sink."

You're on the Team!

Recognize now and forever that your effectiveness in working in health care will be made possible by the efforts, cooperation, and collaboration of others. To maximize the patient outcomes you hope to achieve, you must involve others. The world in which you live and work is far too complex (not to mention constantly changing) for a single health provider to work autonomously.

In addition to the physical therapists (PTs) with whom you work, you will inevitably interface with support staff, occupational therapists and assistants, speech pathologists, nurses, physicians, social workers, case managers, clerical staff, and clergy who will also provide services to your patients and clients.

Collaboration

Assertiveness and cooperation are required for successful collaboration. Collaboration is defined as a problem-solving approach that fully addresses the interests of all involved parties. It promotes a "win-win" solution with each person dedicated to the outcome. The achievement of mutual goals is of higher value than individual objectives. This approach to patient care can be difficult and time-consuming. It requires dedication and team work by all involved. When successful, collaborative outcomes ("win-win") tend to leave team members feeling satisfied, promote trust, and help build stronger relationships among those involved.[1]

The Disciplinary Alphabet Soup

Interdisciplinary, multidisciplinary, transdisciplinary, cross-disciplinary, cooperation, collaboration... The terminology in this growing educational and practice movement is enough to make you dizzy. These words underlie the issues at the heart of the collaborative process. It is important that we understand their meanings. Take a look at how some authors have defined these terms in Table 19-1.

Interprofessional Collaboration in Health Care

The practice of interprofessional collaboration has been identified as a critical skill for educators, health care workers, and social service providers, especially with the increasing complexity of our educational, health, and social service networks. Collaboration involves team building and building integrated service delivery mechanisms to improve outcomes for recipients of health, education, and social services.[2-5]

Culture, language, socioeconomic status, and education distinguish the unique health and social issues each patient or client faces. It is essential for health care providers to be mindful and sensitive to these matters. The needs of victims of domestic abuse, rural or inner city children, families who live in poverty, the elderly who are isolated and dependent on a fixed income, people with no insurance, and persons with lifelong disabilities are so vast that one health care professional cannot begin to address them.

Table 19-1
TERMINOLOGY[2,3,4]

Term	Definition
Discipline	A specific body of teachable knowledge with its own background of education and training, procedures, methods, and content.
Interdisciplinary	The use of methods and language from more than one topic to address common interests or problems.
Multidisciplinary	The juxtaposition of several disciplines side by side, focused on one problem where each discipline works alone.
Cross-disciplinary	The view of one discipline from the viewpoint of another (ie, the biomechanics of performing arts).
Transdisciplinary	A process creating new solutions beyond the scope of the individual disciplines.
Interprofessional	A shared experience that aims to help professionals to work together more effectively in the interests of their clients and patients.
Intraprofessional	A specialized approach within a professional group, using a common perspective.

In addition, our health care and social service systems are tricky to navigate for even those who know the way. It is very easy for critical information and pressing needs to fall through the cracks. Clearly, discipline-specific practice does not work. The needs of a client do not stop at the role boundaries of an individual health care provider.

Consider the following example:

> Mr. Feldman was discharged to his home following an open reduction of a hip fracture. The ambulance drivers brought him into his apartment and put him into his bed. He looked at the floor on which he had spent the night after falling on his way to the bathroom. The door shut and he wondered, "Wasn't someone supposed to bring me a hospital bed?" How do I shop for groceries? What am I going to do?" He had forgotten what the social worker at the hospital had told him and his papers were left on the countertop in the other room. Even the telephone was in the other room. He felt scared and alone.

Interprofessional collaboration involves professionals from different disciplines creating systems which help to meet the complex needs of a patient such as Mr. Feldman. It involves the following elements:[2]

* Interventions (treatment) and case management approach that focuses on individual patient needs.

* Referral systems to link patients and clients to a network of professionals, agencies, and services to meet specific needs.

* Clear and effective communication among all disciplines.

* Procedures that enhance the sharing of information and resources among all involved parties.

* Service locations available to provide more access to patients and clients.

* Mechanisms for linking/collaborating with other service providers.

* Outcome-oriented evaluation systems.

Keys to Success in Collaboration

Working well with others requires several key behaviors. Review Table 19-2 and see how you rate your *collaboration quotient*.

If you score 13 to 15, congratulations! You are a Master Collaborator. Your communication skills, patience, commitment, and nonjudgmental attitudes are key to successful collaboration.

If you score 8 to 12, you need to be aware that communication is the key to successful collaboration. Put your efforts into an outcome, not your personal needs. Hold others accountable for their commitments, instead of passing them off as unreliable or disinterested.

If you score below 8, your focus is on yourself and your experience, not the group outcome. Although

Table 19-2
COLLABORATION QUOTIENT

Collaboration Quotient	SCORE
Consider your experiences when working on a team or on a group project in responding to the following questions.	**Always = 0** **Frequently = 1** **Sometimes = 2** **Never = 3**
Have you experienced communication problems with one or more members of the group?	
Have you taken action before consulting others, just to "get it done"?	
Have you expected others to recognize the value of your contributions?	
Have you missed scheduled group or team meetings for any reason—even if it's a "good" reason?	
Have you resented the limited cooperation or lack of productivity of some group members?	
Total	

your contributions may be valuable, you cannot do this alone. You need help in changing your perspectives. Examine how your behavior contributes to the outcomes of the group. Participate fully in all class activities related to team building and group dynamics.

Being A Team Player

Jade, a PTA student, wrote in her class journal., "I never considered what others thought that we did. I was really shocked to hear that they thought we just adjust crutches. Why would I need to get a two year college education and a license to do that?" The exercise in our last class helped to open my eyes to what others think, in addition to helping me understand my thoughts about others."

Communicate, Communicate, Communicate!

There is no substitute for open, honest communication. Include all group members in written communications. Make sure that all group members are heard. Make a special effort to reach out to those who seem to be less vocal or less involved. Be certain you are hearing what colleagues are saying instead of creating a rebuttal in your mind while they are still speaking.

Perspective-Taking

Perceptions of our unique role on the health care team are formed as a result of personal, academic, and clinical experiences. Those with whom we work have perspectives that are based on their unique experiences. Individuals may perceive the same situation in dramatically different ways based on these differences.

Take another's perspective. What does the client experience when telephoning into the office to change an appointment? What does the clerk who works for an insurance company experience when patient-related documentation is incorrect or incomplete? Looking at the situations you experience from another perspective increases your empathy.

"It must have been (exciting, difficult, frustrating, upsetting...) for you when..." is a good starter to indicate your awareness of another's perspective.

Table 19-3
KEYS FOR PROMOTING TEAMWORK[6]

1. Establish clearly defined and agreed upon goals.
2. Establish roles and responsibilities of each team member.
3. Be aware of and avoid "win/lose" behaviors.
4. Listen actively and empathetically to each other.
5. Avoid absolute statements (eg, "You'll never...").
6. Involve all that will be affected in any decision that is made.
7. Make decisions by consensus versus majority vote, drawing straws, bargaining.
8. Avoid "winning strategies" in yourself and from others.
9. Act in good faith.
10. Employ "best for all" versus "getting your way" philosophy.

Adapted from Newman PD. Interdisciplinary teams/role delineation. *Oklahoma City Community College Course Materials. PTA 2113 Systems/Problems in Health Care*; 2003.

Acknowledge the Contributions of Others

Although you might disagree with a particular suggestion or approach, make sure that other group members know that you heard them and respect their input. A statement such as "What I like about what you said...." " is an effective opener for then proposing a different perspective.

Meeting, Schedules, and Systems

Mutually agreeable meeting times and locations and creating effective communication systems will bring about success. Make every effort to attend meetings as they are scheduled. Read pertinent e-mail or memos in a timely way and provide return communication. Your commitment to being a constructive team player will not only facilitate positive patient outcomes but will be a positive reflection on your profession.

Identifying and Challenge Your Assumptions

Your assumptions about other group members can interfere with group activity. We all have stereotypes, biases, and our own ideas about others. Others have their own stereotypes, biases, and ideas about us. Spend group time up front to get to know other group members and LISTEN.

Identify for yourself what stereotypes you hold about members of other professional groups, clients, patients, ethnic, gender, or age groups. There are many interesting group exercises that can assist you to examine your biases. Acknowledging that you hold biases is the first step to limiting their power over your thoughts and actions.

Break Down Role Boundaries

Our beliefs about our roles determine the ways that we act and what we expect of others. Role conflicts occur when we perceive that we are not able, in some way, to perform our role. Learning more about the way that other professionals view a problem is a key step to successful collaboration. Help others to see and hear you in the way that you would like to be seen and heard. See Table 19-3 for tips on promoting team work.

What is Your Role?

Examine your ideas about what physical therapists do. What about physical therapist assistants (PTAs)? Did these ideas evolve as you gained more exposure to the field? Have those ideas changed after reading the first few chapters of this book? What do others think that physical therapists do? Do members of your team know the difference between a PT and a PTA? You will not find out unless you ask. And then educate others as to what areas of care physical therapy can influence. It will be up to you to participate legally and ethically as a PTA consistent with your state practice act, company policies, *Standards of Ethical Practice* for the PTA, and physical therapy practice standards.

The Role of Education in Promoting Collaboration

Consider the educational experiences that may help you to acquire these skills and perspectives. Not all health care programs include specific training in these skills within the curriculum. Increasingly, physical therapy educators are becoming aware of these needs and are instituting learning opportunities that enhance these skills.

Recent authors in health care summarized the situation well:[7]

> Changes in the nation's health and education systems have mandated that professionals work together in a more cost-effective, collaborative manner. Academic institutions need to provide training to enable graduates to work in interdisciplinary settings, such as school-based health centers, so they can learn the skills needed to work in a truly collaborative manner. Basic knowledge about team building, communication skills, negotiation, conflict resolution, and family-based models of practice needs to be combined with opportunities for group work and decision making. This approach fosters the transformation of a group of individuals from different disciplines to a truly collaborative functioning team.

Summary

Successful collaboration depends on our perspectives and actions towards others. Spending time to work on the collaborative process is an investment with tremendous returns. Developing skills and experience in collaborative processes can change the way we think and the ways in which we deliver services to our patients and clients. The diversity of our population and complexity of our social service and health care systems requires interprofessional collaboration to insure that our clients and patients have access to and receive appropriate services.

References

1. Drench M, Noonan AC, Sharby N, Ventura SH. *Psychosocial Aspects of Health Care.* Upper Saddle River, NJ: Prentice Hall; 2003:347-348.

2. California State University, Fresno. Interprofessional Collaboration Program web page. Available at: http://www.csufresno.edu/interprof. Accessed September 1, 2003.

3. Jacobs HH. *Interdisciplinary Curriculum: Design and Implementation.* Alexandria, Va: Association for Supervision and Curriculum Development; 1989.

4. Soothill K, Mackay L, Webb C. *Interprofessional Relations in Health Care.* London: Edward Arnold; 1995.

5. Hooper-Briar K, Lawson H. *Serving Children, Youth and Families Through Interprofessional Collaboration and Service Integration. A Framework for Action.* Oxford, Ohio: The Danforth Foundation; 1994.

6. Newman, PD. *To Promote Teamwork—Interdisciplinary Teams/Role Delineation,Course Materials, PTA 2113.* Oklahoma City, Okla: Oklahoma City Community College; Fall 2003.

7. Papa PA, Rector C, Stone C. Interdisciplinary collaborative training for school-based health. *J Sch Health.* 1998;68(10):415-419.

PUTTING IT INTO PRACTICE

1. Review your college catalog or Web site. What other health profession education programs exist at your college? What are the required semester hours of study and the names of the courses? How are these programs similar to the PTA program? How do they differ?

2. Examine the physical therapy curriculum at a program in your state either by locating written program materials or on-line at the University's Web site. It may be helpful to interview a current student or new graduate from that program.

   What does this graduate education program include regarding group dynamics, team building, inter-professional collaboration?

   What/how does the PT learn about the role of and how to appropriately utilize the PTA?

3. Reflect for a moment and comment below on your strengths and challenges as a group/team member:

   My strengths as a team member:

   What challenges me when working as a team member?

CHAPTER 20

Student Involvement in the American Physical Therapy Association

American Physical Therapy Association

The American Physical Therapy Association (APTA) is an organization of over 63,000 physical therapists, physical therapist assistants, and students. The APTA offers several categories of membership for students in physical therapist or physical therapist assistant educational programs.[1] Student membership is offered at a fraction of the active membership costs, making it one of the best deals in your career.

For Students in Physical Therapist and Physical Therapist Assistant Programs

Student membership requires enrollment in a physical therapy education program that is accredited or is seeking or granted candidacy status by the Commission on Accreditation in Physical Therapy Education. *Student affiliate membership* requires enrollment in a physical therapist assistant education program that is accredited or is seeking or granted candidacy status.

For Physical Therapists

Active membership is offered to physical therapists who have graduated from physical therapy education programs that have met approval standards defined by the Commission on Accreditation of Physical Therapy Education. Membership is also open to physical therapists from other countries that have an equivalent education, as certified by an authorized agency, state board, or institution, and have citizenship, legal residence, or a legal permit to work in the United States.

For Physical Therapist Assistants

Affiliate membership is offered to physical therapist assistants who have graduated from US physical therapist assistant education programs that have met approval standards defined by the Commission on Accreditation of Physical Therapy Education.

Twenty-seven states have Physical Therapist Assistant Special Interest Groups (PTA-SIG's) in existence.[2] These serve as a means of facilitating camaraderie and communication among PTAs at the local and state level.

All PTA members are automatically members of the *National Assembly of Physical Therapist Assistants* which is a component and membership group of the APTA. The National Assembly promotes and protects the specific interests of physical therapist assistants. In addition to providing unique networking and continuing education opportunities, it provides a unified voice in representing the needs and interests of the affiliate members within the profession.[2] More information can be found on the National Assembly Web page: http://www.apta.org/components/nationalassembly.

Take a look at Table 20-1 for some recent examples of issues affecting the current and future role of the physical therapist assistant that the National Assembly has examined and influenced.

All membership categories require members to sign a pledge to be guided by the Code of Ethics of the APTA.

Table 20-1

PRESSING ISSUES[3]

* Entry-level educational degree—should changes in the entry-level of the physical therapist require a change from the Associate Degree for the PTA?

* Scope of work—what is and should be the level of knowledge and skill of the PTA? Which tests, measures and interventions can a physical therapist assistant safely and effectively perform?

* Recognition of enhanced proficiency—in what meaningful way can the APTA encourage and recognize greater competency and proficiency in the career development of the PTA?

* Voting rights—in what way does governance within the APTA affect practice issues and relationships?

* Licensure in all 50 states—how can the APTA assist with obtaining changes in states that do not regulate physical therapist assistants?

Adapted from APTA. The future role of the physical therapist assistant (RC 40-01). *House of Delegates Handbook*. Alexandria, Va: American Physical Therapy Association; 2003:96-129.

Figure 20-1. APTA career starter program for new graduate physical therapist assistants.

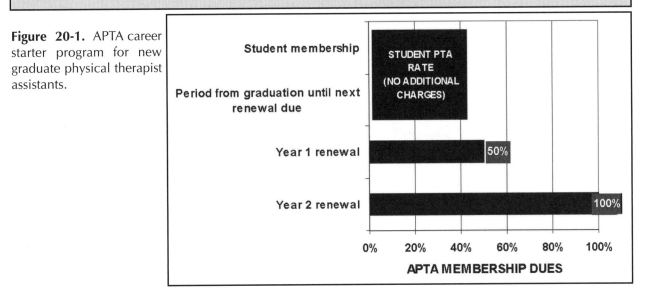

APTA Career Starter Dues Program

At the encouragement of his program director, Jeremy joined the APTA as a student affiliate member in December of the first year of the PTA program. He renewed his membership the following December as he finished classes and looked forward to his final semester of clinical internships. After graduation, on the last day of May, Jeremy's student affiliate membership converted to affiliate membership. In December, Jeremy received a membership renewal invoice for one half of the usual affiliate membership rate. One year later, Jeremy received his annual renewal invoice for the customary affiliate membership rate.

There is a helpful plan to assist students with the financial burden of membership upon entering the profession. As with all APTA dues, student dues expire 1 year from the renewal or join date. On the last day of the graduation month, membership automatically converts to *active* (PT graduates) or *affiliate* (PTA graduates) for the remainder of the 12 months of membership. Once that time expires, the new graduate can join at 50% of the standard dues rate for that membership class. At the conclusion of that year, full membership dues are applicable.[4] See Figure 20-1 for clarification of how this process works. The discounted student membership rate program insures that new graduates will have the continued support of the APTA and access to valuable news and information while establishing themselves in their careers.

Benefits of APTA Membership

APTA membership is one of the best investments that students can make in their future. Through APTA publications and student programs, you will have access to the latest developments in the profession, sources of financial aid and building networks for future employment and professional activities.[1,2,5]

Information on New Developments and Research

* APTA monthly publications include *Physical Therapy* and *PTmagazine of Physical Therapy*. These two publications include articles and information on the latest events in the profession, conference announcements, the latest research, and current professional issues.

* The APTA Web site (www.apta.org) and the student assembly Web page (www.aptastudent.org) are valuable sources for information that students can use for everything from class projects to future job searches.

* *PT Bulletin Online*, (www.apta.org/Bulletin), a weekly electronic newsletter, features current news and classified employment listings.

* *The Flash*, a biannual publication, is a news bulletin containing articles and information written by students from across the country. Twice a year, in the Fall and Spring, *The Flash* is distributed to APTA student liaisons. There are also monthly e-mail newsletters that are distributed to APTA student liaisons in each educational program.

* *The Voice* is a quarterly newsletter comailed within *PT* and the *Journal* to all affiliate members. In it includes a message from the president of the National Assembly.

* *Hooked on Evidence* is a project to promote evidence-based practice by providing clinicians a user-friendly database containing current research articles related to the effectiveness of physical therapy interventions. While considered a "work in progress," there are currently 1128 articles archived. Clinicians from around the country are involved in this grassroots effort. This is a member's only benefit which can be located at www.apta.org/hookedonevidence/search.cfm.

Financial Aid for Students

There are several scholarship, loan programs, and competitive financial awards available for students in physical therapist and physical therapist assistant programs, as well as physical therapists who are enrolled in graduate programs. Specific research-related funding is available through the Foundation for Physical Therapy.[7] More information is available on the APTA Web site at www.apta.org.

Scholarships and awards may also be available through your state chapter of the APTA. To search for your state chapter, go to www.apta.org/chapters. Membership in your professional association may also make you a more viable candidate for scholarships and student awards offered at your college or community.

Mentors and Networking

The APTA is the gateway for developing collegial networking through chapter and district meetings, national conferences, and the National Student Conclave (an annual meeting for students of physical therapy). Membership gives you access to policymakers, researchers, expert clinicians, and leaders in the field. Whether through the organized mentoring program "Members Mentoring Members" available to members of the APTA or with an esteemed role-model close to home, developing a relationship with an experienced clinician can help guide your career development and will inevitably serve you well.

Areas of Clinical Focus

Within the APTA structure, there are 19 specialty groups called "sections" that focus on particular areas of physical therapy practice, such as pediatrics, acute care, or geriatrics. Involvement in a section gives you access to specialized publications, directories of other members with similar interests, and opportunities to learn about state of the art new trends and ways to develop your expertise after graduation.

Professional Books and Conference Discounts

APTA membership also entitles members to discounted rates on all APTA publications and conferences. Special "member" prices also apply to T-shirts, promotional items, and public relations materials about the physical therapy profession. Further, students who volunteer for a few hours to help at state and national conferences can often attend at a markedly reduced rate.

Insurance Plans

Most clinical facilities and academic programs require that students enroll in a malpractice insurance program prior to beginning the clinical education portion of the curriculum. APTA-affiliated malpractice plans offer professional liability insurance to students at a low cost. In addition, the APTA has negotiated reasonable rates on many other forms of auto, home and life insurance.

Leadership Skills

Students can actively participate in district, state chapter, and national activities through student special interest groups (SSIG), the Student Assembly (SA), and the National Student Conclave. These valuable learning opportunities offer critical insights into professional organizational and governance processes. There are scholarship programs available for internships in government affairs as well. These experiences develop leadership skills for future career opportunities.

Land That Position

The APTA sponsors a Career Center at the Annual Conference and the Combined Sections Meeting that offers guidance on resume writing and interviewing skills. Employers and recruiters often exhibit at these meetings and at the National Student Conclave.

APTA membership should be listed on *your resume*. APTA membership and voluntary student activity in the profession reflects a commitment that is recognized by employers and professionals across the country. It indicates that you are in touch with the latest educational and research information. As a member of the APTA, you will have pledged to uphold the Standards of Ethical Practice of the Affiliate Member. This holds you to a higher standard of behavior which is well respected by employers and colleagues alike!

Student Leadership and Involvement

Here are some of the many ways that students can get involved in activities that promote the profession of physical therapy.

On-Campus Organizations

Serve in the leadership of an on-campus organization that promotes physical therapy education or awareness. Established physical therapy student organizations can usually receive financial support from student organization funds. Such groups sponsor physical therapy awareness and disability awareness events, fund-raising, lecture series, and serve as a valuable resource for the campus community.

Fund-Raising Activities

Work on a fund-raising event. There are many potential fund-raising projects that directly support student interests in the physical therapy profession. Campus organizations that support physical therapy students, political action committees, and foundations for research are all in need of support.

Campus and District/State APTA Association Activities

Every campus has funds and mechanisms for donations for student scholarships or resources to support student attendance at professional conferences and other activities. Students can become actively involved in raising funds to support their activities as students. Students may also become involved in district and statewide APTA fund-raising efforts for particular initiatives and organizations.

Political Action

Public policy, state, and federal legislation plays a major role in the future of the physical therapy profession. Political action committees, (like PT-PAC) are critical to insure that legislators are well-informed about the physical therapy profession. Support of political action groups insures that the physical therapy profession will have a strong voice in the state and federal legislative processes.

Physical Therapy Research

The Miami Marquette Challenge is an annual fund-raising competition between physical therapy and physical therapist assistant academic programs that donates funds to the Foundation for Physical Therapy. These funds are used to support physical therapy research. There may be similar organizations in your state or local community as well.

Observe the APTA House of Delegates

Students may observe the annual APTA House of Delegates. This session has been historically held in conjunction with the annual conference in June each year. Students can see organizational governance in action on the floor of the House of Delegates. The APTA Student Assembly elects two student members who attend the House of Delegates as nonvoting participants.

Table 20-2

SAMPLE MOTION PROPOSED BY STUDENT ASSEMBLY AT 2003 APTA HOUSE OF DELEGATES[8]

Mentoring of Professionalism in Academic and Clinical Education
RC 32-03

"It is the responsibility of all academic and clinical faculty, clinical instructors and professional mentors to actively promote to physical therapist students the importance of professionalism as a critical component of a doctoring profession. Professionalism requires ongoing membership and active participation in APTA and support of its standards, policies, positions, guidelines, and Code of Ethics. Academic and clinical faculty, clinical instructors, and mentors of physical therapist assistant students shall promote behaviors that are consistent with APTA's standards, policies, positions, guidelines, and the Standards of Ethical Conduct for the Physical Therapist Assistant and that support the importance of ongoing membership and active participation in APTA."

Reprinted from APTA. New and revised association positions focus on patient access, professionalism. *PT.* 2003;11(9):65, with permission of the American Physical Therapy Association. This material is copyrighted, and any further reproduction or distribution is prohibited.

Volunteer at State and National Conferences

Attending a conference is one of the best ways to see and hear the latest information, meet other students and potential employers, and develop a collegial network. Student members often receive discounted registration rates. Students who volunteer may receive additional benefits. Call well in advance to offer your services.

Join the APTA Student Assembly

The APTA Student Assembly (APTA-SA) was formed 1991 to address the needs of student and student affiliate members. There are now over 10,000 student physical therapist and physical therapist assistant members of the APTA-SA.[5] Students share similar needs and interests in answering the challenges, issues, and pressures placed on them by their learning environment. Students share challenges such as financial and time constraints, school pressures, and concerns about future employment. The APTA-SA includes both student and student affiliate members and provides a strong base of support for future professional development.

The APTA-SA serves several functions in providing information for Assembly members, promoting the role of students in the physical therapy profession, encouraging student membership, and representing the interests of APTA-SA members to APTA leadership and components. The APTA-SA sends both a PT Student delegate and PTA Student delegate to the APTA House of Delegates, which is the policy-making body of the physical therapy profession. Although they cannot vote, they can bring motions and do represent the student assembly on important issues. An example of an important motion proposed by the Student Assembly in 2003 is printed in Table 20-2.

There are many leadership opportunities for APTA student members on the SA board of Directors. A new slate of candidates is nominated and elected annually. Interested candidates can contact the Nominating Committee.

The APTA-SA has a Web page at www.aptastudent.org. A popular feature is a student assembly bulletin board that enables students to post messages concerning everything from good sites for clinical affiliations to requesting roommates for conferences. This site includes information on the latest developments, student members by name, student issues, awards, and contact information for the APTA-SA Board members and Nominating Committee.

Serve as the APTA Student Liaison on Your Campus

Student liaisons link the APTA-SA with physical therapy and physical therapist assistant students around the country. Student liaisons disseminate information received from the Board of Directors of the APTA-SA to their classmates via public announcements, a centrally-located bulletin board and monthly e-mail letters. This information includes developments in the world of physical therapy as it relates to students. It provides a vehicle for students to communicate with each other as well. *The Flash*, the biannual publication for students, is distributed through student liaisons.

Student liaisons must currently be enrolled in either an accredited or developing physical therapy/physical therapist assistant program and be a member of the APTA. Information about becoming a student liaison and an application form can be downloaded from www.aptastudent.org.

Join or Start a Student Special Interest Group

Student special interest groups (SSIG) are groups of student and student affiliate members who are organized on a state-wide basis in conjunction with APTA state chapters. SSIGs promote membership in the American Physical Therapy Association and represent the interests of SSIG members to the APTA state chapter leadership. SSIGs frequently communicate by newsletters, organize meetings, educational sessions and social events in conjunction with chapter conferences.

There are leadership opportunities to serve as officers of SSIGs as well. There are 19 APTA state chapters with SSIGs. A list of which states and the steps to form a SSIG are outlined on the APTA Student Assembly Web page at www.aptastudent.org.

APTA National Student Conclave

The National Student Conclave is an annual weekend conference, sponsored by the APTA and designed to support students, expose them to advances in the field, and introduce them to the APTA governance process. It is a tremendous networking and educational opportunity that should not be missed.

Students attend educational sessions regarding career strategies, interviewing skills, legislative initiatives, and clinical sessions in areas such as orthopedics, home health, and sports physical therapy. There is an exhibition area and many employers recruit students at this event. A popular event is the Mock House of Delegates, where students learn about the APTA governance process and parliamentary procedure. In addition, social events top off the conference activities with talent shows and receptions. Take a look at information from the Conference brochure at a recent student conclave.

This annual meeting occurs in the fall (usually October) and all student and student affiliate members are invited to attend. A typical program format is illustrated in Table 20-3.

Student Awards

There are several awards that recognize outstanding students in the physical therapy profession. Information about these awards and nomination forms are available through the APTA Web site (www.apta.org) or the APTA-SA Web site (www.aptastudent.org). In addition, many state chapters reward students with scholarships as well. Be sure to ask your program faculty and/or look at your chapter's Web site for more information. Is there someone deserving of recognition in your educational program?

* Outstanding PT Student
* Outstanding PTA Student
* Outstanding Student Liaison Award
* Outreach for Cultural Diversity Award
* Miami-Marquette Challenge
* Dorothy Briggs Scientific Inquiry Award
* Mary McMillan Scholarship Awards
* Minority Scholarship Awards for Academic Excellence
* APTA Section Student Awards (eg, Oncology Section Student Research Award)

Summary

Student membership in the APTA offers many benefits including access to the latest research and health policy developments in the field, connections to mentoring networks, opportunities to learn about specific clinical areas of interest through section membership, and discounts on conference registration, APTA publications and group insurance programs. Numerous opportunities exist for students to organize on-campus activities and take leadership roles in the APTA through the Student Assembly and Student Special Interest Groups.

References

1. APTA. Step into your future with APTA: the benefits of belonging to the American Physical Therapy Association. American Physical Therapy Association Web page. Available at: http://www.apta.org/membership/Benefits. Accessed September 13, 2004.

2. APTA. National Assembly fact sheet. Available at: http://www.apta.org/Components/nationalassembly. Accessed September 13, 2004.

Table 20-3

NATIONAL STUDENT CONCLAVE PROGRAM FORMAT

What paths will your future take?

Events include:

* Interactive, expert-led clinical sessions
* Workshops on resume writing, networking skills, and job-search strategies
* Exhibit area with employers and recruiters from across the country
* Student Assembly Board of Directors elections
* And so much more!

NSC: Start Here. Go Anywhere!

The 3-day National Student Conclave helps prepare you for the future by focusing on the ever-changing physical therapy job market. Learn about the dynamic pathways that your future can take via career opportunities, new practice techniques, and available work settings—all while you interact with APTA leaders and physical therapy experts.

Schedule of Events include Résumé Critiquing and Mock Interviews, Ethical Dilemmas & the New Grad, Hooked on Evidence: How to Contribute and Use It In Practice, Physical Therapists and Physical Therapists Working Together, Reimbursement: CPT Coding, Risk & the New Grad... and 10 different clinical sessions to choose from presented by experts within the Specialty Sections.

---

3. APTA. The Future role of the physical therapist assistant (RC 40-01). *House of Delegates Handbook.* Alexandria, Va: American Physical Therapy Association; 2003:96-129.

4. APTA. Bylaws of the APTA as amended June 2002. Article X Finance Section 3 Dues A (8). Available at: http://www.apta.org/pdfs/governance/bylaws.pdf Accessed September 13, 2004.

5. APTA. *Student Assembly* Web page. Available at: http://www.aptastudent.org. Accessed September 14, 2004.

6. APTA. Hooked on Evidence project. Available from: http://www.apta.org/hookedonevidence/search.cfm. Accessed September 14, 2004.

7. APTA. Foundation for physical therapy Available at: http://www.apta.org/foundation. Accessed September 14, 2004.

8. APTA. New and revised association positions focus on patient access, professionalism. *PT.* 2003;11(9):65.

PUTTING IT INTO PRACTICE

1. Who is the APTA student liaison for your program? What are their responsibilities?

2. When and where is the next Student Conclave? How many students from your program have attended in the past few years? Will any attend this year?

3. Access the Student Assembly Web page at www.studentapta.org. Is there a Student Special Interest Group in your state? List the contact person below:

4. Does your program participate in fund-raising for the Miami-Marquette Challenge? Generate several fund-raising ideas and write them here. How can you initiate and/or add to the efforts of fund-raising for the Foundation for Physical Therapy?

5. Check the Student Assembly Web page at www.aptastudent.org. Is there a student in your program who would qualify for a student award? List the requirements and application/nomination deadline below.

CHAPTER 21

Attending Conferences

> Kelly saw the announcement for the state chapter American Physical Therapy Association (APTA) conference and heard other students talking about attending. It was a 3-hour drive and then she would have to stay in a hotel. She worried, "I've never been to a conference before. I have no idea what to do there."

Why Attend Conferences?

Conferences provide multiple opportunities for students to hear about new developments in the field, network with colleagues, try out new equipment, and make essential contacts for a first position.

Access to Information and Research

The latest information, trends, and developments are communicated at conferences long before they are in textbooks and often even before they are in journal articles. Although access to information is almost instantaneous in the electronic age of Internet and e-mail, conferences provide an opportunity to hear about and discuss these types of findings. Many conferences also feature equipment vendors and publishers. You may have an opportunity to try out a new piece of equipment, peruse the latest publications and make purchase decisions at discount, just because you've made the contact at the conference.

Sharing Experiences and Ideas

The greatest advantage of attending a conference is the opportunity to share your experience and interact with others. You will meet others who share your experiences as a student in an academic program have questions about job searching. You will meet potential employers who can assist you in developing your career goals and exploring various physical therapy opportunities. You may have a chance to meet the authors of your textbooks and reading materials, talk with leading researchers in the field and explore new areas that haven't been covered in school.

Networking With Others

There is really no better place to meet potential employers, future colleagues with similar interests, or students and faculty from other colleges and universities. In addition, your chances of finding someone who knows someone that can help you are far greater than when you circulate solely among your own contacts. Become a master networker and use conferences to both develop and strengthen your network.

Bigger Picture of Profession and Opportunities

Job-hunting is always a concern for students. Students, however, are often confined by images of the physical therapy that they have personally seen and experienced. Conferences open up a much wider view, including different geographical areas, different treatment techniques, and types of practice and provide a means for comparing and seeking future opportunities.

Types of Conferences

There are many types of conferences, seminars, and workshops. Often, students are offered a discounted registration, especially if they offer to assist with some aspect of the conference administration.

Continuing Education Courses

Continuing education courses are held frequently all over the country. There are many continuing education companies that sponsor multiple speakers. Most speakers are specialized and many courses are

---
Table 21-1

SAMPLE CONTINUING EDUCATION COURSE LISTING

Title: One Step Ahead: Prosthetics and Amputee Rehab

Description

A dynamic three-day presentation featuring acute care of the amputee, prosthetic componentry, biomechanics of gait, beginning to advanced prosthetic gait training, functional skills, and running gait. 2.1 CEUs for PTs, PTAs and ATCs. Cost $450.00.

When: From: 25-Apr To: 27-Apr

Where: Anytown, USA

Sponsor: Advanced Rehabilitation Therapy, Inc

Instructor: Joe Instructor, PT, PhD

Topic Area: Other

Contact Information

Name: Jane Instructor

Email: jinstructor@email.net

Phone: 305-555-0855

Fax: 305-555-4107

Address:

7641 SW 126 Street

Anytown, USA 33156

---

held in a series. Take a look at the following Web site for a sample of the courses that are offered in your area. Site visitors can sort listings by area, subject, dates or instructor: www.apta.org/Bulletin/Course_Listings.

Table 21-1 illustrates a sample course listing from this site.

An additional site for courses specifically for physical therapist assistants (PTAs) is available on the National Assembly Web site: www.apta.org/Components/nationalassembly.

Table 21-2 displays a course in a series, "Rev Up Your PTAbilities" offered through the National Assembly of Physical Therapist Assistants.

Continuing education courses frequently offer continuing education units (CEUs). Some states require licensed physical therapists (PTs) to attend continuing education courses which offer CEUs to meet state license renewal requirements. Check on the requirements in your state.

It is important to differentiate between contact hours of continuing education (CE) and CEUs. A contact hour is defined as a 50-minute period of organized learning activity.[1] One CEU is equivalent to 10 contact hours of continuing education.[1]

Some states require continuing education for license renewal. Consider the continuing education needs of therapists who live in a state that requires 2.4 CEUs per 24-month period. For example, a day-long continuing education course that runs from 9:00 AM to 12 NOON and 1:00 to 4:00 PM would award 0.6 CEUs for attendees. PTs would need to attend four such courses over the 2-year period to meet their state requirements for license renewal.

Special Interest Areas (Problem-Centered)

Some conferences are focused on particular problems as a way of bringing together many experts to contribute to the resolution of an important issue. It might be a clinical issue, such as lymphedema management or an administrative issue such as the implementation of a new government affairs regulation such as the Health Insurance Portability and Accountability Act (HIPAA). Frequently, the proceedings of such a conference are a valuable reference for future direction.

Table 21-2

EXAMPLE OF CONTINUING EDUCATION FOR PHYSICAL THERAPIST ASSISTANTS

Rev Up Your PTAbilities

Orthopedic and Adult Neurologic Interventions

August 22-23, 2003

Aurora, OH

Join your PTA colleagues for 2 days of discussions focused on Orthopedics and Adult Neurologic Interventions. These three courses will enhance the abilities of the PTA to carry out the interventions identified in the PT's plan of care for patients with orthopedic and/or neurologic impairments.

August 22, 2003
Orthopedics: Total Joint Replacement With a Focus on Current Updates

Friday, August 22, 8:30 AM-5:00 PM

Presenter: Steven G. Lesh, PT, PhD, SCS, ATC

Session Description

This 1-day course is designed to provide the PTA a brief review and update on the surgical and clinical management of patients who have undergone total joint arthroplasty. Current total joint arthroplasty issues will be discussed related to the shoulder, elbow, knee, hip and MP joints. Particular attention will be given to the application of evidence-based intervention strategies selected by the PT for the patient following joint arthroplasty. PTAs that are working in the outpatient, acute care, skilled nursing, or home health environments will discover new and progressive interventions.

Session Objectives

After successfully completing this course, the PTA will be able to:

1. Describe clinical advances in total joint arthroplasty procedures to correct joint deformity and promote enhanced patient function.
2. Discuss the rehabilitation needs identified by the PT for the patient who has undergone a total joint arthroplasty procedure.
3. Explain the postsurgical goals established by the PT for the patient with a total joint arthroplasty.
4. Relate the PTA's role in implementation of intervention strategies found in the Guide to Physical Therapist Practice.
5. Discuss potential evidence-based intervention strategies selected by the PT for patients who have undergone a joint arthroplasty.

August 23, 2003
Adult Neurology: Comparison of PNF and NDT

Saturday, September 20, 8:30 AM to12 NOON

Presenters: Venita Lovelace-Chandler, PT, PhD

Course Description

This course is designed to provide the PTA with an update on PNF and NDT intervention strategies for adult patients with neuromuscular impairments. Current evidence that supports selected intervention strategies will be presented, especially those typically implemented by the PTA.

continued

Table 21-2 continued

EXAMPLE OF CONTINUING EDUCATION
FOR PHYSICAL THERAPIST ASSISTANTS

Course Objectives

After successfully completing this course, the PTA will be able to:

1. Compare and contrast the principles of NDT and PNF.
2. Discuss evidence-based intervention strategies for patients with neuromuscular impairments.
3. Identify selected components of interventions from NDT and PNF that would typically be implemented by the PTA.
4. Determine career development and future educational needs related to NDT and PNF through self-evaluation.
5. Relate the PTA's role in implementation of intervention strategies found in the *Guide to Physical Therapist Practice*.

Facilitating Gait: Using Neuro-Developmental Treatment (NDT) Principles

Saturday, August 23, 1:00 PM to 5:00 PM

Presenter: Jennifaye V. Brown, MSPT, NCS

Course Description

This course is designed to provide the PTA with current knowledge and skills to improve hemiplegic gait using neuro-developmental techniques (NDT). Current research outcomes to support neuro-developmental techniques will be discussed. Normal versus abnormal movement analysis will be reviewed. Therapeutic intervention will address the upper extremity, trunk, and lower extremity transitioning from sitting to completing one gait cycle. Specific treatment interventions will be discussed and demonstrated via media analysis.

Course Objectives

After successfully completing this course, the PTA will be able to:

1. Discuss the NDT philosophy as it relates gait facilitation.
2. Recognize the causes of abnormal movement displayed during hemiplegic gait.
3. Describe techniques to effectively facilitate the phases of gait.
4. Relate the PTA's role in implementation of intervention strategies found in the *Guide to Physical Therapist Practice*.

CEUs are available. 1.3 CEUs or 13 contact hours will be awarded for the 2-day course. .65 CEUs or 6.5 contact hours will be awarded for attending the 1-day course.

APTA's 2-day *Rev Up Your PTAbilities* seminar for PTAs is an exceptional learning opportunity, your chance to participate in discussions designed specifically to meet your particular needs as a PTA. It's an important investment in your future. Make plans now to attend for one day or, better still, for both. You'll be glad you did!

Advance Registration Fees:

APTA Member One day $125*	Nonmember One day $208
APTA Member Two days $195	Nonmember Two days $325

Onsite Registration Fees:

APTA Member One day $175	Nonmember One day $292
APTA Member Two days $225	Nonmember Two days $375

* APTA members save 40% off nonmember fees. If you're not already a member, join APTA today!

continued

Table 21-2 continued

EXAMPLE OF CONTINUING EDUCATION
FOR PHYSICAL THERAPIST ASSISTANTS

Hotel Accommodations

The Bertram Inn and Conference Center

600 North Aurora Rd

Aurora, OH 44202

TEL: 330/995-0200

FAX: 330/562-9163

Room Rate: $89/night

To obtain the special rate, please indicate you are with "American Physical Therapy Association (APTA)" Reservation deadline to receive rate is August 7, 2003.

Shuttle Transportation: The hotel will provide complimentary ground transportation to and from the airport. Participants must contact the hotel before arrival, identify themselves as a participant in the American Physical Therapy Association *PTAbilities* course, and ask to speak with "Dawn." She will take flight information and arrange for airport transfers. Dawn is available Monday through Friday from 8:30 AM to 5:30 PM.

Course Registration Deadline: August 1, 2003

For further course details, registration, and hotel information, visit www.apta.org, or contact APTA's service center at 800-999-2782 x3395.

Cancellation Policy

Cancellation for the seminar must be received 72 hours before it begins. Requests for refunds must be made to APTA in writing prior to the seminar and will be subject to a 20% service charge per registration. APTA reserves the right to cancel the seminar up to two weeks prior to its start date. In the event of cancellation due to circumstances beyond our control, APTA is at no time responsible for expenses incurred by registrants, including but not limited to costs of airline tickets, other travel, food, or room.

Adapted from APTA. *Rev Up Your PTAbilities*. Alexandria, Va: American Physical Therapy Association. Available from: http://www.apta.org/Components/nationalassembly/PTAContinuingEd/Course1/PD. Accessed September 21, 2003.

State or Chapter Conferences

State chapters of the American Physical Therapy Association usually sponsor annual or semiannual conferences that include educational programming, social events, equipment exhibits and organization business meetings. Such conferences are usually fairly low cost and most convenient for students to attend. Many offer special events for students as well. All state chapters are listed at www.apta.org/Components/chapters.

National Conferences of the APTA

There are two national conferences of the American Physical Therapy Association each year. Students are encouraged to attend both conferences. Students who volunteer to provide services at the conference often receive a discounted registration.

Both of these meetings publish a *Call for Papers* during the preceding summer. More information about the meetings listed below can be found on the APTA Web site at www.apta.org/Meetings.

Combined Sections Meeting

This is a 4- to 5-day meeting of all 19 sections of the APTA, which includes special programming specific to each section. Many clinical trends, new developments, and instructional courses are offered at this conference. In addition, each section holds business meetings for its membership. Each section also sponsors an original paper platform and/or poster session. This is an exciting conference because it always features in-depth, practice-oriented information. This meeting is held usually in early to mid-February.

Annual Conference and Exposition of the APTA

This is a larger conference which includes the annual House of Delegates meeting, which is followed by a 4- to 5-day meeting of the APTA membership. There are many social events, educational and special interest sessions, exhibits, research presentations, and career networking opportunities. This meeting is held usually in early to mid-June.

International Physical Therapy Conferences

The World Congress of Physical Therapy (WCPT) meets every 4 years in a different country. This conference includes representatives from many nations who meet each quadrennium to discuss and plan for physical therapy needs on a global basis. There are numerous social events, educational and research sessions, and many opportunities for networking with international colleagues.

Interdisciplinary Conferences

There are many conferences that include clinicians from several disciplines. These conferences are usually focused around a particular clinical area or a specialty interest. PTs and PTAs frequently attend such conferences on issues such as spinal cord injury, pain management, rehabilitation technology advances, and pediatrics. Attending an interdisciplinary conference not only helps participants understand how individuals from other disciplines approach a problem, it enables an interdisciplinary dialogue to begin that ultimately improves service delivery (see Chapter 19 on interprofessional collaboration).

Strategies for First-Time Conference Attendees

Before attending a conference, there are several ways that you can maximize your time and resources.

* *Read abstracts and conference program and highlight interest.* Conference abstracts for several meetings are published in advance of the conference. If not, a package of conference abstracts is usually available at registration. It is well worth the time to read through the abstracts to see what is involved in each session.
* *Plan attendance at specific sessions.* Highlight and plan to attend those sessions that interest you. Going to the conference with a plan will help you to focus your efforts and maximize your

time use. You will know where you want to be, which will make it much easier to ask directions and arrive there! Don't wait until the last minute, as some sessions require preregistration and fill up quickly. Latecomers are often left out.

* *Make an overall schedule of events.* Outline conference events you intend to attend on an hour by hour basis for the duration of the conference. Conferences usually run 10 to 20 competing events at a time. It is difficult to choose, but committing yourself in writing will minimize your confusion. Go through conference programs and note the room and building in which each session will be held. Conference sessions are sometimes in different hotels, blocks away from each other or from your hotel. You'll need to plan to get there.

At the conference:

* *Arrive early at popular sessions.* Arrive early at each session you plan to attend. There are usually limited handouts and seats. Popular sessions fill up quickly and those who don't fit are usually left out.
* *Sit up front.* Choose your seat to maximize what you can see. There are a lot less distractions toward the front of the room. Another reason to arrive early!
* *Exchange business cards.* You will meet dozens of new colleagues. Ask for the business cards of speakers, researchers, and potential employers with whom you wish to stay in contact. You may want to prepare some business cards, as well with your name, address, phone, and e-mail address. Office supply stores offer business cards very inexpensively. Don't pass up the opportunity to make and keep a contact.

How to Submit an Abstract

Call for Papers

A *Call for Papers* is published 6 to 9 months prior to the conference. It may be called a *Call for Proposals* or a *Call for Abstracts*. Several categories of submissions may be included such as research, special interest of theory presentations, video, or multimedia technology programs.

Research reports are presentations of original scientific data collected by the author. *Special interest presentations* cover important issues or new developments in education, administration, or clinical practice. *Theory presentations* address a theory, idea, concept, or model that describes a foundation for administration, education or clinical practice. *Multimedia presentations* are demonstrations of computer or video-based programs that serve an educational or research purpose.[2]

Participants who submit an abstract generally are given the choice of how to present—by a *platform* or *poster presentation*. A *platform presentation* is a delivered address to an audience, in a meeting room at a podium. Conference participants attend the platform session, which is usually one of several papers, each lasting 15 minutes.

A *poster presentation* is a display that is mounted on a large bulletin board, but not presented orally to an audience. In a poster presentation, the content is summarized using brief written statements and graphic materials such as photographs, charts, graphs, and/or diagrams. The poster is usually displayed for most of the conference. Conference participants may visit posters during designated hours to interact with the authors.

A *multimedia presentation* is generally defined by the format of the presentation, such as video or computer. A presenter is given a time to interact with conference participants similar to the arrangements for a poster session.

Deadlines

A firm deadline for receipt of proposals is established. Look carefully at the instructions and see if the date is for receipt or postmark of the materials. It is a good idea to either send an abstract well in advance or by express mail to insure delivery by the designated deadline. Don't miss the deadline!

Guidelines for Submission

The conference abstract must be formatted in a prescribed way. This is detailed in a *Call for Abstracts*. Careful preparation of the abstract is critical, as abstracts will be published as submitted.

Preparing a Presentation

Susan received the conference packet late on a Friday afternoon. Her abstract had been accepted. Now what? She excitedly called her copresenters one by one to tell them the good news. She scheduled a planning session during the next week. Although she was excited, she worried, "I hope someone will be interested in this topic!"

After an abstract is accepted for presentation at a conference, presentation planning must begin. The presentation must be carefully crafted with the anticipated audience in mind. See Table 21-3 for presentation design.

Poster Presentations

Check on the Size of the Display Space

A typical display space is 4 x 6 feet (title should be about 4 to 5 feet long, and 8 to 12 inches tall). Conferences typically provide a bulletin board type of display on which to mount the presentation. Bring push pins with you.

Map Out Your Plan Ahead of Time to Scale

Set up a mock poster in the allowable space, with each of the elements displayed. It will be much easier to see your plan and make needed adjustments this way.

Make it Visually Interesting!

Use photos, graphs and other illustrations in your presentation. Be aware that visual interest will draw participants to your poster. Let pictures tell the story as much as possible, with words to explain the pictures.

Use high contrast materials, either light background with dark letters or dark background with white letters. Use color to create interest, but be sure that your message is readable from 5 feet away. A computer presentation program will be helpful to layout the text for the presentation.

Use Text Sparingly

Limit your text to a simple description of the problem, purpose, subjects, methods, results, and conclusions. Label and explain photographs, graphs, and tables. Use 24-point font and larger, and limit the content on a page to 7 or 8 lines. Check the Table 21-3 for some design guidelines.

Do not display pages or a table from a written paper. In addition to being illegible from a distance, this material is far too complex to understand in just a few minutes.

During the Assigned Poster Session

You will be assigned a time during the conference for the poster session. Stand next to your poster during this time.

Table 21-3

DOS AND DON'TS OF PRESENTATION DESIGN[4]

Do....

* Use a landscape view, rather than portrait view for slides for best projection.
* Plan for projection of your presentation. Test your computer and LCD projector set-up prior to the presentation.
* Keep the presentation moving (plan for 30 seconds to 1 minute maximum per slide).
* Use a sequence of information that is logical and builds on itself.
* Define technical terms before using them.
* Use a title at the top of each slide (such as Introduction, Methods, Results).
* Keep it simple, clear, and concise.
* Use a maximum of 7 lines of text in the space below title of slide.
* Use phrases, not sentences.
* Use upper and lower-case letters; they are easier to read than capitalized text.
* Use simple transitions from one slide to another (fade).
* Use dark background with light letters (purple/yellow; blue/white, etc).
* Use photos to show methods and set-up.
* Create simple tables with a maximum of 3 columns and 3 or 4 rows.
* Use line diagrams or graphics if feasible.
* Create simple graphs and charts and label them clearly.
* Use pie charts to display demographics or proportions.
* Use bar graphs to display differences between groups or over time.
* Use line graphs to display multiple points over time.
* Display only one dependent variable per graph.
* Label the x and y axes on all graphs.

Don't ...

* Display results of different dependent variables on the same slide, unless there is a reason to compare them by your experimental design.
* Use more than two types of fonts, colors, and styles. Keep the font type, font color, and style consistent throughout the presentation.
* Use a font smaller than 18 points in a projected slide program.
* Use a light background with colored letters.
* Use ALL CAPITALS. This is more difficult to read.
* Use tables with more than 3 columns or 4 rows.
* Try to scan in a complicated graph from a written paper.
* Use multiple types of transitions from one slide to another. It may be entertaining for you as a designer but it will distract your audience to see your text fly in from the right, bottom, top, or appear in a checkerboard pattern.

Be aware that participants may not have an understanding of your subject matter. Draw participants to your poster with questions like, "Do you have a program for... in your practice?" Explain your poster briefly and let participants take a look at your findings. Offer to answer questions. Remember that you know far more about your project than participants who visit your poster.

Be sure to bring a supply of business cards and exchange cards with conference participants. If a participant asks for additional information, be sure to write their request on the back of their card. Don't rely on your memory. You may finish the session with dozens of cards.

Provide Materials

Not all participants can attend a poster session when the authors are present. Therefore some poster presenters find it helpful to provide a flyer, business cards, or some other means for participants to see and take away a summary of the poster, with contact information for the authors. Simple materials can be made available in an envelope attached to the poster display board.

Platform Presentations

Platform presentations are typically delivered in conference rooms with a podium and a microphone. The sessions are organized with 3 or 4 papers in succession. Time is limited to 15 to 20 minutes with a few minutes for discussion. Session moderators introduce participants and keep time.

Preparation and Presentation Design

Computer-based programs are readily available to help presentation design. Think carefully about the visual impact and sequence of the material you present. Table 21-3 lists a few tips for presentation design.

Presentation Materials

Indicate to conference organizers what equipment you will need for your presentation. If you are doing a computer-based presentation, it is a good idea to bring your own laptop computer with the presentation preloaded and a set of overhead projector transparencies as a back-up. Technology is not fool-proof. A back-up plan is better than floundering when equipment fails.

You may distribute written material to accompany your presentation. Many speakers give participants a summary of their slide presentation. You may want to consider this option depending on the length and complexity of your talk. Make 50 to 100 copies of materials, more if it is a very large conference.

The moderator of your session may contact you in advance for information about your background. Bring a copy of all materials that you have sent and received in relation to the conference presentation in the event that something is lost or misplaced.

Practice Sessions

Write down what you are going to say and practice it until you do not need to look at it. Practice is critical. Practice, revise, and practice again. Practice speaking slowly and allow the audience to see and read each slide. Practice using a pointer to point out notable features on graphs or tables. Refer to colors of lines or bars on the graph. Time the presentation and allow for questions from the audience. Remember that the audience knows far less about your work than you do.

At the Conference

Check the size and location of the room in which you will present. If possible, attend another presentation in the room so that you can see how speakers get to and leave the podium and how the lighting and projection system works. Although someone else will be responsible for controlling this equipment, you may be able to plan for visuals more effectively when you see the conditions under which you will present.

Dress appropriately in comfortable clothes and shoes. Conference organizers may request that you meet session moderators in advance of your session, often in a Speaker Preparation Room. These rooms typically have audiovisual equipment available so that you can preview your presentation. Use the few minutes before the session wisely. Be sure that all equipment is functioning in the room. Go to the podium and make sure that you know how to turn on equipment to begin your presentation.

Plan to leave copies of written materials at the back of the room. Inform the conference room assistant that you will have written materials accompany your presentation and he or she may be able to direct participants to these materials as they enter the room.

While Giving Your Presentation

Thank the moderator for the introduction and greet the audience. Make eye contact with at least one member of the audience. Breathe and be conscious of your speed of presentation. Don't dwell on small mistakes that you may make; the audience understands that you may be nervous. Finish the presentation and say, "Thank you. Are there any questions?"

Always repeat the question. Then answer it simply. If it is too complex for a simple answer, state, "That's an interesting question. I'd like to talk with you a little further about that after the presentation, if you're available."

One of the greatest fears that new speakers have is not being able to answer a question. If you don't know the answer to a question, tell the participant that you would like to refer to the written manuscript and you will speak with them after the pres-

Table 21-4		
TYPICAL CONFERENCE EXPENSES		
Expenses (4-day conference)	Average Costs	To Cut Costs
Conference registration	$300	Volunteer to assist at the conference and registration fee will be markedly discounted or provided by the organizers.
Hotel (4 nights@ $150.00)	$600	Share a room with other students or look on student list-serves for students in the area who will offer housing to other students.
Round trip airfare	$500	Look for student discounts and lower fares from alternate departure cities.
Meals ($35.00 per day)	$140	Visit exhibit halls and exhibitor parties. While networking, you can often eat for free!
Ground transportation (shuttle to hotel)	$30	Share a cab with other conference participants to often beat "per-person" shuttle rates. Check in advance with taxi driver.
Incidentals	$100	Be prepared to find some "great deals" on books, equipment, and other musts at the conference. And have some fun, too!
Presentation materials	$100	Ask your college or employer to assist you with the preparation costs of presentation materials.
Total	$1770.00	A motivated student can reduce costs by $600 to $800 by using the above tips.

entation. This is an opportunity to get valuable feedback. Spend the time to understand and discuss a point that a participant is making.

Congratulate yourself and go out for lunch or dinner to celebrate!

What Will It Cost?

Conference expenses are fairly predictable and fall into several categories. Table 21-4 shows a typical budget for attending an out-of-state conference.

How Do I Pay for It?

Conference participation is a valuable part of your education. Budget for it and plan to attend. If you have an abstract accepted for a conference presentation, there are many potential means of support.

College and Program Support

Ask for support! Some educational programs have limited funds to support student travel to confer-

ences, especially when representing the program. Ask about available programs, scholarships, and aid that may support such expenses. If not readily available, a motivated student may be able to create such funds by meeting with department and college administrators.

District and State American Physical Therapy Association Funds

Contact your district and chapter offices of the APTA. See if they are able to support your travel and conference expenses in some way.

Loans and Grants

Seek other sources of support to augment your available resources. This is an important investment. The contacts you will make and the addition of a presentation to your resume is worth the expense of attending a conference.

Summary

Conferences provide multiple opportunities for learn new information, share ideas and experience, network with other colleagues and gain additional perspectives of the profession. Successful conference presentations result from careful planning and attention to detail. Students should seek opportunities and support to both attend and present at conferences.

References

1. Corexcel. CEU's and contact hours. Available at: http://www.corexcel.com/html/ceus.contacthours.ceus.htm. Accessed September 24, 2004.

2. APTA. Rev up your PTAbilities. Available at: http://www.apta.org/Components/nationalassembly/PTAContinuingEd/Course. Accessed September 24, 2004.

3. APTA. Complexities of compliance seminar. Available at: http://www.apta.org/documents/public/courses/hipaacomplianceregform.pdf. Accessed September 21, 2003.

4. Curtis KA. Making poster and platform presentations. In: *Student Research Manual*. Fresno, Calif: California State University, Fresno; 2000.

PUTTING IT INTO PRACTICE

1. Find out Call forAbstracts deadline and the dates and location of:
   A.   The next Chapter conference of the American Physical Therapy Association in your state
   B.   The next Combined Sections Meeting of the American Physical Therapy Association
   C.   The next Annual Conference and Exposition of the American Physical Therapy Association

	Call for Abstracts Deadline	Conference Dates, Location
Chapter conference		
Combined Sections Meeting		
Annual Conference and Exposition		

2. Find out about potential sources of support for conference presentations in your college or program. If you were to present your research, to whom would you apply for financial assistance to attend the conference?

   Prepare a budget to estimate your costs of attendance at one of the above conferences.

3. Explore the availability of continuing education conferences in your area. Go to www.apta.org/Bulletin/Course_Listings.

   Look for courses listed in your state. How many did you find?

   How many are within 100 miles of where you live?

   What are the average registration fees per day of instruction? Give a range from the lowest to the highest.

   Which courses specifically mentioned PTAs as participants?

4. Check the continuing education courses listed at the National Assembly of Physical Therapist Assistants Web site: http://www.apta.org/Components/nationalassembly/PTAContinuingEd.

Where and when are the next courses scheduled?

How many are within 100 miles of where you live?

What are the average registration fees per day of instruction? Give a range from the lowest to the highest.

PART SIX

First Steps Into the Profession of Physical Therapy

CHAPTER 22

Preparing for Licensure

Leticia looked at the travel brochures and was anxious to see the world after she completed her physical therapist assistant education. She wondered, "Will it be complicated to get my license in another state?"

State Laws for Licensure and Registration

Each state licensing board has its own criteria that applicants must meet to apply for physical therapist (PT) and in some states, physical therapist assistant (PTA) licensure. There are more than 40 states that require licensure, registration, or certification of the PTA.[1] Graduates of accredited programs should review the materials distributed by the licensing board in the state(s) to which they intend to apply to determine the specific eligibility requirements in each state.[2]

The Federation of State Boards of Physical Therapy provides a Web site and extensive resources that explain the licensure process. However, each state administers and controls the licensure process in that state.

Federation of State Boards of Physical Therapy

509 Wythe Street
Alexandria, VA 22314
Telephone: (703) 299-3100
Fax: (703) 299-3110

Examinations:
Telephone: (703) 739-9420
Fax: (703) 739-9421

To access the State Board of Physical Therapy in your state. Visit www.fsbpt.org/directory.cfm.

The national examination is only one part of the process involved in licensing a therapist to practice. Eligibility for licensure is determined after review of many documents in addition to the National Physical Therapy Examination score. In fact, passing the examination does not guarantee licensure.[3] Licensing requirements may also include an extensive review of educational preparation and transcripts, recommendations of licensed physical therapists, passing a test of state law, screening (fingerprints) for a criminal record and review of prior convictions. Although it varies by state, the application process and fees required to obtain initial licensure will cost the candidate hundreds of dollars.

Once determined eligible by the state licensing authority, the candidate's materials are forwarded to the Federation of State Boards of Physical Therapy (FSBPT). The FSBPT sends the candidate an "authorization to test" letter, which includes instructions for examination scheduling at one of 300 local testing centers in the US, US territories, and Canada. The candidate must sit for the examination within 60 days of the date on the "authorization to test" letter.[4] Test center fees are paid at the time that the examination is scheduled.

Internationally-Educated Therapists

State laws governing the licensure of physical therapists educated outside the United States also varies by state. All internationally-educated therapists will require prescreening of their credentials and English proficiency evaluations (such as TOEFL,

TSE, TWE) before being able to apply for licensure to practice.[5] After passing criteria for credential review and English proficiency and meeting all other criteria for state licensure, candidates may sit for the National Physical Therapy Examination. In some states, applicants must also complete a period of supervised clinical internship.

Additionally, work authorization is required for employment in the United States. Physical therapists may apply for a "temporary" nonimmigrant visa, called the H-1B visa, that permits practice as a PT only.[5] There is an annual cap for H-1B visas.

Requirements are different for Canadian citizens. Citizens of Canada must request a TN visa at the Canadian-US border. This type of visa requires that applicants offer proof of Canadian citizenship, show a valid US license to practice physical therapy, and possess a letter of employment or contract. The TN visa is valid for 1 year. It must be renewed annually.[5]

There is currently no educational preparation comparable to PTA education as accredited by the Commission on Accreditation for Physical Therapy Education (CAPTE). However, individual state licensure boards may provide a process that grants application by individuals who can demonstrate "equivalent" preparation through a combination of academic and clinical experiences.

> *Mustafa had been scraping by to make ends meet since having to quit his job to attend full-time clinicals. Now that graduation was approaching, he wondered if he would be able to work as a PTA before he actually completed the licensure exam. Would someone hire him not knowing for sure that he would be able to pass?*

Physical Therapist and Physical Therapist Assistant Practice by Licensure Applicants

Again, state law varies as to what PT and PTA license applicants may legally do while waiting to take and hear the results of the examination. Some states permit supervised practice by applicants; others do not. It is important that applicants understand their legal status during the period of application and waiting period before a license is issued. Most states require documentation indicating the name of the licensed PT taking responsibility for the applicant. The physical therapy practice act will specifically sanction the number of applicants one PT can be supervise, as well as, the specific type of supervision

required[6] (see Chapter 12). The licensure board that governs physical therapy in each state can provide this information.

The National Physical Therapy Examination for Physical Therapists and Physical Therapist Assistants

The National Physical Therapy Examination (NPTE) is a computerized test, consisting of 225 multiple-choice questions for physical therapists and 175 questions for PTAs. Candidates for the PT and PTA examination are allowed 4.5 hours and 3.5 hours, respectively.[7] Candidates are examined individually and must call to schedule an examination date and time.

The examinations are developed by a committee of physical therapy practitioners. Test questions assess the knowledge and abilities required of physical therapists and PTAs. These questions are developed to reflect a comprehensive analysis of the practice of physical therapists and PTAs.

Raw exam scores are converted to a scale that ranges from 200 to 800 points. The FSBPT national minimum passing score is 600 points for both the PT and PTA examination. Since July 1996, all states have adopted the FSBPT passing score.[4]

Exam content for the PTA examination includes three major areas:

1. Tests and Measures (Data Collection) including:

   Group I: Strength, ROM, posture, body structures, cognition, reflex, and sensory integrity (11.3%);

   Group II: Cardiovascular/pulmonary system, integumentary system, functional status (10%).

2. Intervention including:

   Nonprocedural interventions (18.7%); procedural interventions

   Group I: Exercise and manual therapy (10.7%)

   Group II: Transfer and functional activities, gait training, assistive and adaptive devices and modification of environment (11.3%)

   Group III: Physical agents and modalities (13.3%)

   Group IV: Airway clearance techniques; wound care; and promoting health, wellness, and intervention effectiveness (6.0%).

3. Standards of Care (18.7%)[7]

A practice examination and assessment tool for the PTA examination is under development by the Federation of State Boards of Physical Therapy. You can check on its status at www.fsbpt.org/handbook/review.htm.

Table 22-1

SAMPLE QUESTIONS FROM NATIONAL PHYSICAL THERAPY EXAMINATION

Physical Therapist Assistant Examination

1. A patient falls and sustains a deep laceration on the right forearm, causing extensive bleeding. After putting on gloves the PTA should FIRST:

    a. Apply direct pressure over the wound.

    b. Elevate the right arm higher than the heart.

    c. Apply ice over the wound.

    d. Place a tourniquet proximal to the wound.

2. A patient is doing exercises for abdominal muscles, involving lifting the arms, legs, and head. The patient is unable to prevent lumbar hyperextension. The PTA should determine that:

    a. The back extensors need strengthening.

    b. The exercises are too difficult for the patient.

    c. Additional resistance is needed.

    d. The exercises are too easy for the patient.

3. Which of the following patients is MOST in need of a wheelchair with removable arms in order to be trained in transfer activities?

    a. A patient with an amputation at the distal end of the femur.

    b. A patient with left hemiparesis.

    c. A patient with a cauda equina lesion.

    d. A patient with a T4 spinal cord lesion.

ANSWERS TO SAMPLE QUESTIONS: 1.a; 2.b; 3.d

Reprinted with permission from Federation of State Boards of Physical Therapy. Available at: http://www.fsbpt.org/download/2003CandidateHandbook.pdf. Accessed October 28, 2004.

Table 22-1 depicts sample questions from the PTA examination.

Preparing for the Examination

Gather and Organize Your Resources

Textbooks, class notes, articles, and reading materials you received during school provide a good foundation for examination review. Take care to review the State Practice Act as well. Be sure that your information is current and reflects existing laws in the jurisdiction in which you will practice.

Review Class Notes

Start with your class notes, which are organized by subject area. Look for areas of overlap and begin with a review of terminology. Note indications, contraindications, precautions, and specifications for treatment procedures.

The examination is problem-based, which will require you to review with applications in mind…

Ask yourself:

* What is the clinical application of this information?

* If I was given this information about a patient, what difference would it make in my problem-solving or implementation of treatment?

Be sure to consider all of the following content:

* Information given regarding the condition and/or pertinent medical history of the patient. Be especially aware of "red flags" that may make a treatment choice contraindicated or otherwise unsafe.

* Careful attention to outcomes of your choices, including cost-effectiveness and need to defer to the physical therapist.

* Interventions, including indications, contraindications, precautions by diagnosis or system, and intended response(s) with regard to goal achievement.

* Ethical and legal considerations.
* Documentation requirements.
* Psychosocial aspects of illness, injury, and disability.

Develop a Realistic Study Schedule

Begin your preparation several months in advance. A study group is a useful way to approach this examination. Determine weekly review content and plan study for several hours prior to each group session.

Make use of patients that you have worked with on clinical internships. Remembering information is easier when you anchor it to something or someone meaningful. You may be more motivated when reviewing classroom notes or reading textbooks about a particular condition or treatment approach with a particular patient in mind.

Use Active Information Processing Strategies

Your retention is better if you use an active strategy to process information rather than just re-reading books or notes (see Chapter 9). Take notes from your notes or record key information onto an audiotape. Discuss the information with others periodically to further improve your retention. Review your notes and/or audiotapes at least once weekly.

Take Practice Exams

Practice exams are available through many sources. Be sure that you have covered the content areas included in these examinations.

Review strategies for taking multiple-choice examinations (see Chapter 7). Remember that this is a timed examination. In general, your first answer is the best. Watch for exclusionary words or phrases such as *only, except, never,* or *always.* If English is not your first language, beware of common errors (Chapter 14).

Take a look at Table 22-1 for some sample questions.

Courses, Study Guides, and Computer Programs

There are many review courses available. Although these courses are expensive, they may save the applicant time in identifying key information for review. A course does not take the place of necessary study time and no course provides a fool-proof mechanism to pass the examination. Review books are less expensive and often provide accompanying computer disks to simulate test-taking conditions.

Preparation Resources

A partial listing of examination preparation resources is provided at the following Web site: www.apta.org/Govt_Affairs/state/state_resources/license_exam.

What Happens If I'm Not Successful?

The national first-time pass rate for PTA graduates from accredited programs averages 75%.[9] This means that three of four graduates from PTA programs pass the licensure examination on the first attempt. Individual programs have higher and lower first-time pass rates than the national average. The Commission on Accreditation for Physical Therapy Education monitors program pass rates in consideration of accreditation status. Your program director can provide statistics related to licensure trends.

State licensing boards determine how often and over what time period a candidate may take the examination, if not successful on the first attempt. Re-examination requires reapplication including fees. Superceding state rule, the FSBPT stipulates that no candidate may take the examination more than four times in any 12-month period.[4]

If you are not successful, think about the content that presented the most difficulty. Ask your colleagues, supervisors and faculty with assistance in organizing your studies. Use strategies for active information processing. Enlist the support of others to insure that you will be successful on a subsequent try.

Summary

Licensure to practice as a PTA requires that a candidate meet specific criteria as outlined in each state's physical therapy practice act. The practice of the PTA is not yet regulated in all 50 states. Check with the state licensing board to receive applications and regulatory information.

When criteria are met, the applicant may sit for a computerized national examination administered in a testing center by individual appointment. The candidate must be aware of laws governing his or her practice activities during the licensure application period.

References

1. APTA. Consumer page: who are PTAs? Available at: http://www.apta.org/Consumer/whoareptsptas/Profile_Asst. Accessed September 9, 2004.

2. Federation of State Boards of Physical Therapy. Eligibility. Available at: http://www.fsbpt.org/exams/NPTEEligibility.asp. Accessed September 24, 2004.

3. PT Board of California. Instructions for completing the application for physical therapist or physical therapist assistant examination and/or licensure. Available at: http://www.ptb.ca.gov/license/inst.pdf. Accessed September 9, 2004.

4. FSBPT. Frequently asked questions. Available at: http://www.fsbpt.org/exams/questions.asp. Accessed September 24, 2004.

5. APTA. Information for internationally educated therapists. Available at: http://www.apta.org/Advocacy/internationalaffairs/info_for_intl_edu_pt. Accessed Septemeber 9, 2004.

6. Oklahoma Board of Medical Licensure and Supervision. Forms and resources for PTs and PTAs. Available at: http://www.okmedicalboard.org/display.php?content=pt_forms:pt_forms&group=pt. Accessed September 24, 2004.

7. FSBPT. Examination structure. Available at: http://www.fsbpt.org/exams/content.asp. Accessed September 24, 2004.

8. APTA. Licensure examination candidate resources. Available from: http://www.apta.org/PT_Practice/ptlicensure/license_exam [members only page]. Accessed September 24, 2004.

9. FSBPT. *Summary of Scaled Results School Report for Oklahoma City Community College 2001-2003*. Oklahoma City, Okla: Oklahoma City Community College; 2003.

PUTTING IT INTO PRACTICE

1. Find the Web site for your state licensing board. Download materials and read them to answer the following questions:

   A. What materials are required as part of the application packet?

   B. What is the fee required with the application?

   C. What limitations are placed on practice of first-time applicants during the application period? (look especially for descriptions of terms of temporary licenses or PTA license applicant practice or prohibition of practice by applicants)

   D. What are the policies and fees for repeating the examination if not successful the first time?

2. Review your college catalog and list the required courses in your curriculum that meet each of the following content areas:

	Course Numbers
Tests and measures	
Nonprocedural interventions	
Procedural interventions, including indications, contraindications, precautions, and intended response	
Ethical and legal considerations	
Psychosocial aspects of illness, injury, and disability	

CHAPTER 23

Entering the Job Market

Mel began his job search. He looked over the Sunday paper and saw three ads for part-time physical therapist assistants. They were all in out-patient clinics that seemed to be run by large corporations. He worried, "Which one will be the best for me?" He planned to call each of them on Monday morning. Is this a good strategy?

Looking For a Job

Employer needs change rapidly with health care policy and reimbursement modifications, despite growing societal needs for physical therapy services. While there were numerous job openings for each graduate in the early- and mid-1990s, physical therapist assistants (PTAs) had to compete for available positions in the late-1990s and into the new millennium. Job availability is favorable once again for physical therapists and PTAs; however, vigilant activism against laws restricting access and reimbursement for physical therapy remains an ongoing legislative priority for the profession.[1]

The classified ads are not the place to start a job search. Employers of PTAs advertise in professional publications, Web sites, and/or listservs or draw applicant pools from those who have initiated previous contact.

Let's start with a different mind-set...

New graduates are *beginning their careers in physical therapy*. Although it is possible to "find a job" in the field of physical therapy, graduates who are more creative and initiate their career path with a strategy in mind are likely to be far more satisfied with the results.

Let's approach this important decision by first asking a few questions:

Create a Picture of Your Ideal Life

What is most important to your life? Consider the following:

* What is most important to you in your personal life?

* What is most important to you in your career?

* What are your personal goals? Your career goals?

* How long do you envision yourself staying in one position or one location?

Envision the Ideal Organization

What are the things you consider to be most important in an organization in which you will work?

Consider the following:

* What goals or mission of an organization would be most attractive?

* What would this organization contribute to society?

* What size would this organization be?

* What experience will you gain?

* Where is the optimal location of your ideal workplace?

* What are the working conditions?

* With what kinds of people would you most like to work?

* What are the needs of this type of organization in the current social and health care climate?

What Do You Have to Offer?

Consider the following:

* What unique skills, abilities, and experiences will you bring to the workplace?

* What new programs are you interested in helping develop?

* What will colleagues gain by working with you?

✻ What will clients or patients gain by working with you?

✻ How can you improve the efficiency of the organization?

Now that you have an idea of what you want, it will be easier to ask for help and focus your efforts. Before you write a resume or send a letter, use the essential strategies of networking and informational interviewing.

Networking

> Nia looked at the small stack of business cards she had saved from last year's state APTA conference. She had written to a few of her contacts. How could she work those into a potential job offer?

Networking is an essential way to develop contacts and establish relationships that can be a source of information, collaboration, and future opportunity. There are some key principles that will maximize the effectiveness of your networking efforts.[2,3]

Organize Your Contacts

Be aware of the contacts you already have and organize them in a way to fully take advantage of these resources. Consider your contacts within the field from school, former instructors and students, your former and current colleagues and supervisors, and even people who you met at your affiliation sites.

Then, think of the network of your contacts and the entire scope of people who are available to you. Don't overlook social and family contacts, such as church, community, and others with whom you share special interests. Your potential network is very large.

Use an address book or computer database. Collect business cards and keep them in an organized file. Maintain physical therapy contacts in a way that you can retrieve the addresses and phone numbers easily.

Build Your Clinical Contact Base

Take care to cultivate clinical contacts through your academic and clinical education. Consider who could best address and respond to your specific questions and interests. Both academic and clinical faculty have a broad overview of the physical thera-

py field and can assist in directing you toward helpful contacts.

Stay Visible

Establish your visibility among your contacts. This requires an active commitment to establishing and maintaining contact. Keep in touch.

Your network is only available to you if you use it. Decide what you need and where you want to go in the future. Let contacts know of your interests and goals. You, undoubtedly, will be extremely busy while in school. Utilize opportunities provided by your program to establish and nurture contacts. For example, attend local APTA chapter meetings, PT month, or fundraising events. Have a faculty member, clinical instructor or classmate introduce you to someone you are interested in working with upon graduation. Follow-up is critical if you are interested in landing that job.

Printing business cards will be well worth your investment. Keep your business cards with you at all times. Write notes on the back of your business card as a brief reminder of what you talked about or what information you would like the other person to give you. Your card is a very important impression of yourself to leave with someone.

Ask for Help

Ask for help, information, advice, and other contacts. Listen and learn from others. Mingle in many circles. Make an effort to stay in touch frequently. Ask members of your network to go to lunch or dinner. Thank others for their help.

Acknowledge and Promote Others

Acknowledge and promote the accomplishments of others. Share resources and information. Help others in your network succeed in their interests and reach their goals through your contacts. Find out their areas of interest and expertise and periodically review and update your contact lists.

Make Referrals and Help Others

Refer others to people with whom you have contact. Share resources willingly. Send articles of interest to people in your network. Support the skills, expertise, and accomplishments of others. Let others know of your efforts to promote them.

Make your relationships ones of mutual benefit. This is especially helpful if you are networking with competitors.

Informational Interviewing

Students have multiple opportunities to gather information that will support their future job search. Student PTAs are in a unique position of working with colleagues during clinical internships who have the responsibility to assist their career development.

Talk with these clinical contacts to broaden your network, get advice on your resume and look into opportunities in certain geographical areas.[4] Get the names of their colleagues, school friends, fellow committee members, and previous students to contact. Ask for help in approaching your job search.

Developing Your Résumé

> Stacy worried that the only jobs she'd seen on the physical therapy list serve were in hospitals. She prepared a résumé which indicated her interest in employment in outpatient facilities and then sent her résumé with a cover letter to each facility.

A résumé is a "short account of one's career and qualifications prepared typically by an applicant in a position."[4] A résumé, by itself, will not land a job, especially in a tightening job market that is influenced by personal connections. Some ideas, however, about what a résumé may do for you....

* It may serve as a calling card, by giving an employer your contact information.

* It serves a valuable purpose as a self-inventory, which will enable you, the job seeker, to assess and present your strengths and experience.

* In fact, your résumé, may actually provide an outline for an interview. You have outlined your accomplishments and capabilities and your résumé provides a potential employer with a focus for matching your skills with their needs.

* Lastly, your résumé may serve as a valuable reference for the employer in considering your candidacy for a position among a pool of applicants.[2]

Your résumé must be first-class, without errors, current, concise, and clear. It should catch the employer's attention and provide a clear match for your skills with an available position. It should demonstrate your competence, experience, and skills in descriptions of actions and achievements and show how you can apply your expertise in a position

you are seeking. It should demonstrate your worth to an employer, whether in dollars, contacts, or visibility.

There are several types of résumés (Table 23-1 and Table 23-2).

The Chronological Résumé

This is a standard résumé format. It is simple to prepare and provides a chronological description of student education and experiences by places, dates, and events. The career objective is employee-focused and global. This résumé may be effective for sending out to prospective employers who have not advertised specific job openings.

Is there anything about the résumé in Table 23-1 that sets apart this applicant? Even though this applicant has earned a bachelor's degree in a related field, worked as a physical therapy aide, and maintained good grades, her experience does not jump off the page. Those accomplishments are not presented as unique or different than many other newly graduated PTAs. This type of résumé fails to illustrate in what way her unique experience will add to the organization. Her cover letter will be very important to present these points (Table 23-3).

Debra read the following job ad.

> June 26, 2003 (Center City Women's Bulletin)
>
> University-based medical center seeks dynamic PTA to join interdisciplinary women's health team. The team will focus on collaborative treatment of women's health issues including aquatic therapy. Leadership and aquatic experience desirable. Contact N. Royal, University Medical Center, 1001 University Drive, Center City, IL 62667.

She prepared a position-focused résumé and wrote a cover letter outlining her interests.

The Position-Focused Résumé

The position-focused résumé encourages the author to address the specifics of the employment listing. This type of résumé specifically outlines the applicant's skills and related accomplishments specific to the requirements and preferences outlined in an employment listing for an available position. See Debra's résumé in Table 23-2.

Table 23-1
CHRONOLOGICAL RÉSUMÉ

Shara Straightforward

College address:	Permanent Address:	
Street Address	Street Address	Include all contact addresses and include applicable dates for temporary addresses.
City, State, Zip	City, State, Zip	
Home Phone	Home Phone	
Fax		
E-mail		

Career Objective

An entry-level position in a physical therapy out-patient clinic.

> Can be as general or specific as you like.

Education

Mid-State College, Center City, IL
Associate of Applied Science in PTA, 2003

> College or University Name, City, State, Degree, Major, Year (GPA is optional).

Mid-State University, Center City, IL
Bachelor of Science, Health/Wellness, 2000

Work Experience

Physical Therapy Aide, Middletown Physical Therapy, Middletown, IL. January 2001-August 2002

- Prepared treatment area and assisted with routine therapeutic exercise classes
- Performed inventories, and ordered supplies and patient education materials
- Created a database of area resources for patient referrals

> List in reverse chronological order, most recent first (Title, Employer, City, State, Dates). List related positions prior to physical therapy education or list related positions in the health or human service fields. Give a brief description of your work-related duties.

Clinical Internships

Tri-City Sports Rehabilitation, Tri-City, IL. March 24 to May 2, 2003.

Performed tests & measures and physical therapy intervention within PTs plan of care for recreational and elite athletes. Presented in-service to 15 staff members on use of a wobble board for knee rehabilitation.

St. Johns Hospital, Eastbrook, IN. January 21 to March 14, 2003

Performed tests & measures and physical therapy intervention within PTs plan of care for diverse population in acute hospital setting. Co-treated with OTs, COTAs and speech pathologists. Presented in-service to 30 staff members on lymphedema treatment.

> List in reverse chronological order, most recent first (Facility, City, State, Dates).
> Brief description of clinical responsibilities and accomplishments.

Licensure

Eligible for licensure; will take examination July 2003.

> License number, state, and date or indicate your application status.

Honors and Activities

Student Member, American Physical Therapy Association
National Student Conclave, Birmingham, AL 2002
Dean's List – all 4 semesters PTA program

> List community activities, clubs, professional organizations, honors, and awards. Include dates.

References

References available on request.

> Either list those persons whom you have asked to serve as references or write "References available on request."

Table 23-2

POSITION-FOCUSED RÉSUMÉ IN RESPONSE TO PUBLISHED EMPLOYMENT LISTING

Debra Dynamic	Include all contact addresses and include applicable dates for temporary addresses.
College Address: Permanent Address:	
Street Address Street Address	
City, State, Zip City, State, Zip	
Home Phone Home Phone	
Fax	
E-mail	
Objective	Focus on specifics of employment listing.
Participate on interdisciplinary women's health team. Develop and implement aquatic therapy interventions under direction of licensed physical therapist.	
Related Skills and Accomplishments	Relate to major themes of employment listing.
Women's Health Activities:	Using action verbs and quantifiable terms, describe your related experiences and skills. What are you trying to show?
• Developed, coordinated, and implemented Water Exercise Program, Middletown YWCA, 1999-2002.	
• Participated in organization of Lymphedema Network conference in June, 2000.	I have experience in the Women's Health field and have perspectives which go well beyond physical therapy.
• Provided peer counseling to over 10 women experiencing rape or domestic abuse. Started a support group for women with abuse history at Middletown YWCA.	
Collaborative and Communication Skills:	Yes, I work well with a team. I get things done.
• Practiced as a member of interdisciplinary rehabilitation team at Warm Springs Rehabilitation Center during 7-week internship focusing on neurological rehabilitation and Southland Women's Center focusing on women at a community health clinic.	
• Coauthored and edited quarterly newsletter for student communications during Physical Therapist Assistant Program.	
Leadership and Organizational Experience:	I take on leadership roles and I'm capable of organizing and directing work-related responsibilities.
• Served for 2 years as American Physical Therapy Association Student Liaison and physical therapist assistant club president, organizing fundraising and social events.	
• Recruited, trained, and supervised approximately 50 lifeguards and aquatic instructors for Aquatics Program at Middletown YWCA.	
• Secured funding and organized support group for abused women at Middletown YWCA.	
Licensure	License number, state, date or indicate your application status.
Licensed physical therapist assistant #000000 IL (Date)	
Education	University Name, City, State, Degree, Major, (Year GPA is optional)
Mid-State College, Center City, IL	
Associate of Applied Science in PTA, 2003	

continued

Table 23-2 continued

POSITION-FOCUSED RÉSUMÉ IN RESPONSE TO PUBLISHED EMPLOYMENT LISTING

Other Certifications Water Safety Instructor, American Red Cross, 1998 *Work Experience* Peer Counselor (part-time), Women's Resource Center, YWCA, August 2001 to January 2003. Provided one-on-one peer counseling relating to rape and domestic abuse. Aquatics Supervisor, YWCA, Middletown, IL, December 1998 to August 2001. Recruited, trained and organized lifeguards and water instructors for various aquatics classes and projects in large non-profit organization.	List in reverse chronological order, most recent first. (Title, Employer, City, State, Dates). List related positions prior to physical therapy education or list related positions in the health or human service fields. Give a brief description of your work-related duties. List in reverse chronological order, most recent first.
Clinical Internships Warm Springs Rehab Center, Warm Springs, IL, March 8 to May 5, 2003. Participated in interdisciplinary care of persons with neurological involvement. Southland Women's Center, Southland, IL, January 18 to March 5, 2003. Participated in interdisciplinary education and intervention for women with osteoporosis, balance issues and stress incontinence in community -based women's health clinic.	Facility, City, State, Dates. Brief description of clinical responsibilities and accomplishments. List in reverse chronological order, most recent first.
Honors and Activities Student Liaison, American Physical Therapy Association 2001 to 2003. President, Student Physical Therapist Assistant Organization 2001 to 2003. Dean's list 1997 to 1999, 2001 to 2003.	List community activities, clubs, professional organizations, honors and awards. Include dates.
References References available on request.	Either list those persons whom you have asked to serve as references for you or write, "References available on request."

What to Include?

Most students have acquired valuable experiences while in college and/or with previous responsibilities. Voluntary and work experience, leadership roles, projects, and accomplishments often relate directly to employer needs. Employers want to see that you are a self-starter, have had experience, and can work well with others. Also, if there were large gaps in your activity, you may want to account for those gaps in time with a brief explanation, such as "Part-time college enrollment to fulfill requirements of PTA degree."

What Not to Include?

Although many résumés include a section on personal information traits, you do not need to include personal information, such as age, marital status, number of children, citizenship, ethnicity, or your assessment of your personality. In fact, it is illegal for an employer to ask any question that is unrelated to the position for which you are applying. Why create opportunities for biases to enter the picture?

Table 23-3

SAMPLE COVER LETTER—UNSOLICITED

Shara Straightforward, SPTA
556 W. Highland Ave
Center City, IL 62666
(888)-554-1017

	Your current address and telephone at the time of writing the letter
June 1, 2003	Date letter is sent.
Stephen Simpson, Owner Four Corners Physical Therapy 1500 Reisner Drive Center City, IL 62667	Name, correct title, and address.
Dear Mr. Simpson:	Never write "To Whom It May Concern."
Several of my colleagues in the physical therapist assistant program had the opportunity to work with you during their clinical training. Your clinic's reputation for excellent clinical services in orthopedic and sports physical therapy is well known at Mid-State College. I am writing to inquire about potential clinical openings in the next few months. My résumé details my experiences before and during my education program. One recent experience confirmed my interests in working in an out-patient sports physical therapy practice setting.	Include the purpose of writing this letter. Personalize your letter to the person reading it.
My interest in orthopedics and sports medicine has been long-standing. I completed a bachelor's degree in Health & Wellness from Mid-State University in 2000.	What have you found most meaningful and motivating? Who, where, and how did you have this experience? Personalize this section.
I recently had the opportunity to work with Jerri Jacobson, PT at Tri-City Sports Rehabilitation Clinic during one of my internships. I worked with several athletes who were preparing for competition in the Olympic trials. This experience taught me a great deal about working with elite athletes.	What additional experiences support your qualifications? How did you acquire such outstanding skills? Show your enthusiasm in your achievements and accomplishments.
I am an active student member in the American Physical Therapy Association and I represented Mid-State College at the National Student Conclave in Birmingham, Alabama in 2002.	
Should you anticipate an opening for a physical therapist assistant, please let me know. I am interested in part-time, full-time, or per diem opportunities. You can leave me a message anytime at (888)-554-1017 anytime or reach me at email: sstraightforward@aol.com.	Take action. Remember that the employer has needs that must be met. Be straight forward and indicate your availability to talk. If you don't hear, call periodically and indicate your continued interest.
Thank you for your consideration. I hope to hear from you in the near future.	
Sincerely, Shara Straightforward, SPTA Enclosure: résumé	

Preparing Your Résumé

Keep your résumé up-to-date as you go through the PTA program. There may be scholarships, part-time employment, projects, or leadership opportunities that arise. A current and accurate résumé will assist you to succeed in these opportunities.

After you have prepared a résumé, ask a colleague to look it over. It may also be helpful to ask for feedback from human resource personnel or administrators in a clinical affiliation or from faculty members. Your College's Career Placement Center usually offers services which can support your résumé preparation and job search.

Make certain that there are not typographical or grammatical errors in your résumé. Print the document with a high-quality printer and high-quality paper. Take the original to be copied on heavyweight paper at a copy center. It costs only a few cents more per page and the results are certainly worth it. You want your résumé to work for you. To do that, it must stand out. This is the first impression a potential employer will make of you!

Cover Letter

A cover letter is a critical part of your search for employment. The cover letter must accompany your résumé and needs to show how your individual qualities and experiences set you apart from the rest of the applicants. It should focus on your strongest qualifications, experience and how you will contribute to the employer's organization. Use the following guidelines:

* Your letter, whether unsolicited or in response to a published employment listing, should be addressed to a specific person in the organization, by name and correct title. If you need to, call and ask for spelling and title information. Call and say, "I would like to send a letter to the Director of Physical Therapy; could you help me with the correct spelling and title for this person?" Use a proper business format in writing the letter, providing your return address, the date, and the address of the recipient. An employment ad might direct you to an individual in the Human Resources Department of a large organization. If so, make initial contact with and write your cover letter to that person.

* The introduction of your letter should indicate your purpose in writing and refer to what attracted you to send the letter and résumé. If appropriate, refer to a published employment listing by date and publication and to the job title

listed. If you made a contact at a conference, mention the conference. Even if a specific position isn't advertised or available at the current time, indicate what types of positions you are seeking (staff PTA, full-time, part-time, per diem) Summarize your qualifications and experience in the first paragraph.

* Continue to highlight your experience and qualifications that qualify you for this position in the next few paragraphs. If an employment listing gives several qualifiers, be sure to address each of those. Use action verbs to describe accomplishments and experience. Use your strongest qualifiers in this section. You can refer the reader to other qualifications in your résumé. Try to stay under four paragraphs (one page) in your letter.

* Conclude the letter with a request to schedule an interview. Suggest dates and times that you will be available. This is especially effective if you know that you will be traveling to the employer's location at your own expense and only in town for a few days. Give your telephone number and the dates and times when you can be reached.

Table 23-3 shows the cover letter written by Shara Straightforward in search of possible future openings in practice settings she desired. She sent her résumé (see Table 23-1) with each personalized cover letter.

Table 23-4 shows the cover letter sent by Debra Dynamic in response to the published employment listing. She also sent the résumé (see Table 23-2) that addresses the specifics of this published employment listing.

Interviewing

Make a Good First Impression

Your first impression is made in a matter of moments. Be careful to make the best impression. Although it might seem obvious, here are a few "musts":

* Dress conservatively in clean and pressed business attire, shoes, and socks/stockings.

* Avoid excessive or obvious jewelry and accessories, after-shave, or perfumes.

* Take care with your grooming: hair, beard, and nails.

* Take a shower or bathe.

* Brush your teeth and use mouthwash if needed.

* Use deodorant.

Table 23-4

SAMPLE COVER LETTER–RESPONSE TO PUBLISHED LISTING

Debra Dynamic, PTA *222 W. Hill Street* *Center City, IL 62666* *(888)-555-6666*	Your current address and telephone at the time of writing the letter.
June 27, 2003	Date letter is sent.
Nancy Royal, Director Rehabilitation Services University Medical Center 1001 University Drive Center City, IL 62667	Name, correct title, and address.
Dear Ms. Royal:	Never write "To Whom It May Concern."
Throughout my physical therapist assistant education, I have been impressed with the scope of the clinical services and innovative programs offered at University Medical Center. I am writing to apply for the physical therapist assistant opening on the women's health team, published in the *Center City Women's Health Bulletin* on June 26, 2003. My résumé details my involvement in the women's health field for the past 5 years in a variety of capacities, including both physical and mental health. I'd like to highlight how one of my clinical internships greatly contributed to my experience base and further interested me in the women's health field.	Include the purpose of writing this letter. Summarize your experience in a sentence and introduce the next paragraph.
My assignment to the Southland Women's Center in Southland, IL provided me with a unique opportunity to work with Caroline Coughlin, DPT and a team of other physical therapists, nurse practitioners and physicians. Through this experience, I gained expertise in Women's Health, a growing and important aspect of physical therapy. In addition to the physical therapists, I worked with gynecologists, nurses, and social workers and thoroughly enjoyed this specialty area. I monitored women with osteoporosis and young mothers following childbirth with therapeutic exercise programs. This experience, combined with my previous work, motivated me to seek a career opportunity in women's health.	What have you found most meaningful and motivating? Who, where, and how did you have this experience? Personalize this section.
My leadership and organizational experience also enhances my potential to contribute to program implementation in this area. Through my work at the YWCA and at the Women's Resource Center I have developed outstanding organizational and communication skills. I earned my Water Safety Instructor certification in 1998 and have 5 years of experience in the aquatics field.	What additional experiences support your qualifications? How did you acquire such outstanding skills? Show your enthusiasm in your achievements and accomplishments.
I look forward to discussing your needs and my qualifications for this position. I am available at (888)-555-6666 everyday until 10:00 am and you can leave a message at this number anytime. Thank you for your consideration. I hope to hear from you in the near future.	Take action. Remember that the employer has needs that must be met. Be straight forward and indicate your availability to talk. If you don't hear, call Ms. Royal and inquire about the timetable for the employment search. Indicate your continued interest.
Sincerely, Debra Dynamic, PTA Enclosure: résumé	

Prepare for the Interview

Do your homework and learn as much as possible about the organization and individuals with whom you will be interviewing. Identify the needs and fears of your potential employer. The employer may not know the role or potential contributions that a PTA can make to the organization.

Are PTAs currently employed? Have there been previously? Has the current staff worked with PTAs? If you can allay misconceptions and explain how your presence will meet the employer's needs, you will be more likely to be hired.[2]

Although it may seem that you are the one who needs the job, try to step outside your perspective for a moment. Put yourself in the employer's shoes. The employer may be replacing someone who has left or developing a new position. The employer has an unmet need that created an open position. What, specifically, is the nature of that need? Is it for a certain skill set, temperament, organizational function? Are there trends in this practice setting which require knowledge and skills which you have? Think specifically about the projects you have done and papers you have written. How will you fit into the employer's needs?

Also consider the employer's fears. Although you may be the one who is nervous and afraid that you won't be able to pay back your student loans, your potential employer is also afraid. The employer's fears may center around making a poor decision, about whether your inexperience will spell trouble for the organization, and about whether you will need excessive help and supervision to come up to speed. The employer might be worried that you will take this job for the time being and move onto something better if it comes along. Your job in this interview is to help your potential employer feel comfortable that you can handle the responsibilities of the position and that you are a great choice.

Now, how do you find out what are your potential employer's needs and fears? Informational interviewing, of course. Talk with someone in a similar position in a similar organization. Consult your faculty regarding trends in the field. Consult with employees in similar organizations that you may know through your contacts and networks. Find out as much as you can about the position, why it is open, and who had the job last.

Practice responding to potential interview questions directly and concisely. Make good eye contact. Breathe deeply. Imagine yourself succeeding and things going well.

Your interviewer may bring up a salary figure. Do not commit to anything at this point. You have not been offered a position, yet! Indicate your interest in knowing the range of salary being considered for this position. It is unwise for you to ask about salary and benefits early in the interview.

Finish Strongly

Leave a good impression. Thank your interviewer and express continued interest. Find out when a hiring decision will be made. Make yourself useful in providing a list of references without hesitation.

Be certain that you have permission of each reference you have listed.

Follow-Up Immediately

Go home and immediately write a follow-up letter to your interviewer. Thank your interviewer and restate the areas you would like to emphasize about your background and interests. Be sure to emphasize what you, uniquely, will be able to contribute to the organization. As appropriate, indicate your willingness to travel between facilities, work various hours, or be flexible in waiting for a full-time position to develop.

The Job Offer

When the job offer comes, then you can start negotiating. Look at the terms of employment and the benefits offered. Full health and dental benefits are often valued at 25% to 30% of the total salary package. Negotiate a higher starting salary if you will have to pay benefits yourself. Although a starting salary may be lower than you expected, perhaps there is the potential of career advancement or administrative and program development experience that will strengthen your future career opportunities. Make a list of the tangible and intangible benefits.

Remember that this is your first position in the profession of physical therapy. Make the most of the opportunities available to you.

Summary

Entering the job market as a new graduate can be challenging. It does not have to be painful or traumatic. Preparing for a career in physical therapy can be an exciting time of self-discovery. Networking and informational interviewing can both assist greatly in developing potential employment contacts and opportunities. Thoughtful résumé preparation and construction of appropriate cover letters will encourage doors opening for employment opportunities. Prepare for interviews and approach them with a positive outlook. Get off to a great start!

References

1. APTA. Job listings. *PT Bulletin On-Line.* Available at: http://www.apta.org/bulletin/job_listings. Accessed September 9, 2004.

2. Curtis KA. Career survival skills. Presented at: Cedars-Sinai Medical Center Invited Presentation. Annual Conference, American Physical Therapy Association; June 1998; Las Vegas, Nev.

3. Curtis KA: Wanted: a few good therapists. *Rehab Management.* 1989;2(4):18-22.

4. Bolles RN, Bolles D. *2000 What Color is Your Parachute?* 30th ed. Berkeley, Calif: Ten Speed Press; 2000.

PUTTING IT INTO PRACTICE

Consult your textbooks and the American Physical Therapy Association Web site to answer the following questions about the physical therapy profession:

1. Interview a partner or colleague and write a brief response to each of the following questions. Give your notes to your partner or colleague.

   Your ideal life

   What is most important to your life? Consider the following:
   - What is most important to you in your personal life?
   - What is most important to you in your career?
   - What are your personal goals? Your career goals?
   - How long do you envision yourself staying in one position or one location?

   Envision the ideal organization

   What are the things you consider to be most important in an organization in which you will work? Consider the following:
   - What goals or mission of an organization would be most attractive?
   - What would this organization contribute to society?
   - What size would this organization be?
   - What experience will you gain?
   - Where is the optimal location of your ideal workplace?
   - What are the working conditions?
   - With what kinds of people would you most like to be working?
   - What are the needs of this type of organizations in the social and health care climate?

   What do you have to offer?

   Consider the following:
   - What unique skills, abilities, and experiences will you bring to the workplace?
   - What problems can you help to solve for the organization given your unique skills?
   - What new programs are you interested in helping to develop?
   - What will colleagues gain by working with you?
   - What will clients or patients gain by working with you?
   - How can you improve the efficiency of the organization?

2. Identify your network

   Use the circle below to represent yourself. Write names and draw lines from your circle to individuals whom you would consider in your network, who are readily accessible to you for information, help and advice. Next, write new names and draw lines to individuals, organizations and other entities to which your contacts have access. You should have a page filled with ideas and potential contacts. Circle those whom you feel may be of greatest benefit for information or providing potential contacts in your job search.

   Faculty   Clinical
   Instructors

   (**YOU**)

   Organizations   Family/Friends

3. Informational interviews

Who, in your network, could provide you with information about the current needs, employment climate and trends in the practice sector or geographical location in which you would most like to work? (This is not a person whom you are asking for a position. This is a person whom you are asking for advice in how to approach your job search. You are asking for contacts, access to networks and information which will help you to succeed.) Make a list below of your best choices:

Call one of those contacts and schedule a convenient time to talk or take this person out for lunch or coffee.

Develop a list of questions below:

4. List your strategies for approaching the job search.
   What did you learn from your informational interview?

What new contacts will you make?

What individuals, events, groups or networks can you approach next?

To whom will you send letters and résumés?

CHAPTER 24

Challenges for
the New Graduate

> Portia was excited—she was finally going to begin using all she had learned and worked so hard for the past 2 years on patients—and get paid for it! She looked forward to starting at the skilled nursing facility. It was close to home and had an excellent reputation.
>
> Six weeks later... Portia had difficulty getting up in the morning. She felt exhausted and depressed. It seemed that so few people really cared about what happened to these patients. She took it so seriously; why was she the only one who cared?
>
> Then there was the physical therapy. She found it hard to believe that she and her colleagues had studied about the same career. Why weren't they doing the things they had learned? It seemed like everyone was just cutting corners and trying to get by with the bare minimum of care. Her supervisor seemed only to care about her productivity and her patients were discharged from rehab way too soon. She decided to look for a new job in a few months.

Portia, like many new graduates, is experiencing reality shock.[1] What happened here? Did the skilled nursing center take a turn for the worse? Did Portia have a few bad experiences? It is unlikely that either of these are the cause of Portia 's feelings.

Role Stress

New graduate physical therapists (PTs) and physical therapist assistants (PTAs) often experience role stress.[1] One source of stress is the conflicting values of work and school. This conflict has been called *reality shock*. It is a fairly predictable phenomenon which was first described in the nursing profession in the mid-1970s.[2,3]

What Happens?

Students have often studied and excelled in an idealized environment, where individualized, comprehensive patient-centered care is required, theoretical problem-solving skills are highly valued. In contrast, the work environment demands safe, efficient care, organization and efficiency, delegation to others, teamwork, cooperation, and accountability. Long work days, less sleep, and information overload contributes to the stress in the working world today.[4]

Reality shock often occurs due to the unexpected differences between the values of the academic world and the working world.[2,3] The behaviors required in the work environment conflict with the idea of individualized patient care that students practice in school. The time-consuming and ideal model of patient care presented in school is incompatible with the clinical environment that requires PTs and PTAs to work within established time and resource constraints. See Table 24-1 for examples of conflicts between school and work values.

In addition to experiencing many difficult conflicts between school and work values, new graduates often leave the PTA program with the impression that there is one correct way to accomplish a task, approach a problem, or address a conflict. In striving to answer test questions correctly, students often believe that their answer is the answer, without recognizing that their answer may be one answer and that there may be many others as well.

Further, remember that graduate PTAs are often comfortable in the world of textbooks and practice sessions where clinicians are more comfortable in reality and recognize what it takes to survive in that world. Consider the following situation:

Table 24-1

CONFLICTS IN SCHOOL AND WORK VALUES

School Values	Work Values
I was required to manage my time, plan my projects, and make my own schedule.	You're responsible to see a patient every 30 minutes.
I was rewarded for being thorough and complete in my work.	You must prioritize because you can't do everything in the limited time available.
I was encouraged to reflect, read articles, and consider the rationale for all decisions.	You need to follow the protocol as it's written. This is how we do it here.
I was at the top of my class; I have a great memory and strong intuition to know what's right to do.	You need to get feedback from the rest of the team before taking action and, of course, work within legal and ethical boundaries.
I was encouraged to communicate frequently with the PT.	Some PTs do not appreciate being "interrupted" and don't seem to understand your role or their responsibilities regarding supervision.
If I was bored or tired, I could tell the faculty I had a "crisis" and would not make it to class or had to leave early.	You have a responsibility to your patients and colleagues. If you are detached, late, or absent, everyone is short-changed.
I learned all these great exercises to use in aquatics. you ever hear of my professor?	You'll need to focus on patient education because Did you have only one visit.
These exercises would be perfect for this patient's problem.	These exercises require too much assistance and equipment; the patient lives alone.
School was my first priority. I was never late to class.	In addition to arriving on time, you're also responsible for the safety and well-being of all of your patients and for facilitating communication with the PT.

> Roxie, a new graduate PTA, consulted Quinn, an experienced PTA who had specialized in neurology, regarding the most appropriate treatment for a young man with a brain injury. They watched the patient's gait together to determine the most appropriate way to normalize his movement patterns. Quinn commented on the patient's muscle tone and difficulty flexing the left knee during the push-off phase of gait. He suggested that Roxie work with the patient in the kneeling position to try to normalize his tone. Roxie was surprised to hear Quinn suggest that over gait training with a cane. Roxie asked Quinn why he wouldn't work on his ambulation since that would be more functional?

Both Roxie and Quinn are functioning in their comfort zones. Roxie is trying to make sense of this complex and overwhelming problem using what she remembers from school and seems to be more functional. Quinn is working in the practical reality of observations and possible interventions that the patient can safely practice himself. He is thinking about the future and projecting an effect of an intervention and eventual recovery. Roxie does not think like Quinn at this point in her career (see Chapter 9). The result of this interaction for both Roxie and Quinn may be frustration.

Doing It All is Not Easy

And finally, we have to keep in mind that the new PTA's role requires skills in several areas that are emphasized in many PTA curricula, including time management, caseload management, documentation for reimbursement, and interpersonal relationships. The complex demands in the clinical environment may leave new graduates overwhelmed and exhausted.

Interestingly, new graduates have often been protected from the realities of clinical practice during clinical education. Student PTAs are typically responsible for a reduced caseload, infrequently responsible for completing documentation while working with multiple patients and often see the most interesting "teaching cases." It is not surprising that new graduates are stressed when expectations suddenly change with employment!

Table 24-2
COMMON CAUSES OF ROLE STRESS AND BURNOUT

Cause	Feelings That Precipitate Role Stress and Burnout
Work overload	I can't possibly get all of this paperwork done.
Understaffing	I'm here alone! How can I see all of these patients this afternoon?
Repetitive tasks	If I get delegated to yet another ultrasound, I'll scream!
Underutilization of technical skills and problem solving	It seems hard to believe it requires a degree to turn on a whirlpool!
Role ambiguity	It makes it so hard to work when I'm constantly worried that the PTs don't understand my role and legal responsibilities of appropriate supervision.
Role conflict	One therapist treats me with respect and delegates appropriately; the other one treats me like an aide to do ultrasounds and clean up after her.
Inappropriate helping behavior	I know that I could motivate this patient… if he'd just come for his therapy appointments. I think I'll call and remind him about the schedule of the buses that go by his house.
Unrealistic expectations	I could stay on schedule if the nurses would just do their jobs and have the patients ready when they're scheduled.

Burnout

Burnout is a state of emotional and physical exhaustion that results from intense and persistent stress. This is especially prevalent in the helping professions because of the intensity of the work and the emotional and psychological bonds formed with the people being served.[5,6]

The level and manifestations of burnout vary among individuals; however, no longer enjoying or being motivated by work is a universal symptom. Burnout may result in a loss of concern for people, ineffective communication, and/or poor job performance.[5-7]

Burnout has been documented widely in the profession of physical therapy, often starting during the student years.[7-11] Therapists report feelings of emotional exhaustion, often related to work overload with conflicting time and resource constraints.[7,10] Many issues can contribute to feelings of burnout. Look at the list in Table 24-2 and see if you can identify any common feelings or situations.

So what can we do?

Resolving Reality Shock Productively

By developing awareness and skills that allow them to adapt to and take an active role in the work environment, new graduates feel better about their work, their colleagues, and their career in physical therapy.

New graduates who master the skills required for the clinical role are likely to be more satisfied. In contrast, graduates who are unable to resolve the conflicts they face may find themselves dissatisfied and in a constant search for the perfect job. The consequences of unresolved conflict are serious. Check the list in Table 24-3.

Validating Feelings and Conflicts

Role conflict is a normal process that evolves from a predictable set of circumstances. It occurs across professions and even when changing professions. The workplace is likely to require performance that is in *direct conflict* with the recent graduate's experiences in school.

Graduates must recognize that this stressful period is part of the process of assuming their new roles and joining an organization.[12,13] There are sources of support and strategies that will help graduates to adapt to the realities of clinical practice.

First, recognize that the feelings presented in Tables 24-2 and 24-3 are real. Individual reactions to role conflict may range from disappointment and confusion to outrage. The action that you take as a result of a feeling is what's important. This is where there is a choice.

Second, realize that we often feel frustrated and angry when circumstances that affect us are out of

---

Table 24-3

THE COSTS OF ROLE STRESS

Therapist Feelings	Maladaptive Response	Better Response
There must be a better job out there. My friends from school don't have to put up with this.	Early turnover and job-hopping from one dissatisfying situation to another.	Sharing feelings with colleagues and supervisors. Changing strategies to deal with challenges. Suggesting improvements in working conditions.
I had no idea clinical practice would be this boring.	Leaving the field or pursuing a career change.	Seeking new challenges. Joining a committee, become actively involved in your professional association.
All I've seen for weeks are backs, necks, hips, and knees.	Boredom, depersonalization, treating people like "backs," "necks," "hips," and "knees."	Adopting the point of view that each patient is unique, regardless of their diagnosis. Grouping patients with similar problems to provide similar services and education more efficiently.
I am not making the salary I deserve.	Doing the bare minimum to get by.	Requesting a raise after showing that your work is exemplary and outcomes exceed expectations.
I'm getting nowhere. I've been working on this positioning program for months and it seems like someone on the night shift always forgets.	Giving up. Feeling like it's not worth the effort to try; someone always drops the ball.	Finding out what happened and working individually with staff members who have responsibilities. Expecting accountability and responsibility.
Hospital policy prevents me from spending more than 45 minutes per day with this patient.	Blindly following the rules... the patient will have to suffer because of this policy. Why doesn't the administration consider the patient's needs and not just the bottom line?	Recognizing that there are exceptions to rules. Presenting the patient's needs to your supervisor with a plan to for meeting them. Consider alternatives such as co-treatment with occupational therapy.
No one cares about the patients as much as I do.	Spending free time after work and on weekends doing paperwork and related job duties. Assuming that others are doing a poor job.	Making appropriate referrals to community agencies. Set personal boundaries and time to revitalize.

---

our control. Lashing out is a coping mechanism that absolves us of responsibility for the problems we face. Decisions that impose massive cost containment and restrictive regulations may leave physical therapists and PTAs feeling powerless. However, individual physical therapists and PTAs can be responsible for their own thoughts and attitudes, interactions and actions with their patients and colleagues.

Rather than judging your colleagues and co-workers as wrong, lazy, incompetent, thoughtless, or insensitive, recognize that there are thoughts and beliefs that also motivate their behaviors. Focus your energy on changing what is changeable and on the areas in which you have some control and influence.

Making Good Choices

The choices that present themselves in a day of work are endless. You may not feel that you are accomplishing everything that you "should" be doing. Eliminate this from your expectations. Then, concentrate on what is most important for your responsibilities to run smoothly, and other staff to be able to work effectively with you.

Survival Skills

There are key activities that will lead to a productive and satisfying career in the profession of physical therapy. These survival skills are essential to cope with the many demands of clinical practice.[13] They include:

* Addressing highest priority patient needs
* Using effective interpersonal skills with patients, coworkers and supervisors
* Choosing effective time management and documentation strategies
* Continue your education and networking with supportive colleagues

Time Management

Managing your time can be a challenge throughout your physical therapist assistant education and career. Review some of the key elements of time management in Chapter 11. Table 24-4 lists many useful time management strategies in the clinical setting.

Peer Support Networks

One of the most effective coping strategies to deal with reality shock is to develop strong support networks of colleagues who face similar challenges. It is especially important that new graduates have contact with experienced colleagues who can offer support to help deal with difficult patients, productivity pressures, communication with coworkers and other issues about which new graduates express concerns.

Peer support helps to decrease role stress. When workers have positive interpersonal interactions with their co-workers, they tend to feel more satisfied about their work.[14] Create networks of peers who are able to support each other. Organize social events, informal networking and make an effort to both seek and offer this essential support.

Mentors

A mentor is an experienced clinician who is able to validate your experiences and feelings, share strate-gies, and offer guidance and advice that assists with early career development. Mentoring is a process that enables an individual to develop personal and professional growth as a result of a special relationship with another individual who serves as a guide.[16] This differs from a clinical supervisor in that a supervisor has direct responsibility for your performance.

If there is not a program in place through your employer, you can seek a mentor either through clinical networks in your area or with the mentoring program offered by the American Physical Therapy Association. You can read more about this at www.apta.org/advocacy/womeninitiatives/members-mentor.

Choose Your Battles

Although it may seem that most of the requirements, policies, and procedures in the clinical environment are out of your control, think carefully about where and how your time will be best spent. Take action where it counts. Choosing your battles means working smarter and applying effort in areas which are both important and changeable. Remember the important ways in which you contribute to the future of physical therapy as described in Chapter 3. Be proactive and believe in your self! Table 24-5 gives guidelines for choosing issues for maximum effect.

Summary

New graduates face predictable challenges and frustrations as they move from the more controlled environment of education into the workplace. The choices that one makes determine one's experience during this stressful time. Practicing effective survival skills, such as time management, seeking peer and mentor support and actively choosing when, where, and how to apply effort for change are essential early career strategies. New graduates who develop awareness and skills that allow them to adapt to and take an active role in the work environment are more satisfied with their work, their colleagues, and the profession of physical therapy.

References

1. Deckard G, Present R. Impact of role stress on physical therapists; emotional and physical well-being. *Phys Ther*. 1989;69:713-718.
2. Kramer M. *Reality Shock*. St Louis, Mo: Mosby; 1974.

Table 24-4

TIME MANAGEMENT STRATEGIES IN THE CLINICAL SETTING FOR THE NEW GRADUATE

1. Develop a system. List goals and set priorities.

If applicable, make sub-goals and give each a target date. Keep your list in plain view, over the desk or on a bulletin board or your clipboard. (You may want to do this in conjunction with your supervisor.)

2. Give yourself a time to think and handle problems.

This might involve a few minutes before starting your morning and afternoon schedules. Plan on this and make this time a priority, just as important as all your other scheduled responsibilities.

3. Schedule daily paperwork time and a time to return phone calls.

Have what you need to do ready to go, so that you can use this time most effectively. Do not compromise on this time more than once a week, no matter how busy you are.

4. Make a daily TO DO list (every day at the same time; on one piece of paper).

Post this in a conspicuous place or carry it on a clipboard you have with you all the time.

5. Ask yourself "What is the best use of my time right now?" FREQUENTLY!

6. For memos, announcements, paperwork:

A.   Handle each piece of paper you receive only once:
   1. Get rid of it ASAP
   2. Either:
      • Take action (respond, place on to do list, etc).
      • Pass it on to others.
      • Read it, absorb it, and destroy.
B.   For patient-related documentation
   1. Document once, while seeing the patient. Copying over your notes wastes time.
   2. Use pre-printed forms or computerized documentation systems when possible to help organize your notes and insure thorough documentation.
   3. Dictate if available. Once you get used to doing this, it takes less than one-quarter the time of writing the same information!
   4. During daily treatment, include documentation time while the patient is being seen.

7. For phone calls you make or receive:

A.   Use your "on-hold" time to your advantage to do other paperwork or sort mail and papers.
B.   Make several phone calls at once.
C.   If it is not convenient to receive a phone call, request that a message be taken. Ask reception personnel to find out from the caller when the best time is for you to return the phone call or give the caller a good time to call you back.
D.   Make a list of questions or points you want to cover during the phone call. Make records of all phone calls in the same location. A daily planner or desk log works well.

8. Do this now.

Adapted from Curtis KA. *Training New Staff for Clinical Survival.* Los Angeles, Calif; Health Directions, 1987.

Table 24-5
WORKING SMARTER

Is it important to me, a patient, my colleagues, and the organization in which I work?	Can I/We Influence the Desired Outcome Here?	
	YES	NO
YES	The highest priority for action. Plan carefully and strategize a series of approaches that are likely to result in the desired outcome.	Find out who can influence the desired outcome. At what level is a policy or decision being made? Serve as an advocate for patients. Take community-based action. Write letters, make phone calls. Involve your Representative or Senator at the state or federal level.
NO	Focus your time and energy on outcomes that make a difference in people's lives.	Do not bother... It is not important and it's out of your control.

---

3. Schmalenberg, C., Kramer, M. *Coping with Reality Shock: The Voices of Experience*. City: Nursing Resources; 1979.

4. Mayo Clinic Staff. Managing workplace stress: plan your approach. Available at: http://www.mayoclinic.com/invoke.cfm?id=HA00017. Accessed September 8, 2004.

5. Malugani M. Battling burnout: health professions are at high risk. Available at: http://healthcare.monster.com/articles/burnout. Accessed September 24, 2004..

6. Levine J. Throwing in the towel: are you experiencing burn-out? Available at: http://daycare.about.com//library/weekly/aa042301a.htm. Accessed September 24, 2003.

7. Waldrop S. Battling burnout: maintaining enthusiasm in a challenging environment. *PT*. 2003;11(6): 38-45.

8. Balogun JA, Hoeberlein-Miller TM, Schneider E, Katz JS. Academic performance is not a viable determinant of physical therapy students' burnout. *Percept Mot Skills*. 1996;83(1):21-22.

9. Kolb K. Graduating burnout candidates. *Phys Ther*. 1994;74(3):264-265.

10. Donohoe E, Nawawi A, Wilker L, Schindler T, Jette DU. Factors associated with burnout of physical therapists in Massachusetts rehabilitation hospitals. *Phys Ther*. 1993;73(11):750-761.

11. Wandling BJ, Smith BS. Burnout in orthopaedic physical therapists. *J Orthop Sports Phys Ther*. 1997;26(3):124-130.

12. Smith DM. Organizational socialization of physical therapists. *Phys Ther*. 1989;69(4):282-286.

13. Schwertner RM, Pinkston D, O'Sullivan P., et al. Transition from student to physical therapist. *Phys Ther*. 1987;67(5):695-701.

14. Cooper B. Beat burnout! *PT*. 2003;11(4): 29-31.

15. Curtis KA. *Training New Staff for Clinical Survival*. Los Angeles: Health Directions; 1987.

16. APTA. Mentoring program. Available at: http://www.apta.org/advocacy/womeninitiatives/membersmentor. Accessed September 9, 2004.

PUTTING IT INTO PRACTICE

1. Read each of the following and identify the feelings of the graduate. Discuss a strategy or response that addresses the problem presented:

   A. I'm not being given the opportunity to use any of my resources or my education. I don't have my own patients or any responsibility for anything important. I've done a lot more as a student than I'm doing now! There's nothing I've done to make them think that I'm unsafe or incompetent.

   B. I had some training in how to run treatment groups, but doing it is a totally different story. We're so short-staffed that there's no one I can go to for ongoing support and feedback after each group. I'd really like to know what I'm doing wrong and how I can get all of the patients more involved.

   C. I learned how to do this procedure in school. They did it a different way during my clinical affiliations. Now they do it a different way here. To top it all off, the nurses on the floor do it even another way. I just don't know what's right!

   D. Before I came here, I worked in a much larger facility. I know that part of the experience I had is because of the size of the place, but it really doesn't seem that the standards of care here are anywhere near as high. I'm really worried that something awful is going to happen to one of my patients, especially on the evening and night shift.

   E. It seems that my supervisor never talks to me except to tell me what is going wrong. There's no comment on all the good things I'm doing!

   F. There's an experienced member of our staff who outright lies about the things he's doing. I covered some of his patients this weekend. He says that he's done all these wonderful things and the patients looked at me like I was crazy when I asked them about those same things.

   G. The thing that I find most disturbing is the attitude of the staff toward the patients. I've been working with very severely involved patients and it just doesn't seem like anyone cares whether they do the best job possible. I hope that I never turn into someone like that!

   H. I'm so nervous when I have to ask this one PT to change something. I know exactly what I want to say and then it just comes out sounding like I don't know anything.

2. Identify a person who could serve as a mentor. Keep in touch during your first few years of practice.

CHAPTER 25

Planning for Life-Long Learning

Senovia looked at the brochures for continuing education courses. They all looked so good and they were all so expensive. She thought, "I've just finished my Associate's degree. There is so much that I still need to learn, but how can I pay for all of this?"

Life-Long Learning for the Physical Therapist Assistant

Entry-level education is just the beginning. Learning does not end at the conclusion of the physical therapist assistant educational program. Life-long learning involves continuing to question, read, and apply information that facilitates growth. It requires reflection and processing of experiences and integration of new developments into existing knowledge and practices.

Changes in policy requires changes in attitudes, practices, and sometimes, organizational structures. New developments, new technology, and collaboration also offers opportunities to grow and enhance the foundation gained during formal education. Life-long learning assures that clinicians use up-to-date and relevant information about teaching and learning, technology, administration, and clinical practice parameters.

Standard 5 of the *Guide for Conduct of the Physical Therapist Assistant* (see Appendix 2) indicates that physical therapist assistants (PTAs) shall achieve and maintain competence in the provision of selected physical therapy interventions. This involves three considerations, competence, self-assessment, and development (Table 25-1).

The Information Age

Information and knowledge are changing at a pace never before experienced. We are bombarded daily by e-mail, the Web, voicemail, fax, newspapers and magazines, professional journals, television, unsolicited mail, and telemarketers calling us in our homes and businesses. Information overload has been well-documented. For the first time in history, our capabilities for generating information are far greater than the human capacities to process all the information produced.[1]

Within the physical therapy field alone, we have seen the emergence of dozens of research journals, on-line publications, list-servs, and bulletin boards. How does one know what is most important? How does a practicing PTA access, sift through, prioritize, and decide to use the abundant information that is out there? There are several strategies that can guide career development.

A Career Development Plan

Set goals for career development. What interests do you have? Where do you see your career going in the next new months? The next year? In 5 years?

Self-Assessment

Let's look first at what you find interesting, exciting, and challenging. Consider yourself doing each of the activities in Table 25-2 in the next few years. What intrigues you? In which areas did you score the highest?

The career directions that you choose should be consistent with your interests. Interests can change with changes in responsibility and job requirements, as well. Therefore, what interests you now may not be what interests you for the future. You may want to return and repeat this inventory periodically to assess changes in your interests.

Table 25-1

STANDARDS SUPPORTING PHYSICAL THERAPIST ASSISTANT LIFELONG LEARNING

Standard 5:
A physical therapist assistant shall achieve and maintain competence in the provision of selected physical therapy interventions.

5.1 Competence

A physical therapist assistant shall provide interventions consistent with his/her level of education, training, experience, and skill.

5.2 Self-assessment

A physical therapist assistant shall engage in self-assessment in order to maintain competence.

5.3 Development

A physical therapist assistant shall participate in educational activities that enhance his/her basic knowledge and skills.

Adapted from APTA. *Guide for Conduct of the Physical Therapist Assistant.* Alexandria, Va: American Physical Therapy Association; 2001.

There are many career directions and paths one can take. The questions in Tables 25-3 and 25-4 may help you to prioritize your path and direction.

Continuing Education Courses and Conferences

José lived in Florida, a state that has a continuing education requirement for license renewal. How would he find courses that counted toward his license renewal requirements?

Courses, Seminars, and Workshops

There are numerous opportunities for PTAs to participate in short- and long-term seminars, courses, conferences, on-line, and home study courses. States that require continuing education for license renewal publish a specific listing of the types of organizations, courses, conferences, and activities that count toward meeting these requirements. Continuing education courses must meet specific criteria and often undergo evaluations to be able to offer continuing education units (CEUs). Check on your state's requirements.

High quality continuing education courses are well-founded in educational principles and use qualified course faculty and appropriate instructor to stu-

dent ratios and effective learning activities. Promotional materials often provide sufficient information to evaluate a course. Seek feedback from others who have taken the course as well. The guidelines presented in Table 25-5 may assist in decision making of which courses to consider taking.

Popular continuing education courses are available in many cities on different dates. The schedule of courses is often known months in advance. Call the continuing education provider to check on upcoming schedules and dates to plan ahead. Courses are publicized by brochures, on-line listings, and print listings in professional publications. American Physical Therapy Association (APTA) members often receive substantial discounts.

A listing of continuing education courses is available in *PT Bulletin On-line* at www.apta.org/bulletin/course_listings.

On-Line Continuing Education Series

There are various on-line continuing education courses offered through the American Physical Therapy Association and Sections. An online continuing education index is available at www.apta.org/Education/Continuing_Education.

The National Assembly of Physical Therapist Assistants (NAPTA) also offers continuing education courses specifically for the PTA. Check their Web site at www.apta.org/ Components/nationalassembly/PTAContinuingEd.

Table 25-2
SELF-ASSESSMENT OF CAREER INTERESTS[2]

Physical Therapist Assistant Career Interest Inventory

1	2	3	4	5	6	7
Not Interested						Extremely Interested

Using a scale from 1 to 7, rate your interest in each of the following activities:

_____ 1. Organize and teach an in-service session for physical therapist assistant students.

_____ 2. Read physical therapy journal articles and discuss clinical applications with colleagues.

_____ 3. Learn and apply new treatment techniques.

_____ 4. Help plan staffing requirements in your area for the next 2 months.

_____ 5. Help teach an orientation for new employees to prevent back injuries.

_____ 6. Attend a professional conference.

_____ 7. Discuss a patient's specific equipment needs.

_____ 8. Serve on a committee to design new programs to meet department needs.

_____ 9. Provide coaching or mentoring to high school students who are seeking a career as a physical therapist assistant.

_____ 10. Take an on-line course for physical therapist assistants.

_____ 11. Serve on a state task force to define clinical practice guidelines for the physical therapist assistant.

_____ 12. Research costs/features of needed equipment for your department.

_____ 13. Help teach a continuing education course

_____ 14. Save articles of interest from journals.

_____ 15. Discuss the best way to meet an individual patient's needs with the physical therapist.

_____ 16. Supervise (as permitted by state law) and evaluate performance of physical therapy aides.

_____ 17. Provide clinical instruction to PTA students.

_____ 18. Assist with data collection on physical therapy patient outcomes. Interact in team meeting to discuss patient progress.

_____ 19. Interact in team meeting to discuss patient progress

_____ 20. Help other staff members establish career goals.

_____ 21. Help develop or revise patient education materials (handouts, pamphlets).

_____ 22. Visit other facilities to observe a new or different program.

_____ 23. Advise others on the role of physical therapist assistant.

_____ 24. Give suggestions to increase productivity of a practice site.

_____ 25. Work with APTA district or state chapter to organize and publicize continuing education courses or seminars for physical therapist assistants.

_____ 26. Help to develop a survey for staff members or patients to obtain information.

_____ 27. Communicate patient progress to the physical therapist.

_____ 28. Be involved with interviewing new staff for hiring.

_____ 29. Help develop a videotape, CD-ROM, or Web site to teach new staff or patients.

_____ 30. Read manuals on high-tech equipment used in patient treatment.

_____ 31. Learn clinical protocols for treatment.

_____ 32. Help with patient scheduling to accommodate staff illnesses and vacations.

_____ 33. Preview a book or videotape for physical therapist assistants.

_____ 34. Look up books and articles in libraries and bookstores.

continued

Table 25-2 continued

SELF-ASSESSMENT OF CAREER INTERESTS[2]

Physical Therapist Assistant Career Interest Inventory

1	2	3	4	5	6	7
Not Interested						Extremely Interested

Using a scale from 1 to 7, rate your interest in each of the following activities:

_____ 35. Specialize in an area of clinical practice or work with a specific disability group.

_____ 36. Serve on a task force at your clinical facility to develop systems for smooth patient transition from in-patient to out-patient physical therapy.

_____ 37. Be a guest speaker in a physical therapist assistant educational program.

_____ 38. Read and discuss articles with colleagues about patient outcomes in physical therapy.

_____ 39. Receive recognition by patients and colleagues as an excellent clinician.

_____ 40. Help to write or revise departmental policies and procedures.

Enter and tally your scores below:

My Score	Item	My score	Item	My score	Item	My score	Item
_____	1.	_____	2.	_____	3.	_____	4.
_____	5.	_____	6.	_____	7.	_____	8.
_____	9.	_____	10.	_____	11.	_____	12.
_____	13.	_____	14.	_____	15.	_____	16.
_____	17.	_____	18.	_____	19.	_____	20.
_____	21.	_____	22.	_____	23.	_____	24.
_____	25.	_____	26.	_____	27.	_____	28.
_____	29.	_____	30.	_____	31.	_____	32.
_____	33.	_____	34.	_____	35.	_____	36.
_____	37.	_____	38.	_____	39.	_____	40.
TOTAL		**TOTAL**		**TOTAL**		**TOTAL**	
Teaching		Inquiry		Clinical		Administration	

Adapted from Curtis KA. Career planning in physical therapy. Presented at: California Chapter, American Physical Therapy Association Annual Conference; October 8, 1988; Monterey, Calif.

Conferences

Attending conferences may be very helpful to foster career development opportunities. Carefully check the conference program to identify sessions of interest. There may also be preconference courses which meet your needs as well. Review Chapter 21 for information about various types of conferences.

Certificates of Advanced Study

Another option for career development is to pursue university-based education to obtain a certificate of advanced study in a particular area such as health care management, information systems or practice management.

Certificates are non-degree programs that offer clusters of related courses, often designed to meet real-life business and organizational needs. These

---

Table 25-3

CAREER INTEREST INVENTORY SCORING FOR PHYSICAL THERAPIST ASSISTANTS[2]

Percentile Scores

	Low	Moderate	High	Very High
Teaching	10 to 48	49 to 54	55 to 60	61 to 70
Inquiry	10 to 33	34 to 35	46 to 57	58 to 70
Clinical	10 to 54	55 to 60	61 to 66	67 to 70
Administration	10 to 37	38 to 48	49 to 59	60 to 70

Select your two highest areas of interest:

Clinical-Teaching

This is the most common combination. Your interests are combined in working with students and patients. You will also be a natural at helping to develop educational materials for your patients. You are attracted to working with groups and will be an excellent clinician.

Administrative-Clinical

With this combination, you are a great resource for any organization. Keep up on changes in regulations and work proactively with other staff to help your organization adapt to the changing health care environment. You will enjoy creating new systems that enable you to provide clinical services with new challenges that face you.

Education-Inquiry

This combination is particularly well suited for a career that combines teaching and learning. Seek out opportunities to teach in the clinical setting. You may be able to volunteer as a guest speaker at local high schools and colleges to contribute to student learning. Seek a position at an institution that provides clinical education for student physical therapist assistants.

Clinical-Inquiry

Physical therapist assistants with this combination may be happiest in a clinical setting, working collaboratively with physical therapists who are involved in research. Seek opportunities to help with data collection in the course of your clinical day. Explore opportunities for advanced degrees that match your interests.

Administrative-Inquiry

Physical therapist assistants with this combination may be happiest working alone or with others on various projects and tasks. You may be very capable in managing a business or assisting with marketing of a clinical practice. You may need to seek an advanced degree to follow your interests on this career path.

Administrative-Teaching

With this combination of interests, you are well suited to assist with student or patient education programs in either academic or clinical settings. Additional education may be indicated to pursue this career path.

Adapted from Curtis KA. Career planning in physical therapy. Presented at: California Chapter, American Physical Therapy Association Annual Conference; October 8, 1988; Monterey, Calif.

Table 25-4

SETTING CAREER DEVELOPMENT GOALS

Consider your responses to the following questions:

1. What performance goals would you like to meet in the next year? Draw from your most recent clinical performance evaluation or other sources.

2. What do you need to be able to do or need to know to reach the above goals?

3. In what two areas would you like to develop your clinical, administrative, teaching, or inquiry skills in the next year? Be specific.

4. What is the best way for you to develop these areas? (Consider independent study, in-service education at work, mentoring relationships with another person, outside continuing education courses).

5. What resources are available in your current workplace that will help you to develop these areas? (Consider mentors, practice opportunities, in-service classes, employee development programs).

6. What resources are available in the community that will help you to develop these areas? (Consider continuing education courses, university programs, self-study courses, mentors).

7. What career goals would you like to meet in the next 5 years? What type of position would you like to have in 5 years? What additional skills or training do you need to make this career move? What additional responsibilities can you seek now that would prepare you for these goals?

---

courses may or may not offer university credit hours. Check with your local university extension office to see what is available in your area.

Clinical Residencies for Physical Therapists

Celia overheard Janice, a new graduate physical therapist, talking with an experienced staff member. Celia asked her colleague if it she knew anything about the new clinical residency program in pediatrics offered in the department.

Some physical therapists participate in postprofessional clinical residency programs. Clinical residency programs offer an established and organized program of clinical and specialty education. Residency programs enable physical therapists to enhance their preparation in providing clinical services in a specific area of clinical practice. Residents focus on skills such as examination, evaluation, diagnosis, prognosis, intervention, and management of patients. Residency programs often also include experiences in community service, patient education, research, and supervision of other personnel.

Credentialed residency programs must be at least 1500 hours and between 9 and 36 months duration. Following completion of a residency program, a physical therapist (PT) may be eligible and more prepared to sit for the American Board of Physical

Therapy Specialties (ABPTS) examination in a particular specialty area.

Clinical Specialization for Physical Therapists

Nathan had a strong interest in sports physical therapy and had been certified as an athletic trainer prior to pursuing physical therapy education. He wanted most to work with a professional football team. How could he best prepare himself for this career opportunity?

Clinical specialty certification recognizes physical therapists who have demonstrated advanced clinical knowledge and skills in physical therapy specialty areas. Between 1985 and 2003, the ABPTS certified 4686 physical therapists as clinical specialists (Table 25-6). Clinical specialty certification is currently available in seven areas of physical therapy practice.[4] Clinical specialty certification is not available to the physical therapist assistant at this time.

The APTA House of Delegates recently passed a motion, *RC-27: Postentry-level and recognition of enhanced proficiency of the physical therapist assistant,* which ensures that a mechanism will be developed in the near future to recognize enhanced competence in a particular skill set in the physical therapist assistant.[5]

Table 25-5		
CRITERIA TO EVALUATE CONTINUING EDUCATION COURSES[3]		
Keys to Evaluating Continuing Education Courses (before you take them)	*YES*	*NO*
Is there a clear rationale for the course? Does this rationale fit with your career development goals?		
Has the target audience been identified? Do you fit within this description?		
Has the instructional level been identified? Is this level consistent with your prior knowledge and exposure to this material?		
• Basic (1): This level assumes that participants have little information within the areas to be covered so that the focus of the activity is a general orientation and increased awareness.		
• Intermediate (2): This level assumes that the participants have a general familiarity with the topic, so it focuses on increased understanding and application.		
• Advanced (3): This level assumes thorough familiarity with the topic and focuses on advanced techniques, recent advances, and future directions.		
• Various (0): This category indicates that a single level cannot be determined. It is intended for programs in which the instructional level may vary.		
Have learning outcomes been described? What will you learn? Do these outcomes fit with your professional development goals?		
Are objectives achievable, based on the length of the program?		
Are the instructional methods appropriate to achieving the learning objectives? For clinical topics, will you have exposure to case studies, patient demonstrations, or laboratory practice sessions?		
Has the content been outlined and a schedule of presentation provided?		
Are CEUs awarded? Is the CEU provider designated with name, address and telephone number? (CEUs may or may not be required for license renewal, given requirements by state.)		
Is certification or credentialing offered? How many courses are required for certification or credentialing? How is performance evaluated? What additional requirements must be met before or after this course?		
Is registration restricted (important for laboratory and clinical demonstration courses)?		
Are faculty qualifications listed? Do faculty qualifications seem appropriate for course content and learning outcomes?		
Is the course fee listed, with a clear statement about cancellation policies?		
Have other attendees rated the course highly?		

Board-certified clinical specialists use the following initials after the "PT" in their titles to designate their area(s) of specialization:

* CCS (Cardiopulmonary Certified Specialist)
* ECS (Clinical Electrophysiologic Certified Specialist)
* GCS (Geriatric Certified Specialist)
* NCS (Neurologic Certified Specialist)
* OCS (Orthopaedic Certified Specialist)
* PCS (Pediatric Certified Specialist)
* SCS (Sports Certified Specialist)

Table 25-6	
CLINICAL SPECIALTY CERTIFICATION FOR PHYSICAL THERAPISTS[4]	
Specialty Area	*Number of Certified Specialists*
Cardiopulmonary	94
Clinical Electrophysiologic	103
Geriatric	570
Neurologic	374
Orthopaedic	2563
Pediatric	566
Sports	416
TOTAL	4686

Advantages of Specialization

Specialty certification provides a mechanism to validate physical therapist clinical expertise in a practice area. Clinical specialists are often involved in consultation, education, and research in their area of specialization. Although there is not a required salary increase with certification, many clinical specialists assume higher level positions in their organizations that are consistent with their experience and specialty area.

Certification Process

Specialty certification is carried out through electronic testing at various sites nationwide during a specified testing period. Applicants must be meet licensure and specified direct patient care experience requirements to be eligible to sit for the examination. The examination is a multiple-choice test of approximately 200 questions.[4,5] Minimum eligibility requirements are available from the American Physical Therapy Association Specialist Certification Department.

Additional Education

Additional education may be required to meet your long-term career objectives. Explore the career opportunities that may be available by combining a background as a physical therapist assistant with a degree in health science, business, or basic or applied sciences.

When and why to go back to school should be a carefully considered decision. Is an additional degree required for your next career move?

Some physical therapist assistants seek graduate education to become a physical therapist. Physical therapists are educated at the graduate level with either a master's degree or Doctor of Physical Therapy degree. Seek additional information about admission requirements and prerequisite courses by consulting with the physical therapy educational programs in your area. A listing of accredited physical therapist educational programs is available on the American Physical Therapy Association Web site: www.apta.org/Education/accreditation/Dir_Acc_PT_ED_Prog.

Climbing the Clinical Ladder

Consider for a moment that you could combine lifelong learning, your interests, and your job responsibilities into one fabulous package, called your career! Your education and qualifications as a physical therapist assistant offers opportunities to do all this and more.

You can craft your career and create opportunities which match your interests and talents. Consider the activities and roles described in Table 25-7 as ways to develop your experience base in your first few years on the job.

Clinical Ladders for the Physical Therapist Assistant

Some employers and organizations offer career ladders for the physical therapist assistant. These promotional opportunities encourage the physical therapist assistant to advance their skills and knowledge and make an important contribution to the organization in which they work.

Compare the sample job descriptions for the PTA I and PTA II in Table 25-8.

Table 25-7

CAREER DEVELOPMENT ACTIVITIES FOR GRADUATE PHYSICAL THERAPIST ASSISTANTS

Area	Professional Development Activities
Teaching	• Provide clinical supervision for a student volunteer or a student physical therapist assistant.
	• Help to organize a continuing education seminar or class for physical therapist assistants.
	• Seek continuing education or prepare for additional degrees to support your long term career objectives.
	• Present an in-service for staff or students. Offer to help with a guest lecture in a physical therapist assistant class.
	• Develop content for new patient education materials.
Administration	• Help to develop a new program.
	• Attend workshops on new regulations.
	• Serve on a committee or task force in your organization.
Inquiry	• Read and share articles related to clinical responsibilities.
	• Attend presentations at a state or national conference.
Clinical	• Learn how to use a new piece of equipment.
	• Use and help revise clinical pathways and protocols.
	• Gain experience in several clinical areas; collaborate with others and learn about what they do.

Keeping Connected

Tricia took a job in a hospital close to her home. After 6 months, she found herself forgetting some medical terminology. She didn't recognize the names of the drugs her patient was taking. She found herself so busy that it was impossible for her to keep up with learning about her patient's condition. She had lapsed into the habit of just "going with the flow."

One morning, she failed to take her patient's blood pressure while the patient was sitting at the edge of the bed. She felt she could "talk the patient through" her dizziness she complained of and finish the treatment session in time to meet her colleagues for lunch. Her patient fainted and fell to the floor. Luckily, the patient was not injured. She completed an incident report. On discussion later with her supervisor, she realized how many mistakes she had made.

Continue to Think and Reflect

Many practice situations provide new and unexpected challenges. Be careful not to fall into poor habits out of convenience. Your patient's safety comes first. Remember that you are a key member of the patient care team and you are responsible for your patient's well-being.

Continue to challenge your problem-solving abilities. Ask yourself key questions that allow you to use all of the information available to you. Never allow yourself to put a patient in danger because you have not had time to find an answer to a question. If you find your self feeling frustrated or stressed, review some of the strategies presented in Chapter 24.

Push Yourself to Be Your Best

Ask questions of your supervising physical therapist and other members of the health care team with whom you work. Be sure that you understand what you are seeing and reading in a patient's medical record. Seek resources and references in the clinical setting. Attend team meetings and in-service presentations. Ask others if you can observe them to learn more about what they do. Be a team player.

Develop your communication skills. Use effective, clear communication with patients, families, and staff members. Take the time to introduce yourself

Table 25-8

EXAMPLE OF A PHYSICAL THERAPIST ASSISTANT CAREER LADDER[6,7]

	PTA I	PTA II
Basic Function	Perform physical therapy treatments and assist the physical therapist with tests and measurements.	Perform physical therapy treatments to patients with complex medical problems, assist the physical therapist with tests and measurements, assist in the clinical education activities of the physical therapy department.
Distinguishing Characteristics	Under general supervision, assist with physical therapy treatments.	Under general direction, provide physical therapy treatment to patients with complex problems such as burns or behavioral deficiencies; assist in instructing and evaluating students.
Typical Work	Prepare patient and environment for therapy; implement treatment as directed by the physical therapist; report changes in patients' status to therapist; participate in rounds for assigned patients; schedule assigned patients and departmental duties; assist the therapist in performing patient evaluations and tests; write progress notes; assist in completing informational forms; conduct hydrotherapy treatments of patients; maintain a clean, safe working environment; maintain therapeutic equipment; complete charge documents for patient services; may perform clerical duties; perform related duties as required.	Perform all duties of PTA I; provide treatments to patients with more complex problems such as burns,- severe behavioral deficient patients, or intensive care unit patients; provide required physical therapy services in clinics; participate in selected instruction and evaluation of students; assist in developing training programs for physical therapy students; culture whirlpool tanks; maintain necessary supplies and equipment in hydrotherapy; orient new physical therapist assistants, aides, and student helper; orient, instruct, and assign work to volunteers; participate in clinical educa tion meetings with schools providing physical therapy curricula; perform related duties as required.
Minimum Qualifications	An Associate of Science Degree in Physical Therapy from an accredited program that includes patient treatment affiliation. Physical ability to move patients and equipment.	An Associate of Science Degree in Physical Therapy from an accredited program that includes patient treatment affiliation. Eighteen months of experience as PTA I, or equivalent. Physical ability to move patients and equipment.

Adapted from Higher Education Personnel Board. Specification for class physical therapy assistant I, Class code: 6128. Available at: http://hr.dop.wa.gov/lib/ hrdr/highered/specs/6000/6128.htm and Specification for Class Physical Therapy Assistant II, Class Code: 6129. Available from: http://hr.dop.wa.gov/ lib/hrdr/highered/specs/6000/6129.htm. Accessed September 10, 2004.

and establish relationships with the other members of the health care team. The time and effort that you spend in these areas is of critical importance to your competence and clinical role.

Maintain an Active APTA Membership

Some new graduates feel that APTA membership is too expensive and drop their membership after graduation. This is one of the biggest mistakes you can make. APTA membership allows you to receive publications, stay informed on the latest developments, attend conferences at a discount, and pursue many career development opportunities. APTA membership keeps you informed regarding legislative and political action which supports physical therapy.

Another reason to maintain your membership… during recent times of diminishing career opportunities, a greater percentage of APTA members reported employment than non-APTA members.[8] Take advantage of the Career Starter Dues Program and reduced membership fees for your first few years in practice. Budget and pay dues in installments if needed. Do what you need to do to keep your membership active!

Practicing clinicians rely on APTA expertise and credibility for up to date and credible information about developments in the field of physical therapy.

Set a Good Example

Be aware of your attire, and written and spoken communication. Help others understand what physical therapist assistants and physical therapists do. Help others see, by your example, how effective physical therapist assistants can be as a partner with the physical therapist. Take the time to get involved in community activities as well.

Keep Ties to Your College

Be sure to keep in touch with classmates and faculty. They can serve as a valuable network in opening future doors. Those connections can also be a valuable support in your early career experiences. They can provide a bridge from the past to your future. Attend alumni events and help with communications among your classmates.

Summary

Principles of lifelong learning support physical therapist assistant development. Physical therapist assistants should consider their interests in various areas such as clinical practice, inquiry, teaching and administration in planning their career development. Seek opportunities that allow you to combine life-long learning, interests, and job responsibilities. Make the most of your career as a physical therapist assistant!

References

1. Shenk, D. *Data Smog*. New York, NY: Harper and Collins; 1997.

2. Curtis KA. Career planning in physical therapy. Presented at: California Chapter, American Physical Therapy Association Annual Conference; October 8, 1988; Monterey, Calif.

3. APTA. Guidelines for evaluating continuing education programs. BOD 03-97-32-91 (Program 65) [Initial BOD 11-94-41-138]. Available at: http://www.apta.org/Education/Continuing_Education/Guidelines_CEProgs. Accessed September 10, 2004.

4. APTA. Clinical specialization. Available at: http://www.apta.org/Education/specialist/whycertify/OverviewSpecCert/SpecCertOverviewDetail#Clinical%20Specialization. Accessed: September 27, 2003.

5. RC-27, Post entry level and recognition of enhanced proficiency of the physical therapist assistant, House of Delegates, 2003. In: *The Future Role of the PTA*. Alexandria, Va: American Physical Therapy Association., 2003:100.

6. Higher Education Personnel Board. Specification for class physical therapy assistant I, Class code: 6128 Web page. Available at: http://hr.dop.wa.gov/lib/hrdr/highered/specs/6000/6128.htm. Accessed September 27, 2004.

7. Higher Education Personnel Board. Specification for Class Physical Therapy Assistant II, Class Code: 6129 Web page. Available from: http://hr.dop.wa.gov/lib/hrdr/highered/specs/6000/6129.htm. Accessed September 27, 2004.

8. APTA. APTA Physical therapist assistant employment survey Fall 2001: executive summary. Available from: http://www.apta.org/Research/survey_stat/pta_employ_nov01. Accessed September 27, 2004.

PUTTING IT INTO PRACTICE

1. Complete the inventory in Table 25-2. What do the results tell you? Do the results fit with your expectations? What interest areas would you like to emphasize in your career development?

2. What performance goals would you like to meet in the next year? Draw from your most recent clinical performance evaluation or other sources?

   What do you need to *be able to do* or *need to know* to reach the above goals?

3. In what two areas would you like to develop your clinical, inquiry, teaching, or administrative skills in the next year? Be specific.

   What are the best ways for you to develop these areas? Consider independent study, in services at work, mentoring relationships with another person, outside continuing education courses)

   What resources are available in your current workplace that will help you to develop these areas? (Consider mentors, practice opportunities, in-service classes, employee development programs)

   What resources are available in the community that will help you to develop these areas? (Consider continuing education courses, college courses and programs, self-study courses, mentors)

4. What career goals would you like to meet in the next 5 years?

What type of position would you like to have in 5 years?

What additional skills or training do you need to make this career move?

What additional responsibilities can you seek now that would prepare you for these goals?

CHAPTER 26

Working With Your Supervisor(s)

Developing an effective relationship with your supervising physical therapist (PT) is a critical aspect of working as a physical therapist assistant (PTA). In fact, you may answer to multiple supervisors (PTs) with regard to patient care and yet another person who is in charge of administrative issues, such as work assignments, patient load distribution, and performance appraisals.

A compatible PT-PTA team results in a more unified approach to the delivery of high quality and cost-effective physical therapy care. Collaborating within a frenzied health care environment can be challenging. Let's examine some ways to create successful partnerships with the PTs that supervise you.

> *"Oh, here we go again!"* sighed Trevor, an experienced physical therapist as Victoria, the clinic manager, announced to the staff that a new graduate physical therapist assistant would be starting on Monday. *"I'll just continue to see all of my own patients anyway since none of the previous PTAs were worth the time it took to explain everything to them. The only reason they would hire a PTA is to bring in more patients anyway!"*

Barriers to Communication

Communication skills are of critical importance in physical therapy practice. You may wish to review these and the other standards of conduct considered in Chapter 6. Appropriate and effective interaction is a basic competency; yet, misunderstanding and ineffective communication are often the cause of patient complaints and staff disagreements. In fact, the ability to skillfully communicate with patients and colleagues can impact the satisfaction and success of physical therapy clinicians as much or more than any technical skill they possess![1]

Communication, in its simplest form, involves a sender, a message, a receiver, and the context in which the interaction occurs. The meaning of a particular word exists within each individual. The same word can have quite different meanings to the sender of the message than the receiver of the message.

Any or all of the following can filter and distort the exchange of ideas between individuals.

Belief Systems, Values, and Prejudices

- Example: "If I don't do it myself, it won't get done correctly."

Because backgrounds and lifestyles differ, people can have prejudgments and opinions that are not accurate about a given situation. This can cause messages to be distorted and misunderstood.

Personalities and Differing Perspectives

- Example: "What I say doesn't matter anyway so I just won't participate..."

An individual's frame of reference and idiosyncrasies can influence one's confidence and style of communication.

Preconceived Notions

- Example: "Using support staff is risky."

It can be difficult to let go of ideas that have emerged over a long period of time or due to adversity.

Multiple Demands

- Example: "I need to consult the PT about this but I need to see Mr. Jones now before they bring the lunch trays or I won't get to him this morning."

Prioritizing responsibilities of similar importance may seem overwhelming and can result in hasty, incomplete sharing of information.

Distractions in a Busy Physical Therapy Clinic

- Example: "I know that the PT just suggested a change in Miss Traylor's exercise program but I was still focused on what Dr. Foster had just said and now I don't exactly remember."

The inability to fully concentrate on a message has the potential for misinterpretation and can be more time consuming in order to verify the content of the information.

The ways in which people send or receive messages, or even decide to communicate, are influenced by culture and life experiences. This is more completely discussed in Chapter 18. Ineffective or miscommunication occurs when the message being sent is perceived by the receiver differently than it was intended by the sender.[2]

In the scenario described above, Trevor appears to have a preconceived bias about working with a PTA. Unless he communicates this to the clinic manager, Victoria, she has every reason to believe, that the PTA will be an asset to Trevor. Unless honest communication occurs, establishing a positive working relationship may be difficult for this PT-PTA team.

It would be in the best interest of this clinical team for Trevor to openly share his concerns about PTAs with his supervisor, Victoria. This would allow Victoria to deal with Trevor's presumptions directly and before the PTA arrives. Whether or not Trevor admits to his feelings, Victoria may astutely perceive contradictory nonverbal communication from him when the PTA is mentioned. Investigation may lead to discussion and, optimally, Victoria can help create a strategy to salvage an otherwise ill-fated relationship.

It is customary for the PTA to demonstrate competent clinical intervention, proper judgment, and effective communication in order to earn the trust of the PT. This may take a bit more effort in a situation like this, where Trevor may have had less-than-favorable experiences working with another PTA. Building a successful relationship with Trevor may take more energy and effort but it certainly can be accomplished.

Fostering Effective Communication

Although specific strategies to effectively communicate will depend on the individuals and the unique circumstances involved, the guidelines presented in Table 26-1 may be helpful in doing what you can to enhance communication.

Doing More With Less

Cost cutting measures in the delivery of health care have resulted in fewer therapists seeing more patients. Documentation requirements continue to multiply in quantity and complexity. Meanwhile, concerns about litigation continue to rise for health care workers.[3] These concerns can strain the working relationship between the physical therapist and PTA.

Productivity

Pressure to generate revenue may tempt the PT to *over-* or *under*-utilize the PTA. Utilization means "to put to use, especially to find a profitable use for."[5] *Overutilization* occurs when a PT inappropriately delegates interventions to the PTA or is not readily available for consultation or to re-examine a patient as requested by the PTA. For example, the PT may perform evaluations and complete paperwork while expecting the PTA to independently treat the patients for as long as allowable by law. This stretches the limits of what are acceptable standards of physical therapy practice because the supervising PT is expected to be involved in the management of each patient.[6]

Underutilization, on the other hand, occurs when the PT may feel it is more timely and less risky to not delegate at all or only utilize the PTA as an aide. For example, utilizing a PTA to set up equipment and provide modalities with specific directions is an inappropriate use of a competent PTA.

Health System Administration

Clinic managers or health system administrators may urge or require the PT to delegate more to PTAs to lower costs and optimize efficiency of service delivery. This may lead to delegation of interventions that are beyond the competency of the specific PTA, little time for the PT and PTA to confer, and/or an inability of the PT to re-examine the patient as requested by the PTA. This can lead to frustration and discouragement for the PT-PTA team. Of most importance, however, is that when an outside entity controls clinical practice patterns or decision-making, the safety, and quality of physical therapy care may be compromised.

Third-Party Payers

Restrictions imposed by third-party payers may influence the delegation of tasks to the PTA. Some insurance and managed care companies authorize very few physical therapy visits or stipulate that

---

Table 26-1

COMMUNICATION GUIDELINES FOR A SUCCESSFUL RELATIONSHIP[4]

*1. Be **aware** that barriers exist*

Carefully examine the people and environment specific to your situation. What facilitates and/or detracts from effective communication?

*2. Create **unconditional positive regard** and **trust***

Treat others as you wish to be treated. Do your best to gain the confidence of those with whom you work.

*3. Be willing to **receive** and **provide honest feedback***

Above all else, focus on what is in the best interest of the patient. Be humble.

*4. **Listen***

- Pay attention
- Focus on the sender
- Ignore distractions
- "Check it out": The only test of message's success is comprehension
- Avoid constructing your "come back" while the sender is still speaking.

*5. Display **empathy***

Try to put yourself in the other person's shoes. How does it feel for the physical therapist to place his or her trust in you to care for the patient for whom he or she is ultimately responsible? Take steps to demonstrate that you will follow through and can be trusted.

*6. Be **genuine***

Display consistency between your verbal and nonverbal messages. Share what you think/feel at an appropriate time and place.

*7. **Hear** the whole message (verbal and nonverbal)*

Be present. Attend fully to the person with whom you are communicating in that moment before moving on to your next priority.

Adapted from Newman PD. *Systems and Problems in Physical Therapy Course Syllabus*. Oklahoma City, Okla: Oklahoma City Community College PTA Program; 2003:3.

---

services be provided only by a PT. If the patient may only receive a limited total number of physical therapy visits, the transfer of care to a PTA may not be a viable option in the mind of the PT. Specifically, when the third-party payer will not authorize interventions if provided by a PTA, the PT will not have the option of delegating to the PTA. It is important to be aware of the specific stipulations of the third party payers where you are employed.

Implications for the Physical Therapist Assistant

In spite of these or any other pressures, the scope of work, supervisory relationship, and role boundaries of the PTA are **not** susceptible to modification.

Ethical guidelines and standards of physical therapy practice require that the PT and PTA anticipate and respond appropriately to any situation that compromises the best interest of the patient. It would be necessary to discuss concerns with the appropriate parties and discontinue employment if not resolved.

The Physical Therapist-Physical Therapist Assistant Partnership

As an integral member of the physical therapy team, the PTA is uniquely qualified to assist the PT in achieving patient-centered, functional outcomes in an effective, cost-efficient manner.[7]

A thriving PT-PTA team will depend on many factors including:

> *"Hey Scott," yelled the PT, Don from across the gym, "do you know how to do contract-relax to stretch tight heel cords? I need some help with Mr. Frye while I finish Ms. Carter. And grab an ice pack on your way." Although the physical therapist assistant Scott could hardly believe his ears, he took a deep breath and headed to the freezer before going over to work with Mr. Frye. Scott pondered how to approach Don about his academic preparation and 18 weeks of clinical internships including 7 weeks at the Rehab Institute.*

- Mutual respect
- Confidence and trust in one another
- Accurate understanding and appreciation for educational preparation, laws, and standards of practice
- Common goals and enthusiasm for the patient/clients
- Commitment to lifelong learning[8,9]

Given the hectic pace of most clinical settings and the assorted experiences PTs have in working with PTAs, it is likely that the PTA will need to facilitate the communication process. This may include educating the PTs about the academic preparation, licensure, and supervisory requirements of the PTA.

Scope of Work

The scope of work of the PT assistant is determined by the supervising PT on the basis of federal and state laws and regulations, ethical standards, competency and skill level, standards of practice established by the profession, and current performance expectations in the workplace.[10]

Differences of opinion regarding the proper role and utilization of the PTA have persisted among PTs since the inception of a formalized extender of care began in the early 1960s. The role has evolved over the past three decades as a result of marked changes in health care, federal and state laws/regulations, and the needs and expectations of supervising PTs in the workplace.

Progress has been made in achieving profession-wide consensus regarding the educational preparation, accreditation requirements, and state laws that stipulate minimal standards for the PTA. However, the scope of work and delegation guidelines for the PTA remain hotly debated and are handled quite inconsistently in daily clinical practice across the country.[10] For example, while it may be acceptable practice for a PTA in a state with general supervision to suction a patient in the Intensive Care Unit following resisted coughing exercises, it may not be appropriate for a PTA to be working in this way in a state that requires direct on-site supervision. Further information regarding levels of supervision will be discussed later in the chapter.

The American Physical Therapy Association (APTA) delineates the clinical relationship and practice guidelines concerning support personnel in a variety of policies, positions and standards such as the following summary from the *Guide to Physical Therapist Practice*:

> *The physical therapist is ultimately responsible for all aspects of patient/client management. Examination, evaluation, diagnosis, and prognosis are to be performed by the physical therapist. Intervention and aspects of data collection are to be performed by the physical therapist or by a physical therapist assistant under the direction and supervision of the physical therapist.[6]*

This means it is **never** acceptable for the PTA to treat a patient until the PT has conducted an initial examination/evaluation and established the goals and plan of care to be followed.

Other Support Personnel

Other support personnel, such as physical therapy aides, may perform clerical, maintenance, preparation, and clean-up activities. Patient-related tasks delegated to (non-PTA) support personnel may include only specifically selected routine portions of an intervention or treatment session. For example, it is acceptable to allow a physical therapy aide to help a patient onto and set up the parameters of the treadmill as specifically directed by the PT. It is **not** appropriate for the physical therapy aide to have a schedule of patients that they are responsible to treat.

> *Situations in which physical therapists choose to utilize other personnel to provide patient-related care violate the commitment to the physical therapist-physical therapist assistant team.[10]*

For further information about policy and positions related to role and responsibilities in the delivery of physical therapy services go to www.apta.org/governance/HOD. For the complete wording of the *Provision of Physical Therapy Interventions and*

Table 26-2
LEVELS OF SUPERVISION DESCRIBED IN STATE LAWS[13]
A. *General supervision* allows the PTA to practice without the supervising PTA to be continuously on the premises. The supervising physical therapist must be readily available to the PTA at least by telecommunications. Twenty-nine states' practice acts require physical therapists to provide general supervision of physical therapists.
B. *Periodic on-site supervision* defines specific frequencies in which the physical therapist must be physical present. State requirements vary from 50% of the PTA's workweek to a particular number of patient visits to once every 2 weeks. There are 14 states that stipulate periodic supervision.
C. *Full on-site supervision* requires the supervising physical therapist to be on the premises at all times when a PTA is providing patient related care. Nine states require this type of supervision.
Adapted from Thomas B. Supervising personnel in subacute and long-term care. *Advance for Physical Therapists and Physical Therapist Assistants.* 2003;14(17):63.

Related Tasks, HOD 06-00-17-28, see Appendix 6.

Supervision, Direction, and Delegation

Supervision

Supervision is defined as "to have the direction and oversight of others."[11] Supervision is a mutual responsibility between the PT and PTA.[12] Regardless of philosophy, competency, experience, or reimbursement guidelines, the minimally acceptable level of supervision for any clinical setting is as outlined in your state's physical therapy practice act.

See Table 26-2 for the levels of supervision described in various state laws. It is important to remember that the purpose of these laws and regulations is to protect the safety and promote the best interest of those we serve. Supervision will be discussed in more detail later in this chapter with regard to boundaries.

Many states limit the number of PTAs that one PT may supervise at any one time. It is essential that every PTA and PT know and understand the physical therapy laws for each state in which they provide services. Failure to do so can lead to fines and loss of the ability to practice.

Direction

Direction involves "....the relation between something and the course along which it points or moves....direction or advice as to a course of action... the act of managing something..."[11] Consider this definition in the context of physical therapy. It is the PT's responsibility to *direct* the course and progression of the patient/client's plan of care. Regardless of what, if any, aspects of the care the PT chooses to share with the PTA, the PT is ultimately responsible and must be involved in each person's care.

Delegation

Delegation is a function that is based on competence and trust. It is a matter of deciding which parts of a patient's care will be performed by whom. Delegation has been described as a skill that improves with practice but requires a level of fundamental knowledge and practice opportunities during the educational process.[14]

In order to establish the trust necessary for a PT to confidently share the responsibility of patient care, the PTA must:

1. *Demonstrate competence*: Do not be threatened when the PT wants to co-treat with you or have you perform various interventions on him or her. This is a positive sign that this PT wants to know what you can do well in order to trust you to properly care for patients.

2. *Make proper judgments*: Trust is developed by what you do, not by what you say. As you competently carry out the plan of care, regularly communicate pertinent information and alert the PT of the need to re-establish goals and/or the plan of care you will earn respect.

3. *Communicate, communicate, communicate*: Ask questions if you are not sure about something; go the extra mile to seek out the PT to get or give input; never assume anything!

How and what to appropriately direct and delegate in clinical practice continues to be an issue of much debate with the physical therapy profession. In a landmark article published in *Physical Therapy* in 1971, Nancy Watts proposed a taxonomy based on "doing" or "deciding" behaviors required in the practice of physical therapy. Within this systematic approach for the division of responsibility, tasks are analyzed in terms of the process of decision making versus delivering an intervention.[15]

Another study published in *Physical Therapy* in 1990 indicated that the level of complexity of the physical therapy procedures affects the PT's decision to delegate.[16] For example, instructing a patient without any other medical problems to properly use a walker after total hip surgery would be considered less complex than with a doing so with a patient who fell on the treadmill while participating in cardiac rehabilitation following heart surgery.

To delegate typically adds to the delegator's workload at the outset. As trust is established within a PT/PTA team, supervision, direction, and delegation become like a flawlessly choreographed experience that well serves the patients, the clinicians and the health care system.

A study published in *Physiotherapy* in 1998 audited out-patient physical therapy clinics over a 3-year period after specific training was performed on appropriate utilization and delegation. Calculations regarding the cost spent on providing patient care, percentage of time spent by the PTs versus the PTAs performing specific type of treatments, and outcomes from patient satisfaction surveys were analyzed. The study concluded that utilization of PTAs resulted in cost-benefits without loss of quality or reduction in patient satisfaction.[17]

Take a look at Table 26-3 for some well-established guidelines the PT considers when determining whether and what to delegate to the PTA.

The American Physical Therapy Association outlines who can supervise the PTA in various policies and position statements including:

> The physical therapist assistant will provide physical therapy services **only** under the direction and supervision of a licensed physical therapist.[6,7]

This means it is **never** acceptable for the PTA to be supervised or directed by anyone other than a licensed PT including physicians, nurses, occupational therapists, or physical therapy students. Most states have specific statements about this in the physical therapy practice act. Regardless, it is against the ethical and clinical standards of physical therapy practice for a PTA to be supervised by a non-PT. To see the actual wording of your state's practice act, go to www.fsbpt.org

Additionally, the APTA defines supervision, direction and delegation requirements in a variety of policies, positions and standards such as the Direction and Supervision of the PTA, HOD 06-01-16-27, (Appendix 5) which provides guidance about what responsibilities are reserved for the PTs and what factors must be considered when utilizing support staff.[7]

For the complete wording of these and other core documents, go to: www.apta.org/governance/HOD.

Boundaries

Keeping up with and abiding by the laws, regulations, standards of practice and company policies

> Alyson hung up the phone in disbelief from what she had just heard from Sam, a PT, calling from the skilled nursing facility she had just been assigned to across the river. "How on earth am I going to get all the patients seen if I can only treat them when he is on the premises?" Alyson had only worked in her home state since becoming a licensed physical therapist assistant last summer. The new facility is located across the state line.

governing physical therapy practice can make your head spin! This responsibility, however, is part of the commitment of working in health care.

PTAs are responsible for compliance with all laws and regulations. It is unacceptable to allow anyone else to impose policies that conflict with laws, regulations or ethical guidelines. The PTA must be aware of and educate others as necessary when it comes to following all practice standards and regulations concerning supervision and utilization.[8]

State Law

As discussed in detail in Chapter 12, state practice acts differ significantly in many ways. Supervision and utilization of support personnel are among the most variable from state to state. It is critical to fully comprehend the law governing physical therapy in each state that you practice. One state may not even license the PTA and require direct, on-site supervision by the supervising PT. Across the state line may require licensure and stipulate general supervision. You may wish to refer back to Table 26-2 to refresh your memory about levels of supervision.

This is the case with Alyson in the above scenario. She has been working in a state that requires general supervision but is being assigned to a new facility across the state line that requires full on-site supervision. Alyson would be practicing in error if she failed

---

Table 26-3
DELEGATION CONSIDERATIONS[15,18]

Focus	Illustration
Level of education, training, experience, and skill	New graduate? A new setting? Patient mix?
Criticality, acuity, stability, and complexity of the patient	How much and how quickly is in status likely to occur? How serious will be the results if a poor decision is made or an intervention performed poorly?
Ambiguity, observability, predictability of the the patient	How clear or uncertain is this situation? How confidently can you predict the consequences?
Setting in which the care will take place	Will the physical therapist be on the premises?
Federal and State laws	Who can do what? How often? Must be aware of laws/ regulations.
Liability and risk management	What do job descriptions say? Company policies? Has there been a recent incident/lawsuit?
Mission of the service setting	What do the physical therapy services primarily consist of? Treatment? Consultation? Education?
Needed frequency of re-evaluation	How often will examination and assessment be necessary?

Adapted from Watts NT. Task analysis and division of responsibility in physical therapy. *Phys Ther.* 1971;51:23-25 and APTA. *A Normative Model of PTA Education: Version '99.* Alexandria, Va: APTA.

---

to comply with this requirement and practiced as she has been in her home state. For specific information regarding each state's practice act, go to www. fsbpt.org.

Reimbursement Agencies

The Center for Medicare and Medicaid Services (CMS) issues guidelines, updates, and clarifications rulings in the *Federal Register*. CMS has issued many notifications regarding supervision and utilization of support personnel during the delivery of physical therapy services. Once these notifications are published, CMS considers it the responsibility of each individual health care provider to be aware of and follow these rules. This is known as record notice.[19] Failure to adhere to Medicare regulations can lead to fraudulent billing allegations that can result in fines, loss of license and imprisonment. It is important to note that when state law is more stringent than Medicare, state law is obligatory. To view the *Federal Register,* go to www.cms.gov and click on *Quarterly Provider Update.*

Insurance and managed care companies demand compliance with specific rules. These are typically outlined in the contract between the physical therapy provider and the insurance company. Failure to comply with these regulations can result in nonpayment and potential cancellation as an authorized physical therapy provider. Reimbursement agency regulations vary as considerably as state laws. For example, some do not allow physical therapy intervention to be provided by a PTA.

The American Physical Therapy Association provides protection to the PTA by stipulating that:

The physical therapist assistant will not be required or agree to provide care beyond his/her competency, ethical and legal boundaries.[8]

It is essential to be honest with yourself and supervising PTs regarding your proficiency, strengths, and weaknesses in order to provide the quality physical therapy services that every patient deserves. Likewise you must comply with and stay informed regarding all laws and practice standards that apply.

In the unlikely event that a PT pressures the PTA to work outside the scope of legal or ethical boundaries, it is imperative to discuss this with the individual. You may wish to contact the program director or a favorite faculty member from your academic program to talk over your concerns.

Share the documents that you know outline proper practice guidelines with your supervising PTs.

Table 26-4

CONSIDERATIONS WHEN CONFRONTED WITH A POTENTIALLY ILLEGAL OR UNETHICAL SITUATION

Steps to Take
1. Identify the incident or problem.
2. Gather documents pertaining to related legal, ethical and practice standards.
3. Share this information with all concerned parties.
4. Request specific changes in operations.
5. Assist with implementation.

Refer to the Standards of Practice and Ethical Guidelines in the Appendix. If the pressure continues, even if your employment is threatened, alert another supervisor, administrator, and the licensure board if necessary. Ultimately, you are responsible for what you do and do not do in everyday practice. It is therefore up to you to remove yourself from any situation that turns unethical or illegal.

Take a look at Table 26-4 for suggestions on specific steps to take if such a situation arises. Additionally, you may want to review Chapter 12: Legal and Ethical Considerations for further discussion on related issues.

What You Can Do To Promote A Successful Relationship

Although obstacles exist, developing a collaborative relationship that is mutually satisfying and enhances physical therapy care is certainly an attainable goal. In addition to carefully following the Communication Guidelines outlined in Table 26-1, refer to Table 26-5 for suggestions concerning what you must do to shape the evolving relationship with your physical therapy supervisor(s) and prevent unnecessary turmoil.

Summary

Multiple factors influence the working relationship between the PT and PTA. The PTA is a valued contributor to providing cost-effective, quality physical therapy care. It is up to each PT and PTA team to accomplish this in daily practice.

References

1. Davis, C. *Patient Practioner Interaction.* 3rd ed. Thorofare, NJ: SLACK Incorporated; 1998:140.

2. Longest BB. *Health Professionals in Management.* Stamford, Conn: Appleton & Lange;1995:282-287.

3. Waldrop S. Battling burnout: maintaining enthusiasm in a challenging environment. *PT.* 2003; 11(7):39-45.

4. Newman P. *Systems and Problems in Physical Therapy Course Syllabus.* Oklahoma City, Okla: Oklahoma City Community College PTA Program; 2003.

5. The *American Heritage Dictionary of the English Language.* 4th ed. Web page. Available at: http://education.yahoo.com/reference/dictionary. Accessed September 10, 2004.

6. APTA. *Guide to Physical Therapy Practice.* 2nd ed. Alexandria, Va: American Physical Therapy Association; 2001:31-42.

7. Bohmert J. The PT/PTA team: the future begins now. *PT.* 2003;11(9):23-25.

8. APTA. *The Normative Model for Physical Therapist Assistant Education, Version '99.* Alexandria, Va: American Physical Therapy Association; 1999: 203–214.

9. Thuringer B. Building successful PT and PTA teams. *Acute Care Perspective.* 2001;10(4):13.

10. APTA. *The Future Role of the Physical Therapist Assistant (RC 40-01). House of Delegates Handbook.* Alexandria, Va: American Physical Therapy Association; 2003:96-129.

11. WordNet 1.6 Web page. Available from: http://dictionary.reference.com/search?q=Direction. Accessed 09/10/04.

12. AOTA. *Guide for Supervision of Occupational Therapy Personnel in the Delivery of Occupational Therapy Services.* Rockville, Md: American Occupational Therapy Association; 1999.

Table 26-5
THE PHYSICAL THERAPIST ASSISTANT'S ROLE IN DEVELOPING A SUCCESSFUL PARTNERSHIP

* Communicate frequently, clearly, and concisely in writing and/or verbally whenever you determine:
  a. A change in patient status
  b. Re-examination or revisions to plan of care/goal updates are approaching
  c. Clarification is needed
  d. Modification of anything deemed inappropriately delegated
  e. Interventions should not be provided due to changing clinical conditions
  f. Abnormal or questionable patient response to interventions

* Identify a mutually agreeable time and method to communicate (non-emergency) information to each supervising physical therapist.

* Clarify all confusing or unknown medical jargon, abbreviations or wording within the physical therapist's initial evaluation and subsequent documentation.

* Maintain a clear understanding of the state practice act regarding supervision and utilization of the physical therapist. Insure adherence to it.

* Maintain a clear understanding of reimbursement regulations pertaining to supervision and provision of services by a PTA. Insure adherence to them.

* Maintain your membership and actively participate in the American Physical Therapy Association – even if this means simply reading the information sent to you. This is the most prudent way to protect yourself by having readily available access to the most credible information available.

* Stay connected to mentors and supportive colleagues that you know strive to provide legal, ethical, and superior patient care.

* Join your College's Alumni Association. Maintain contact with the program director or one of your favorite faculty members now and then. Educators must stay abreast of changes and typically are involved in what is happening within the field.

* DO NOT ever compromise your ethics or character—even if urged to do so by a supervisor!! If it sounds too good to be true, it usually is…. Listen to your instincts!

13. Thomas B. Supervising personnel in subacute and long-term care. *Advance for Physical Therapists and Physical Therapist Assistants*. 2003;14(17):63.
14. Manthey, M. Trust: essential for delegation. *Nursing Management*. 1990;21(11):28-30.
15. Watts NT. Task analysis and division of responsibility in physical therapy. *Phys Ther*. 1971;51:23-25.
16. Hart E, Pinkston D, Ritchey FJ, et al. Relationship of professional involvement to clinical behaviors of physical therapists. *Phys Ther*. 1990;70:179-184.
17. Saunders L. Improving the practice of delegation in physiotherapy. *Physiotherapy*. 1998;84(5):207-21.
18. APTA. *A Normative Model for Physical Therapist Assistant Education*. Alexandria, Va: American Physical Therapy Association; 1999:198.
19. Kornblau B, Starling S. *Ethics in Rehabilitation*. Thorofare, NJ: SLACK Incorporated; 2000:20.

PUTTING IT INTO PRACTICE

1. Communication tools may help you identify and reflect upon your strengths, weaknesses, and preferences. Visit the Communication Skills test at: http://discoveryhealth.queendom.com/questions/ communication_short_1.html.

    What do the results of this test tell you regarding your ability to communicate on a health care team? What specific steps can you take to improve any areas that are of concern?

2. Interview a physical therapist who has been in practice and supervised PTAs for more than 10 years. Ask about changes regarding:
    A. Utilization of support personnel
    B. Productivity demands
    C. Documentation requirements
    D. Managing the supervisory relationship

3. Investigate what coursework exists regarding supervision, utilization, and delegation of support personnel at a local physical therapy program:
    A. Explore the Web site.
    B. Interview a student currently enrolled in the program.

4. Review the physical therapy practice act for the state in which you plan to work. Are PTAs licensed? How many PTAs can a PT supervise? How many physical therapy aides? Can PTAs supervise physical therapy aides? What type of supervision is required? Does it specify what components of patient care are allowable by the PTA vs what must be performed by the PT?

Appendices

Definition Language, Model Practice Act for Physical Therapy

Model Practice Act for Physical Therapy Language (2002) Federation of State Boards of Physical Therapy

Definitions

B. "Physical therapy" means the care and services provided by or under the direction and supervision of a physical therapist who is licensed pursuant to this [act]. The term "physiotherapy" shall be synonymous with "physical therapy" pursuant to this [act].

C. "Physical therapist" means a person who is licensed pursuant to this [act] to practice physical therapy. The term "physiotherapist" shall be synonymous with "physical therapist" pursuant to this [act].

D. "Practice of physical therapy" means:

1. Examining, evaluating, and testing individuals with mechanical, physiological and developmental impairments, functional limitations, and disabilities or other health and movement-related conditions in order to determine a diagnosis, prognosis and plan of therapeutic intervention, and to assess the ongoing effects of intervention.

2. Alleviating impairments, functional limitations and disabilities by designing, implementing and modifying therapeutic interventions that may include, but are not limited to, therapeutic exercise; functional training in self-care and in home, community or work integration or reintegration; manual therapy, including soft tissue and joint mobilization/manipulation; therapeutic massage; prescription, application and, as appropriate, fabrication of assistive, adaptive, orthotic, prosthetic, protective and supportive devices and equipment; airway clearance techniques; integumentary protection and repair techniques; debridement and wound care; physical agents or modalities; mechanical and electrotherapeutic modalities; and patient-related instruction.

3. Reducing the risk of injury, impairment, functional limitation and disability, including the promotion and maintenance of fitness, health and wellness in populations of all ages.

4. Engaging in administration, consultation, education, and research.

Excerpted from: Federation of State Boards of Physical Therapy. Model Practice Act for Physical Therapy. Available from: http://www.fsbpt.org/pdf/MPA_2002_Language.pdf. Accessed September 10, 2004.

APTA *Standards of Ethical Conduct and Guide for Conduct for the Physical Therapist Assistant*

HOD 06-00-13-24 (Program 17)
[Amended HOD 06-91-06-07; Initial HOD 06-82-04-08]

Preamble

This document of the American Physical Therapy Association sets forth standards for the ethical conduct of the physical therapist assistant. All physical therapist assistants are responsible for maintaining high standards of conduct while assisting physical therapists. The physical therapist assistant shall act in the best interest of the patient/client. These standards of conduct shall be binding on all physical therapist assistants.

Standard 1

A physical therapist assistant shall respect the rights and dignity of all individuals and shall provide compassionate care.

Standard 2

A physical therapist assistant shall act in a trustworthy manner towards patients/clients.

Standard 3

A physical therapist assistant shall provide selected physical therapy interventions only under the supervision and direction of a physical therapist.

Standard 4

A physical therapist assistant shall comply with laws and regulations governing physical therapy.

Standard 5

A physical therapist assistant shall achieve and maintain competence in the provision of selected physical therapy interventions.

Standard 6

A physical therapist assistant shall make judgments that are commensurate with their educational and legal qualifications as a physical therapist assistant.

Standard 7

A physical therapist assistant shall protect the public and the profession from unethical, incompetent, and illegal acts.

Guide for Conduct of the Physical Therapist Assistant

This *Guide for Conduct of the Physical Therapist Assistant* (Guide) is intended to serve physical therapist assistants in interpreting the *Standards of Ethical Conduct for the Physical Therapist Assistant* (Standards) of the American Physical Therapy Association (APTA). The Guide provides guidelines by which physical therapist assistants may determine the propriety of their conduct. It is also intended to guide the development of physical therapist assistant students. The Standards and Guide apply to all physical therapist assistants. These guidelines are subject to change as the dynamics of the profession change and as new patterns of health care delivery are developed and accepted by the professional community and the public. This Guide is subject to monitoring and timely revision by the Ethics and Judicial Committee of the Association.

Interpreting Standards

The interpretations expressed in this Guide reflect the opinions, decisions, and advice of the Ethics and Judicial Committee. These interpretations are intended to guide a physical therapist assistant in applying general ethical principles to specific situations. They should not be considered inclusive of all situations that could evolve.

Standard 1

A physical therapist assistant shall respect the rights and dignity of all individuals and shall provide compassionate care.

1.1 Attitude of a physical therapist assistant

A. A physical therapist assistant shall demonstrate sensitivity to individual and cultural differences.

B. A physical therapist assistant shall be guided at all times by concern for the physical and psychological welfare of patients/ clients.

C. A physical therapist assistant shall not harass, abuse, or discriminate against others.

Standard 2

A physical therapist assistant shall act in a trustworthy manner towards patients/clients.

2.1 Trustworthiness

A. To act in a trustworthy manner a physical therapist assistant shall act in the patient's/client's best interest. Working in the patient's/client's best interest requires sensitivity to the patient's/client's vulnerability and an effective working relationship between the physical therapist and the physical therapist assistant.

B. A physical therapist assistant shall act to ameliorate the patient's/client's vulnerability, not to exploit it.

C. A physical therapist assistant shall clearly identify him/herself as a physical therapist assistant to patients/clients.

D. A physical therapist assistant shall conduct him/herself in a manner that supports the physical therapist/patient relationship.

E. A physical therapist assistant shall not engage in any sexual relationship or activity, whether consensual or nonconsensual, with any patient entrusted to his/her care.

F. A physical therapist assistant shall not invite, accept, or offer gifts or other considerations that affect or give an appearance of affecting his/her provision of physical therapy interventions.

2.2 Exploitation of Patients

A physical therapist assistant shall not participate in any arrangements in which patients/clients are exploited. Such arrangements include situations where referring sources enhance their personal incomes as a result of referring for, delegating, prescribing, or recommending physical therapy services.

2.3 Truthfulness

A. A physical therapist assistant shall not make statements that he/she knows or should know are false, deceptive, fraudulent, or unfair.

B. Although it cannot be considered unethical for a physical therapist assistant to own or have a financial interest in the production, sale, or distribution of products/services, he/she must act in accordance with law and make full disclosure of his/her interest to patients/clients.

2.4 Confidential Information

A. Information relating to the patient/client is confidential and may not be communicated to a third party not involved in that patient's care without the prior consent of the patient, subject to applicable law.

B. A physical therapist assistant shall refer all requests for release of confidential information to the supervising physical therapist.

Standard 3

A physical therapist assistant shall provide selected physical therapy interventions only under the supervision and direction of a physical therapist.

3.1 Supervisory Relationship

A. A physical therapist assistant shall provide services only under the supervision and direction of a physical therapist.

B. A physical therapist assistant shall provide only those physical therapy interventions that have been selected by the physical therapist.

C. A physical therapist assistant shall not carry out any selected physical therapy interventions that are outside his/her education, training, experience, or skill and shall notify the physical therapist.

D. A physical therapist assistant may adjust specific interventions within the plan of care established by the physical therapist in response to changes in the patient's/client's status.

E. A physical therapist assistant shall not perform examinations or evaluations, interpret data, determine diagnosis or prognosis, or establish or alter a plan of care.

F. Consistent with the physical therapist assistant's education, training, knowledge, and experience, he/she may respond to the patient's/client's inquiries regarding interventions that are within the established plan of care.

G. A physical therapist assistant shall have regular and ongoing communication with the physical therapist regarding the patient's/client's status.

Standard 4

A physical therapist assistant shall comply with laws and regulations governing physical therapy.

4.1 Supervision

A physical therapist assistant shall know and comply with applicable law. Regardless of the content of any law, a physical therapist assistant shall provide services only under the supervision and direction of a physical therapist.

4.2 Representation

A physical therapist assistant shall not hold him/herself out as a physical therapist.

Standard 5

A physical therapist assistant shall achieve and maintain competence in the provision of selected physical therapy interventions.

5.1 Competence

A physical therapist assistant shall provide interventions consistent with his/her level of education, training, experience, and skill.

5.2 Self-assessment

A physical therapist assistant shall engage in self-assessment in order to maintain competence.

5.3 Development

A physical therapist assistant shall participate in educational activities that enhance his/her basic knowledge and skills.

Standard 6

A physical therapist assistant shall make judgments that are commensurate with their educational and legal qualifications as a physical therapist assistant.

6.1 Patient Safety

A. A physical therapist assistant shall discontinue immediately any components of interventions that, in his/her judgment, appear to be harmful to the patient and shall discuss his/her concerns with the physical therapist.

B. A physical therapist assistant shall not carry out any selected physical therapy interventions that are outside his/her education, training, experience, or skill and shall notify the physical therapist.

C. A physical therapist assistant shall not perform interventions while his/her ability to do so safely is impaired.

6.2 Patient Status Judgments

A physical therapist assistant participates in patient status judgments by reporting changes to the physical therapist and requesting patient re-examination or revision of the plan of care. See Section 3.1.

6.3 Gifts and Other Considerations

A physical therapist assistant shall not invite, accept, or offer gifts or other considerations that affect or give the appearance of affecting his/her provision of physical therapy interventions or that exploit the patient in any way. See Section 2.1(B).

Standard 7

A physical therapist assistant shall protect the public and the profession from unethical, incompetent, and illegal acts.

7.1 Consumer Protection

A physical therapist assistant shall report any conduct that appears to be unethical or illegal.

7.2 Organizational Employment

A. A physical therapist assistant shall inform his/her employer(s) and/or appropriate physical therapist of any employer practice that causes him or her to be in conflict with the Standards of Ethical Conduct for the Physical Therapist Assistant.

B. A physical therapist assistant shall not engage in any activity that puts him or her in conflict with the Standards of Ethical Conduct for the Physical Therapist Assistant, regardless of directives from a physical therapist or employer.

APTA *Code of Ethics* and *Guide to Professional Conduct*

HOD 06-00-12-23 (Program 17) [Amended HOD 06-91-05-05; HOD 06-87-11-17; HOD 06-81-06-18; HOD 06-78-06-08; HOD 06-78-06-07; HOD 06-77-18-30; HOD 06-77-17-27; Initial HOD 06-73-13-24]

Preamble

This Code of Ethics of the American Physical Therapy Association sets forth principles for the ethical practice of physical therapy. All physical therapists are responsible for maintaining and promoting ethical practice. To this end, the physical therapist shall act in the best interest of the patient/client. This Code of Ethics shall be binding on all physical therapists.

Principle 1

A physical therapist shall respect the rights and dignity of all individuals and shall provide compassionate care.

Principle 2

A physical therapist shall act in a trustworthy manner towards patients/clients, and in all other aspects of physical therapy practice.

Principle 3

A physical therapist shall comply with laws and regulations governing physical therapy and shall strive to effect changes that benefit patients/clients.

Principle 4

A physical therapist shall exercise sound professional judgment.

Principle 5

A physical therapist shall achieve and maintain professional competence.

Principle 6

A physical therapist shall maintain and promote high standards for physical therapy practice, education and research.

Principle 7

A physical therapist shall seek only such remuneration as is deserved and reasonable for physical therapy services.

Principle 8

A physical therapist shall provide and make available accurate and relevant information to patients/clients about their care and to the public about physical therapy services.

Principle 9

A physical therapist shall protect the public and the profession from unethical, incompetent, and illegal acts.

Principle 10

A physical therapist shall endeavor to address the health needs of society.

Principle 11

A physical therapist shall respect the rights, knowledge, and skills of colleagues and other health care professionals.

APTA Guide for Professional Conduct

Purpose

This *Guide for Professional Conduct* (Guide) is intended to serve physical therapists in interpreting the *Code of Ethics* (Code) of the American Physical Therapy Association (Association), in matters of professional conduct. The Guide provides guidelines by which physical therapists may determine the propriety of their conduct. It is also intended to guide the professional development of physical therapist students. The Code and the Guide apply to all physical therapists. These guidelines are subject to changes as the dynamics of the profession change and as new patterns of health care delivery are developed and accepted by the professional community and the public. This Guide is subject to monitoring and timely revision by the Ethics and Judicial Committee of the Association.

Interpreting Ethical Principles

The interpretations expressed in this Guide reflect the opinions, decisions, and advice of the Ethics and Judicial Committee. These interpretations are intended to assist a physical therapist in applying general ethical principles to specific situations. They should not be considered inclusive of all situations that could evolve.

Principle 1

A physical therapist shall respect the rights and dignity of all individuals and shall provide compassionate care.

1.1 Attitudes of a Physical Therapist

A. A physical therapist shall recognize individual differences and shall respect and be responsive to those differences.

B. A physical therapist shall be guided by concern for the physical, psychological, and socioeconomic welfare of patients/clients.

C. A physical therapist shall not harass, abuse, or discriminate against others.

D. A physical therapist shall be aware of the patient's health-related needs and act in a manner that facilitates meeting those needs.

Principle 2

A physical therapist shall act in a trustworthy manner towards patients/clients, and in all other aspects of physical therapy practice.

2.1 Patient/Physical Therapist Relationship

A. To act in a trustworthy manner the physical therapist shall act in the patient/client's best interest. Working in the patient/client's best interest requires knowledge of the patient/client's needs from the patient/client's perspective. Patients/clients often come to the physical therapist in a vulnerable state and normally will rely on the physical therapist's advice, which they perceive to be based on superior knowledge, skill, and experience. The trustworthy physical therapist acts to ameliorate the patient's/client's vulnerability, not to exploit it.

B. A physical therapist shall not exploit any aspect of the physical therapist/patient relationship.

C. A physical therapist shall not engage in any sexual relationship or activity, whether consensual or nonconsensual, with any patient while a physical therapist/patient relationship exists.

D. The physical therapist shall create an environment that encourages an open dialogue with the patient/client.

E. In the event the physical therapist or patient terminates the physical therapist/patient relationship while the patient continues to need physical therapy services, the physical therapist should take steps to transfer the care of the patient to another provider.

2.2 Truthfulness

A physical therapist shall not make statements that he/she knows or should know are false, deceptive, fraudulent, or unfair. See Section 8.2.D.

2.3 Confidential Information

A. Information relating to the physical therapist/patient relationship is confidential and may not be communicated to a third party not involved in that patient's care without the prior consent of the patient, subject to applicable law.

B. Information derived from peer review shall be held confidential by the reviewer unless the physical therapist who was reviewed consents to the release of the information.

C. A physical therapist may disclose information to appropriate authorities when it is necessary to protect the welfare of an individual or the community or when required by law. Such disclosure shall be in accordance with applicable law.

2.4 Patient Autonomy and Consent

A. A physical therapist shall not restrict patients' freedom to select their provider of physical therapy.

B. A physical therapist shall communicate to the patient/client the findings of his/her examination, evaluation, diagnosis, and prognosis.

C. A physical therapist shall collaborate with the patient/client to establish the goals of treatment and the plan of care.

D. A physical therapist shall use sound professional judgment in informing the patient/client of any substantial risks of the recommended examination and intervention.

E. A physical therapist shall respect the patient's/client's right to make decisions regarding the recommended plan of care, including consent, modification, or refusal.

Principle 3

A physical therapist shall comply with laws and regulations governing physical therapy and shall strive to effect changes that benefit patients/clients.

3.1 Professional Practice

A physical therapist shall provide examination, evaluation, diagnosis, prognosis, and intervention. A physical therapist shall not engage in any unlawful activity that substantially relates to the qualifications, functions, or duties of a physical therapist.

3.2 Just Laws and Regulations

A physical therapist shall advocate the adoption of laws, regulations, and policies by providers, employers, third party payers, legislatures, and regulatory agencies to provide and improve access to necessary health care services for all individuals.

3.3 Unjust Laws and Regulations

A physical therapist shall endeavor to change unjust laws, regulations, and policies that govern the practice of physical therapy. See Section 10.2.

Principle 4

A physical therapist shall exercise sound professional judgment.

4.1 Professional Responsibility

A. A physical therapist shall make professional judgments that are in the patient/client's best interests.

B. Regardless of practice setting, a physical therapist has primary responsibility for the physical therapy care of a patient and shall make independent judgments regarding that care consistent with accepted professional standards. See Section 2.4.

C. A physical therapist shall not provide physical therapy services to a patient/client while his/her ability to do so safely is impaired.

D. A physical therapist shall exercise sound professional judgment based upon his/her knowledge, skill, education, training, and experience.

E. Upon accepting a patient/client for physical therapy services, a physical therapist shall be responsible for: the examination, evaluation, and diagnosis of that individual; the prognosis and intervention; re-examination and modification of the plan of care; and the maintenance of adequate records, including progress reports. A physical therapist shall establish the plan of care and shall provide and/or supervise and direct the appropriate interventions. See Section 2.4.

F. If the diagnostic process reveals findings that are outside the scope of the physical therapist's knowledge, experience, or expertise, the physical therapist shall so inform the patient/client and refer to an appropriate practitioner.

G. When the patient has been referred from another practitioner, the physical therapist shall communicate the findings of the examination and evaluation, the diagnosis, the proposed intervention, and re-examination findings (as indicated) to the referring practitioner.

H. A physical therapist shall determine when a patient/client will no longer benefit from physical therapy services.

4.2 Direction and Supervision

A. The supervising physical therapist has primary responsibility for the physical therapy care rendered to a patient/client.

B. A physical therapist shall not delegate to a less qualified person any activity that requires the unique skill, knowledge, and judgment of the physical therapist.

4.3 Practice Arrangements

A. Participation in a business, partnership, corporation, or other entity does not exempt physical therapists, whether employers, partners, or stockholders, either individually or collectively, from the obligation to promote, maintain and comply with the ethical principles of the Association.

B. A physical therapist shall advise his/her employer(s) of any employer practice that causes a physical therapist to be in conflict with the ethical principles of the Association. A physical therapist shall seek to eliminate aspects of his/her employment that are in conflict with the ethical principles of the Association.

4.4 Gifts and Other Consideration

A physical therapist shall not accept or offer gifts or other considerations that affect or give an appearance of affecting his/her professional judgment.

Principle 5

A physical therapist shall achieve and maintain professional competence.

5.1 Scope of Competence

A physical therapist shall practice within the scope of his/her competence and commensurate with his/her level of education, training, and experience.

5.2 Self-assessment

A physical therapist shall engage in self-assessment, which is a lifelong professional responsibility for maintaining competence.

5.3 Professional Development

A physical therapist shall participate in educational activities that enhance his/her basic knowledge and skills.

Principle 6

A physical therapist shall maintain and promote high standards for physical therapy practice, education and research.

6.1 Professional Standards

A physical therapist shall know the accepted professional standards when engaging in physical therapy practice, education and/or research. A physical therapist shall continuously engage in assessment activities to determine compliance with these standards. If a physical therapist is not in compliance with these standards, he/she shall engage in activities designed to reach compliance with the standards. When a physical therapist is in compliance with these standards, he/she shall engage in activities designed to maintain such compliance.

6.2 Practice

A. A physical therapist shall achieve and maintain professional competence. See Section 5.

B. A physical therapist shall demonstrate his/her commitment to quality improvement by engaging in peer and utilization review and other self-assessment activities.

6.3 Professional Education

A. A physical therapist shall support high-quality education in academic and clinical settings.

B. A physical therapist participating in the educational process is responsible to the students, the academic institutions, and the clinical settings for promoting ethical conduct. A physical therapist shall model ethical behavior and provide the student with information about the Code of Ethics, opportunities to discuss ethical conflicts, and procedures for reporting unresolved ethical conflicts. See Section 9.

6.4 Continuing Education

A. A physical therapist providing continuing education must be competent in the content area.

B. When a physical therapist provides continuing education, he/she shall ensure that course content, objectives, faculty credentials, and responsibilities of the instructional staff are accurately stated in the promotional and instructional course materials.

C. A physical therapist shall evaluate the efficacy and effectiveness of information and techniques presented in continuing education programs before integrating them into his or her practice.

6.5 Research

A. A physical therapist shall support research activities that contribute knowledge for improved patient care.

B. A physical therapist shall report to appropriate authorities any acts in the conduct or presentation of research that appear unethical or illegal. See Section 9.

Principle 7

A physical therapist shall seek only such remuneration as is deserved and reasonable for physical therapy services.

7.1 Business and Employment Practices

A. A physical therapist's business/employment practices shall be consistent with the ethical principles of the Association.

B. A physical therapist shall never place her/his own financial interest above the welfare of individuals under his/her care.

C. A physical therapist shall recognize that third-party payer contracts may limit, in one form or another, the provision of physical therapy services. Third-party limitations do not absolve the physical therapist from making sound professional judgments that are in the patient's best interest. A physical therapist shall avoid under-utilization of physical therapy services.

D. When a physical therapist's judgment is that a patient will receive negligible benefit from physical therapy services, the physical therapist shall not provide or continue to provide such services if the primary reason for doing so is to further the financial self-interest of the physical therapist or his/her employer. A physical therapist shall avoid overutilization of physical therapy services.

E. Fees for physical therapy services should be reasonable for the service performed, considering the setting in which it is provided, practice costs in the geographic area, judgment of other organizations, and other relevant factors.

F. A physical therapist shall not directly or indirectly request, receive, or participate in the dividing, transferring, assigning, or rebating of an unearned fee.

G. A physical therapist shall not profit by means of a credit or other valuable consideration, such as an unearned commission, discount, or gratuity, in connection with the furnishing of physical therapy services.

H. Unless laws impose restrictions to the contrary, physical therapists who provide physical therapy services within a business entity may pool fees and monies received. Physical therapists may divide or apportion these fees and monies in accordance with the business agreement.

I. A physical therapist may enter into agreements with organizations to provide physical therapy services if such agreements do not violate the ethical principles of the Association or applicable laws.

7.2 Endorsement of Products or Services

A. A physical therapist shall not exert influence on individuals under his/her care or their families to use products or services based on the direct or indirect financial interest of the physical therapist in such products or services. Realizing that these individuals will normally rely on the physical therapist's advice, their best interest must always be maintained, as must their right of free choice relating to the use of any product or service. Although it cannot be considered unethical for physical therapists to own or have a financial interest in the production, sale, or distribution of products/services, they must act in accordance with law and make full disclosure of their interest whenever individuals under their care use such products/services.

B. A physical therapist may receive remuneration for endorsement or advertisement of products or services to the public, physical therapists, or other health professionals provided he/she discloses any financial interest in the production, sale, or distribution of said products or services.

C. When endorsing or advertising products or services, a physical therapist shall use sound professional judgment and shall not give the appearance of Association endorsement unless the Association has formally endorsed the products or services.

7.3 Disclosure

A physical therapist shall disclose to the patient if the referring practitioner derives compensation from the provision of physical therapy.

Principle 8

A physical therapist shall provide and make available accurate and relevant information to patients/clients about their care and to the public about physical therapy services.

8.1 Accurate and Relevant Information to the Patient

A. A physical therapist shall provide the patient/client information about his/her condition and plan of care. See Section 2.4.

B. Upon the request of the patient, the physical therapist shall provide, or make available, the medical record to the patient or a patient-designated third party.

C. A physical therapist shall inform patients of any known financial limitations that may affect their care.

D. A physical therapist shall inform the patient when, in his/her judgment, the patient will receive negligible benefit from further care. See Section 7.1.C.

8.2 Accurate and Relevant Information to the Public

A. A physical therapist shall inform the public about the societal benefits of the profession and who is qualified to provide physical therapy services.

B. Information given to the public shall emphasize that individual problems cannot be treated without individualized examination and plans/programs of care.

C. A physical therapist may advertise his/her services to the public.

D. A physical therapist shall not use, or participate in the use of, any form of communication containing a false, plagiarized, fraudulent, deceptive, unfair, or sensational statement or claim.

E. A physical therapist who places a paid advertisement shall identify it as such unless it is apparent from the context that it is a paid advertisement.

Principle 9

A physical therapist shall protect the public and the profession from unethical, incompetent, and illegal acts.

9.1 Consumer Protection

A. A physical therapist shall provide care that is within the scope of practice as defined by the state practice act.

B. A physical therapist shall not engage in any conduct that is unethical, incompetent or illegal.

C. A physical therapist shall report any conduct that appears to be unethical, incompetent, or illegal.

D. A physical therapist may not participate in any arrangements in which patients are exploited due to the referring sources' enhancing their personal incomes as a result of referring for, prescribing, or recommending physical therapy. See Section 5.

Principle 10

A physical therapist shall endeavor to address the health needs of society.

10.1 Pro Bono Service

A physical therapist shall render pro bono publico (reduced or no fee) services to patients lacking the ability to pay for services, as each physical therapist's practice permits.

10.2 Community Health

A physical therapist shall endeavor to support activities that benefit the health status of the community. See Section 3.

Principle 11

A physical therapist shall respect the rights, knowledge, and skills of colleagues and other healthcare professionals.

11.1 Consultation

A physical therapist shall seek consultation whenever the welfare of the patient will be safeguarded or advanced by consulting those who have special skills, knowledge, and experience.

11.2 Patient/Provider Relationships

A physical therapist shall not undermine the relationship(s) between his/her patient and other healthcare professionals.

11.3 Disparagement

Physical therapists shall not disparage colleagues and other health care professionals. See Section 9 and Section 2.4.A.

Standards of Practice
for Physical Therapy

HOD 06-03-09-10 (Program 32, Practice Dept.)
[Amended HOD 06-00-11-22; 06-99-18-22; HOD 06-96-16-31; HOD 06-91-21-25;
HOD 06-85-30-56; Initial HOD 06-80-04-04; HOD 06-80-03-03]

Preamble

The physical therapy profession's commitment to society is to promote optimal health and function in individuals by pursuing excellence in practice. The American Physical Therapy Association attests to this commitment by adopting and promoting the following Standards of Practice for Physical Therapy. These Standards are the profession's statement of conditions and performances that are essential for provision of high quality professional service to society, and provide a foundation for assessment of physical therapist practice.

I. Ethical/Legal Considerations

A. Ethical Considerations

The physical therapist practices according to the Code of Ethics of the American Physical Therapy Association.

The physical therapist assistant complies with the Standards of Ethical Conduct for the Physical Therapist Assistant of the American Physical Therapy Association.

B. Legal Considerations

The physical therapist complies with all the legal requirements of jurisdictions regulating the practice of physical therapy.

The physical therapist assistant complies with all the legal requirements of jurisdictions regulating the work of the assistant.

II. Administration of the Physical Therapy Service

A. Statement of Mission, Purposes, and Goals

The physical therapy service has a statement of mission, purposes, and goals that reflects the needs and interests of the patients/clients served, the physical therapy personnel affiliated with the service, and the community.

B. Organizational Plan

The physical therapy service has a written organizational plan.

C. Policies and Procedures

The physical therapy service has written policies and procedures that reflect the operation, mission, purposes, and goals of the service, and are consistent with the Association's standards, policies, positions, guidelines, and Code of Ethics.

D. Administration

A physical therapist is responsible for the direction of the physical therapy service.

E. Fiscal Management

The director of the physical therapy service, in consultation with physical therapy staff and appropriate administrative personnel participates in planning for, and allocation of, resources. Fiscal planning and management of the service is based on sound accounting principles.

F. Improvement of Quality of Care and Performance

The physical therapy service has a written plan for continuous improvement of quality of care and performance of services.

G. Staffing

The physical therapy personnel affiliated with the physical therapy service have demonstrated competence and are sufficient to achieve the mission, purposes, and goals of the service.

H. Staff Development

The physical therapy service has a written plan that provides for appropriate and ongoing staff development.

I. Physical Setting

The physical setting is designed to provide a safe and accessible environment that facilitates fulfillment of the mission, purposes, and goals of the physical therapy service. The equipment is safe and sufficient to achieve the purposes and goals of physical therapy.

J. Collaboration

The physical therapy service collaborates with all disciplines as appropriate.

III. Patient/Client Management

A.

Within the patient/client management process, the physical therapist and the pat-ient/client establish and maintain an ongoing collaborative process of decision-making that exists throughout the provision of services.

B. Initial Examination/Evaluation/Diagnosis/Prognosis

The physical therapist performs an initial examination and evaluation to establish a diagnosis and prognosis prior to intervention.

C. Plan of Care

The physical therapist establishes a plan of care and manages the needs of the patient/client based on the examination, evaluation, diagnosis, progno-sis, goals, and outcomes of the planned interventions for identified impairments, functional limitations, and disabilities.

The physical therapist involves the patient/client and appropriate others in the planning, implementation, and assessment of the plan of care.

The physical therapist, in consultation with appropriate disciplines, plans for discharge of the patient/client taking into consideration achievement of anticipated goals and expected outcomes, and provides for appropriate follow-up or referral.

D. Intervention

The physical therapist provides, or directs and supervises, the physical therapy intervention consistent with the results of the examination, evaluation, diagnosis, prognosis, and plan of care.

E. Reexamination

The physical therapist reexamines the patient/client as necessary during an episode of care to evaluate progress or change in patient/client status and modifies the plan of care accordingly or discontinues physical therapy services.

F. Discharge/Discontinuation of Intervention

The physical therapist discharges the patient/client from physical therapy services when the anticipated goals or expected outcomes for the patient/client have been achieved.

The physical therapist discontinues intervention when the patient/client is unable to continue to progress toward goals or when the physical therapist determines that the patient/client will no longer benefit from physical therapy.

G. Communication/Coordination/Documentation

The physical therapist communicates, coordinates and documents all aspects of patient/client management including the results of the initial examination and evaluation, diagnosis, prognosis, plan of care, interventions, response to interventions, changes in patient/client status relative to the interventions, reexamination, and discharge/discontinuation of intervention and other patient/client management activities.

IV. Education

The physical therapist is responsible for individual professional development. The physical therapist assistant is responsible for individual career development.

The physical therapist, and the physical therapist assistant under the direction and supervision of the physical therapist, participate in the education of students.

The physical therapist educates and provides consultation to consumers and the general public regarding the purposes and benefits of physical therapy.

The physical therapist educates and provides consultation to consumers and the general public regarding the roles of the physical therapist and the physical therapist assistant.

V. Research

The physical therapist applies research findings to practice and encourages, participates in, and promotes activities that establish the outcomes of patient/client management provided by the physical therapist.

VI. Community Responsibility

The physical therapist demonstrates community responsibility by participating in community and community agency activities, educating the public, formulating public policy, or providing pro bono physical therapy services.

Direction and Supervision of the Physical Therapist Assistant

HOD 06-00-16-27 [Amended HOD 06-99-07-11; HOD 06-96-30-42; HOD 06-95-11-06; HOD 06-93-08-09; HOD 06-85-20-41; Initial HOD 06-84-16-72/HOD 06-78-22-61/HOD 06-77-19-37]

Physical therapists have a responsibility to deliver services in ways that protect the public safety and maximize the availability of their services. They do this through direct delivery of services in conjunction with responsible utilization of physical therapist assistants who assist with specific components of intervention. The physical therapist assistant is the only individual permitted to assist a physical therapist in selected interventions under the direction and supervision of a physical therapist.

Direction and supervision are essential in the provision of quality physical therapy services. The degree of direction and supervision necessary for assuring quality physical therapy services is dependent upon many factors, including the education, experiences, and responsibilities of the parties involved, as well as the organizational structure in which the physical therapy services are provided.

Regardless of the setting in which the service is provided, the following responsibilities must be borne solely by the physical therapist:

1. Interpretation of referrals when available.

2. Initial examination, evaluation, diagnosis, and prognosis.

3. Development or modification of a plan of care which is based on the initial examination or reexamination and which includes the physical therapy anticipated goals and expected outcomes.

4. Determination of when the expertise and decision making capability of the physical therapist requires the physical therapist to personally render physical therapy interventions and when it may be appropriate to utilize the physical thera-

pist assistant. A physical therapist shall determine the most appropriate utilization of the physical therapist assistant that provides for the delivery of service that is safe, effective and efficient.

5. Re-examination of the patient in light of the patient's anticipated goals, and revision of the plan of care when indicated.

6. Establishment of the discharge plan and documentation of discharge summary/status.

7. Oversight of all documentation for services rendered to each patient.

The physical therapist remains responsible for the physical therapy services provided when the physical therapist's plan of care involves the physical therapist assistant to assist with selected interventions. Regardless of the setting in which the service is provided, the determination to utilize physical therapist assistants for selected interventions requires the education, expertise and professional judgement of a physical therapist as described by the *Standards of Practice, Guide to Professional Conduct* and *Code of Ethics.*

In determining the appropriate extent of assistance from the physical therapist assistant (PTA), the physical therapist considers: the PTA's education, training, experience and skill level patient/client criticality, acuity, stability, and complexity the predictability of the consequences the setting in which the care is being delivered federal and state statutes liability and risk management concerns the mission of physical therapy services for the setting the needed frequency of reexamination

Physical Therapist Assistant

Definition

The physical therapist assistant is a technically educated health care provider who assists the physical therapist in the provision of physical therapy. The physical therapist assistant is a graduate of a physical therapist assistant associate degree program accredited by the Commission on Accreditation in Physical Therapy Education (CAPTE).

Utilization

The physical therapist is directly responsible for the actions of the physical therapist assistant related to patient/client management. The physical therapist assistant may perform selected physical therapy interventions under the direction and at least general supervision of the physical therapist. In general supervision, the physical therapist is not required to be on-site for direction and supervision, but must be available at least by telecommunications. The ability of the physical therapist assistant to perform the selected interventions as directed shall be assessed on an ongoing basis by the supervising physical therapist. The physical therapist assistant may modify an intervention in accordance with changes in patient/client status within the scope of the established plan of care.

The physical therapist assistant must work under the direction and at least general supervision of the physical therapist. In all practice settings, the performance of selected interventions by the physical therapist assistant must be consistent with safe and legal physical therapist practice, and shall be predicated on the following factors: complexity and acuity of the patient/client's needs; proximity and accessibility to the physical therapist; supervision available in the event of emergencies or critical events; and type of setting in which the service is provided.

When supervising the physical therapist assistant in any off site setting, the following requirements must be observed:

1. A physical therapist must be accessible by telecommunications to the physical therapist assistant at all times while the physical therapist assistant is treating patients/clients.

2. There must be regularly scheduled and documented conferences with the physical therapist assistant regarding patients/clients, the frequency of which is determined by the needs of the patient/client and the needs of the physical therapist assistant.

3. In those situations in which a physical therapist assistant is involved in the care of a patient/client, a supervisory visit by the physical therapist will be made:

   a. Upon the physical therapist assistant's request for a reexamination, when a change in treatment plan of care is needed, prior to any planned discharge, and in response to a change in the patient/client's medical status.

   b. At least once a month, or at a higher frequency when established by the physical therapist, in accordance with the needs of the patient.

   c. A supervisory visit should include:
      1. An on-site reexamination of the patient/client.
      2. On-site review of the plan of care with appropriate revision or termination.
      3. Evaluation of need and recommendation for utilization of outside resources.

Levels of Supervision

HOD 06-00-15-26

The American Physical Therapy Association recognizes the following levels of supervision:

General Supervision

The physical therapist is not required to be on-site for direction and supervision, but must be available at least by telecommunications.

Direct Supervision

The physical therapist is physically present and immediately available for direction and supervision. The physical therapist will have direct contact with the patient during each visit that is defined in the *Guide to Physical Therapist Practice* as all encounters with a patient/client in a twenty four hour period. Telecommunications does not meet the requirement of direct supervision.

Direct Personal Supervision

The physical therapist, or where allowable by law, the physical therapist assistant, is physically present and immediately available to direct and supervise tasks that are related to patient/client management. The direction and supervision is continuous throughout the time these tasks are performed. Telecommunications does not meet the requirement of direct personal supervision.

APPENDIX 6

Provision of Physical Therapy Interventions and Related Tasks

HOD 06-00-17-28

It is the position of the American Physical Therapy Association (APTA) that:

Physical therapists are the only professionals who provide physical therapy interventions. Physical therapist assistants are the only individuals who provide selected physical therapy interventions under the direction and at least general supervision of the physical therapist.

Physical therapy aides are any support personnel who perform designated tasks related to the operation of the physical therapy service. Tasks are those activities that do not require the clinical decision making of the physical therapist or the clinical problem solving of the physical therapist assistant. Tasks related to patient/client management must be assigned to the physical therapy aide by the physical therapist, or where allowable by law, the physical therapist assistant, and may only be performed by the aide under direct personal supervision of the physical therapist, or where allowable by law, the physical therapist assistant. Direct personal supervision requires that the physical therapist, or where allowable by law, the physical therapist assistant, be physically present and immediately available to direct and supervise tasks that are related to patient/client management. The direction and supervision is continuous throughout the time these tasks are performed. The physical therapist or physical therapist assistant must have direct contact with the patient/client during each session. Telecommunications does not meet the requirement of direct personal supervision

Index

WAIT

...There's More!

SLACK Incorporated's Professional Book Division offers a wide selection of products in the field of Physical Therapy. We are dedicated to providing important works that educate, inform and improve the knowledge of our customers. Don't miss out on our other informative titles that will enhance your collection.

Physical Therapist Assistant Exam Review, Fourth Edition
Theresa Meyer, PT
336 pp., Soft Cover, 2000, ISBN 1-55642-589-9,
Order #45899, **$27.95**

Be at the top of your class with this revolutionary study tool. The chapters contain a variety of information that consists of lists, charts, comparisons, outlines, and short definitions, and topics such as physiology, cardiology, oncology, the health care system, and much more.

Quick Reference Dictionary for Physical Therapy, Second Edition
Jennifer Bottomley, PhD², MS, PT
624 pp., Soft Cover, 2003, ISBN 1-55642-580-5,
Order #45805, **$28.95**

This second edition provides quick access to words and their definitions that are encountered on a day-to-day basis. There are 39 appendices included in this user-friendly, handy reference where you can find materials such as selected APTA documents and World Wide Web resources. This the perfect, pocket size companion for school, clinical affiliations, preparation for the licensure exam, and physical therapy practice.

PT Study Cards in a Box
Theresa Meyer, PT
288 Study Cards, 2001, ISBN 1-55642-482-5,
Order #44825, **$50.95**

Physical Therapy Professional Foundations: Keys to Success in School and Career
Kathleen Curtis, PhD, PT
304 pp., Soft Cover, 2002, ISBN 1-55642-411-6,
Order #44116, **$38.95**

The Physical Therpist's Guide to Health Care
Kathleen Curtis, PhD, PT
320 pp., Soft Cover, 1999, ISBN 1-55642-378-0,
Order #43780, **$35.95**

Practical Kinesiology for the Physical Therapist Assistant
Jeff G. Konin, PhD, AT, PT
240 pp., Soft Cover, 1999, ISBN 1-55642-299-7,
Order #42997, **$38.95**

Orthopedics at a Glance: A Handbook of Disorders, Tests, and Rehabilitation Strategies
Nancy Gann, MS, PT, OCS
240 pp., Soft Cover, 2001, ISBN 1-55642-500-7,
Order #45007, **$32.95**

Business Fundamentals for the Rehabilitation Professional
Tammy Richmond, MS, OTR and Dave Powers, MA, MBA, PT
224 pp., Soft Cover, 2004, ISBN 1-55642-593-7,
Order #45937, **$42.95**

Complementary Therapies in Rehabilitation: Evidence for Efficacy in Therapy, Prevention, and Wellness, Second Edition
Carol M. Davis, EdD, PT, MS, FAPTA
416 pp., Hard Cover, 2004, ISBN 1-55642-581-3,
Order #45813, **$44.95**

Special Tests for Orthopedic Examination, Second Edition
Jeff G. Konin, PhD, AT, PT; Denise Wiksten, PhD, ATC; Jerome A. Isear, Jr, MS,PT, ATC-L; and Holly Brader, MPH, ATC, CHES
352 pp., Soft Cover, 2002, ISBN 1-55642-591-0,
Order #45910, **$36.95**

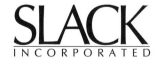